Free!

6/2002

2000

# The
# Power
## of the
# Inner Judge

# The Power of the Inner Judge

## Psychodynamic Treatment of the Severe Neuroses

**Léon Wurmser, M.D.**

JASON ARONSON INC.
*Northvale, New Jersey*
*London*

This book was set in 10 pt. New Baskerville by Alpha Graphics of Pittsfield, NH, and printed and bound by Book-mart Press, Inc. of North Bergen, NJ.

Copyright © 2000 by Léon Wurmser

Originally published in German by Springer-Verlag under the title *Flucht vor dem Gewissen*. Copyright © 1987, 1993 by Léon Wurmser.

10 9 8 7 6 5 4 3 2 1

**Library of Congress Cataloging-in-Publication Data**

Wurmser, Léon
   [Flucht vor dem Gewissen. English]
   The power of the inner judge: psychodynamic treatment of the severe neuroses / by Léon Wurmser.
      p. ; cm.
   Includes bibliographical references and index.
   ISBN 0-7657-0177-4 (alk. paper)
     1. Neuroses—Treatment.  2. Borderline personality disorder—Treatment.  3. Psychodynamic psychotherapy.  I. Title.
     [DNLM: 1. Neurotic Disorders—therapy. 2. Defense Mechanisms. 3. Psychoanalytic Theory.  4. Psychoanalytic therapy—methods.  5. Superego. WM 170 WM 170 W968f 1999]
RC530.W8713 1999
616.85'20651—dc21                                                     99-046506

Printed in the United States of America on acid-free paper. For information and catalog write to Jason Aronson Inc., 230 Livingston Street, Northvale, NJ 07647-1726. Or visit our website: www.aronson.com

# Contents

# Preface

This volume has one overriding purpose: to describe at length how the work with severely ill, but not psychotic, patients can effectively be done by careful analytic work on the defenses and the superego. The method used is quite flexible, but diverges widely from the parallel efforts by Kernberg and Kohut (and their schools) of dealing with the same very broad spectrum of patients. Instead of calling them "borderline patients" I prefer to call them, with Freud (1940b, p. 180), the "severe neuroses"—for a number of reasons that are laid out here in great detail. This markedly different practical approach, as well as theoretical understanding, has shown its efficacy not only in my own work, as presented here, but also in that of many others whom I have been supervising, mostly in Europe.

In order to show such a largely heuristic value it is important to document the work not just in the form of relatively concise, sanitized, strongly abstracted case presentations, but to submit material that is concrete and as close to the actual interaction as is feasible. I try not to spruce it up in ways that would hide or embellish my own errors. The quandaries faced in such difficult treatments deserve to be shared.

There is, as well, a second important aim here, as had been the case in the two major books I have published in English (*The Hidden Dimension* and *The Mask of Shame*); it is to show how this type of work requires a double perspective—one that is patterned after the natural sciences in its generalizing, the other after the humanities in its individualizing. There is therefore a constant weaving together of the strands of clinical theory and of more literary and philosophical study. The original plan, in fact, had been to give both sides equal weight and to combine the clinical works with the literary and philosophical essays under the unifying title *Conflict and Complementarity*. However, that undertaking grew to such size that a separate volume under the title *Broken Reality* (*Die zerbrochene Wirklichkeit*) collected those essays separately. The two works very much belong together, each throwing light on the other.

This American edition, though, is much reduced in size from the German version, first appearing in 1987 under the title *Flight from Conscience*. Most of the originally planned, expanded case presentations have been removed to give it greater compactness. Only two major case studies and two shorter clinical excerpts of the original one dozen have been kept in this work. The remainder will be published in a parallel volume, returning to the original title *Flight from Conscience*.

I would also say that over the intervening ten years my theoretical center of gravity, which had been rather onesidedly on the side of conflict, has shifted to one more in the middle between trauma and conflict. I consider these two concepts indissolubly linked, indispensable, and complementary to each other. With that shift, the issues of affect regulation have assumed much greater importance, as have the elements in the technique that go "beyond interpretation," as Gedö (1979) has postulated. Here also, the complementarity of both adds enormously to the complexity of the task at hand—in understanding, treating, and writing.

I have already mentioned that what is concrete, individual, and thus historical takes at least as much space as what is abstract and general, and thus theoretical. This convergence of the narrative and the theoretical dimensions also means that special care was given to preserve and represent the high complexity of each case and hence also of the ideas guiding the work. I often quote from Lagerkvist's (1966) *Pilgrimen*: "What is simple and unified is not true, can hardly be that. Only what is composite can perhaps be assumed to be that" [*Det enkla och enhetliga är inte sant, kan inte gärna vara det. Bara det sammansatta kan möjligen tänkas vara det*] (p. 230).

This by necessity very detailed study of material from the sessions did not present a huge problem in a different language and on another continent. But a prominent reason why I have waited so long to present such detailed material in this country is the issue of confidentiality, which I have resolved mostly by adding decades of distance. Although all the patients have very generously and kindly consented to my using the material, it became much more important to disguise it, as much as possible, without compromising its authenticity. I hope I have been able to successfully balance both values—truth and nil nocere.

Many of the common concepts of psychoanalytic parlance, like repetition compulsion, masochism, aggression, and narcissism, are treated as valuable descriptive terms; but I have taken issue with the frequently made hasty leap from description to explanation, from phenomenology to causality. This issue of psychoanalytically relevant causality was to be explored much more deeply in *Broken Reality* (1989a). I made therefore a constant effort to get as much away from the clichés of theories and to approach the direct observations as closely as possible, without therewith denying the need for theory. Both Confucius' words, "Learning without thinking is empty, thinking without learning is dangerous," and Kant's statement, "Experience without concepts is blind, concepts without experience are empty" show the necessary conjunction of observation and theory.

It was most important for me to counter the implicit and often quite explicit spirit of judgmentalness that emerges when severely ill patients are dealt with, markedly so in the presentations, too, not only in the clinical exchange. Categories are necessary, but they always tend to be slowly transformed into words of devaluation, as if the origin of the term came back to haunt its logical use: *kategorein* means in Greek "to accuse, to blame."

"Authority" may mean "authoritarian": critical, commanding, prohibiting or allowing, condemning, punishing. But it also may evoke its original Latin meaning of *auctoritas*, "a warrant for growth" (*augere* means "to grow"): to be authoritative as questioning, helping in self-observation, even educative, guiding, "psychagogigal" (like Socrates in Plato's *Phaedrus*). It is such authority and a peculiar form of dialogue that allows what Plato wrote in regard to the philosophical dialogue (in *The Seventh Letter*):

> For it does not admit of exposition like other branches of knowledge; but after much converse about the matter itself and a life lived together, suddenly a light, as it were, is kindled in one soul by a flame that leaps to it from another, and thereafter sustains itself . . . in the course of scrutiny and kindly testing by men who proceed by question and answer without ill will, with a sudden flash there shines forth understanding about every problem. . . . [pp. 809, 810]

If there is, therefore, one consistent emotional attitude going through all my books and my practical work it would be this: to avoid, as much as it is possible, falling into the role of a judging authority, to avoid fulfilling in reality, much less creating, the transference of superego functions, and rather, in Paul Gray's words, to analyze them: "Exploring instead of judging," and conversely to notice the defensive use of "judging instead of exploring" (personal communication). One has to pay for everything: one consequence of this attitude is certainly the greater length of treatment. But then again, such severe pathology always takes a long time of very intense and very patient work. There are no shortcuts.

My German works have, moreover, to emphasize this in opposition to the less intensive and time-limited form of analysis typically practiced in Germany: three times a week and mostly for no more than about three hundred hours. In the meantime the zeitgeist here in the United States has made the one prevailing in Germany look like paradise, ever since the managed care steamroller has more and more disparaged this type of work and this way of understanding of severe psychopathology as seemingly obsolete and hence unacceptable.

One more remark. I have often been questioned, occasionally even ridiculed as pretentious, because of my use of other languages in my texts. I reply to this: all the quotes in foreign languages have been translated (or at least reviewed and, if need be, modified) by myself. Especially with psychoanalytically relevant texts where fine nuances and details of metaphors can be highly pertinent I tried to get as close to the meaning of the original, even if it may sound clumsy. Therefore, it is my strongly held view that the original text should usually be included so that at least some readers can validly compare, especially if the quoted work is otherwise hard to gain access to (in contrast, for example, to Freud's German text). Unfortunately, no translation is fully faithful, and sometimes we encounter in psychoanalytic writings grotesque errors based on inexact translation, as well as other problems, as where it had been impossible to translate with full accuracy (this latter is true for the Nietzsche quote below, for example).

It is impossible to acknowledge all the individuals who have helped me in one way or another during the decades that the growth of this book has taken, both in its original German and now in this strongly reworked version. Most of all, I would like to express my very special gratitude to all my patients who have helped me understand, and who have consented to the use of material from our work. In the Talmud tractate *Ta'anith* 7a, Rabbi Chanina is quoted: "I have learned much from my teachers, and from my colleagues more than from my teachers, and from my students more than from all of them" (*harbeh lamadti merabotai, umechaverai yoter merabotai, umitalmidai yoter mikullan*) (*Steinsaltz Talmud*, vol. XIII, p. 82). In a very deep sense, our patients are students from whom we learn the most, as well as what is of the essence.

Then I am very grateful to Jason Aronson and his team (Norma Pomerantz, Cindy Hyden, and Elaine Lindenblatt) for making this English edition possible, and before them the colleagues and friends at the Springer-Verlag in Heidelberg, especially Tony Graf-Baumann and Heike Berger.

Special gratitude is due to my teachers: Gaetano Benedetti in Switzerland, and Lawrence Kubie, Jenny Waelder-Hall, Paul Gray, and Joe Lichtenberg in this country. From all the friends and colleagues who have supported this work in Europe I only mention André Haynal, Martha Eicke, Jack and Rosmarie Berna, and Verena Wenger in Switzerland, Peter Buchheim, Manfred Cierpka, Günter Reich, Helmut Thomä and Horst Kächele, and Friedrich and Elisabeth Eickhoff in Germany; Marianne Faxén, Mats Fridell, Erich Franzke and Gunnar Windahl in Sweden; and Dieter Blumer, Marion Oliner, Judy Felton, Anne Lewis, and Cibeles Vidaud, in this country; I apologize to all those others who have supported me in many ways over those years, but whom I fail to mention now.

Finally much thanks goes to my family, whose thoughtfulness and support have accompanied my work during trying decades: my wife Zdenka, my sons Daniel, David, and Yory, and their spouses Mimi, Meyrav, and Nina.

What Nietzsche (1873) said about classical philology is, I believe, ever so true for psychoanalysis: "I would not know what meaning [it] would have in our time unless it were to appear in it as untimely, that is, to stand up against the time and thus to have an effect upon the time, and work, it is to be hoped, in favor of a coming time" (*Denn ich wüßte nicht, was [sie] in unserer Zeit für einen Sinn hätte, wenn nicht den, in ihr unzeitgemäß—das heißt gegen die Zeit und dadurch auf die Zeit und hoffentlich zugunsten einer kommenden Zeit—zu wirken*) (II, p. 99).

—*Léon Wurmser*
Towson, Maryland
October 1999

# 1

## Introduction

Ich bin der Geist, der stets verneint.
(I am the spirit that always denies.)
—Goethe, *Faust*, Part I

## SEVEN POLARITIES

### Anxiety and Protection

Last night I had a strange dream. I was driving on a lonely stretch. Around me was desert. I passed a girl. We both stopped. I talked with her, and then we went back to her house. It was uncanny and got more and more devilish. We had sex, and it became wilder and wilder, in overwhelming, crazy passion. Then we were not alone anymore. I was held by the girl and a man and was not able to move. They started cutting me with razor blades on my hands and arms and letting my blood flow. They tested my threshold for pain. It did not hurt. But I turned into one of them. Something took me into its power, something like a vampire, sucking the blood. When you get bitten by it you turn into it. With the razor blades they drained me of my blood, and I changed into these people. . . . We have lost the joy in everything. We chase after success, but we never can relax because we always feel guilty right away.—Our conscience—resentment and despair.[51][1]

These are the words of a young man who sought help for his abuse of alcohol and cocaine following the recent death of his mother. After several months of shallow, unproductive chatting in the analysis he has been sliding into deep despair about the absolute emptiness and meaninglessness of his life, although socially and professionally it seems extremely busy and successful. More and more he is preoccupied with suicidal thoughts. There is a ferocious force in him, a demon who has ambushed him on the desert road of his vacuous existence and has overpowered him. He has changed himself into the demon, the tormentor, identifying with him. He seeks protection from anxiety and abandonment in the chase, in his restless drivenness, in his sucking the lifeblood out of others (especially a long series of girlfriends) and then spitting them out. He has become the one who always does the leaving, instead of being the one who is being left. He does the same with treatment, leaving it and not paying his debts.

3

A 30-year-old ballerina who is entering psychotherapy because of episodes of depressive mood and eating disorders (bulimia, anorexia, and self-induced vomiting) dreams after an attack of binge-eating the following "weird" dream:

> A strangely big lizard man was standing there, and opposite to him there was a little man, a kind of gremlin. I was pregnant, and I thanked the big man for it. Then the two men were strongly looking into each other's eyes, and suddenly the lizard man was in my stomach and was gnawing at me from within.
>
> She is commenting how her attacks of devouring always occur then, when she is attacking herself, when she is feeling "badly about herself." She is eating, she adds, in order to get relief from her self-criticism. I ask whether perhaps the lizard man is her exaggerated conscience, which is gnawing and eating on her: "When you deal particularly severely with yourself you start devouring, but then you become even more severe against yourself." She nods: "It happens when I need all the relief from that inner tension. The devouring soothes me, but then I attack myself even more. It is like taking drugs or getting drunk. At first it is as if I were nurturing myself, were taking care of myself. But then I would be out of it, and one time I almost killed myself with a car accident." It is an *altered state of consciousness*: "Bingeing is the closest I can get to not being here. . . . It is killing consciousness and conscience; it resembles a demon, another personality. Something foreign is bringing me into its power and does violence to me. I become hostile toward my fiancé, icy, almost possessed. I took it so to heart when my mother criticized my haircut (before the impending wedding). It made me totally crazy. I wanted to kill her, smash her face. Then I got very embarrassed and afraid of everything." With that, she has taken over the sharp judgment of her mother. She has, in her words, "such a bad body image"; she can see herself fat like her mother, "such a mush like her, unable to control herself and her surroundings." She tries to lose 5 pounds from her weight of 116, and is very afraid she would get pregnant and have children; "I want to keep control over my body, I want to tame it, but I feel trapped in it. I would prefer to be a man." [8]

On the one side she profoundly fears and hates any likeness with her mother and would like to kill off any identification with her; it is an identity full of shame. On the other side stands her conscience, an incessantly threatening and merciless inner authority, entirely patterned after the menacing voice of a mother she experienced as intrusive and lacking any understanding. The ideal image she has of herself—that of a pure, autonomous, ethereal self, free of any greed—stands in constant and at times deadly conflict with her conscience. Like a poisonous flower, the uncanny figure of the demon grows out of this struggle.

One meaning of the dream lies in her very mixed feelings toward her fiancé; she wants him big, not wimpish and impish. This is gnawing at her;

yet she does not want to hurt him—by canceling the wedding, set in two weeks. The feelings from these conflicts appear demonic to her, and deprive her of her self-control.

"I was in a forest; it was cool and wet," another woman patient has been dreaming.

> The ground was covered by thick green moss, and brooks were rushing through the trees. In the middle, there was pitched a big rosy tent, and, in front of it, a pile of wood. I approached it from below on a carpet of atlas and made my way through gossamer. Suddenly it was my own pyre. My body was lying on top. The dream vanished before I could see my face. I only noticed a very deep gaping wound on my throat. I could not see my face" [63]. "I often woke up as child," says the patient, a young political scientist whom I shall describe later on more in detail as Vera, "and saw in the open door of my bedroom a veiled, dark figure. She was coming close, and I felt her long, cold fingers on my throat and in my face" [75]. "I just had the image: you are sitting there in your chair, entirely muffled up as if you were sitting on a sled in the Russian winter. You go mad, and your eyes get a demonic look—not violent, not that you would strike out, but that you would have lost all your rational thoughts" [157].

She quotes from Blake's poem "Garden of Love":

> And I saw it was filled with graves,
> And tomb-stones where flowers should be;
> And Priests in black gowns were walking their rounds,
> And binding with briars my joys and desires.

What is this strange counterforce? As it happened for these three patients, this question becomes for most of my patients one of life and death, of meaning and desperate meaninglessness—this sense of an inner *doubleness*, of an inner split that cannot be answered by consolations of either a religious or philosophical sort, or by simple explanations of a sociological or psychoanalytic nature—neither by encompassing world designs, great concepts, nor practical suggestions.

Certainly, what most of the more severely ill patients describe as a "demon" or as "something demonic" is finally nothing other than the compelling force of the neurosis, which is able to persist against conscious willpower and to determine actions and feelings to such an extent that all interests and every happiness are being poisoned and each success is destroyed. It is a "counterwill" (*Gegenwille*) crossing the intentions of the conscious personality, as Freud (1892/1893) called that power in his first paper dealing with the psychotherapy of hysteria. Later he described it, with much broader and deeper understanding, as *repetition compulsion*: "The manifestations of a compulsion to repeat . . . exhibit to a high degree an instinctual (*triebhaft*: driving) character and, when they act in opposition to the pleasure principle, give the appearance of some 'demonic' force at work" (Freud 1920, p. 35). He tried to trace it back to the instinctual drive of primary masochism or the death instinct.

Yet, what is this counterforce in the severe neuroses, what is the nature of the repetition compulsion, and, in particular, how is it related to the superego—to the conscious and unconscious inner authority? What is the *perversion of conscience* that leads to the appearance of that "demon"?

Frightening figures and protective figures, in enigmatic doubleness, seem to determine the life of these patients, defying all demands of outer reality. What does this twinship of seemingly fatal dread and protective fantasy mean?

These extremely important questions will not get any easy and simple answers here. Rather, this book is structured so as to present the multilayeredness of *psychic causality*, the complexity and circularity of inner life: "There is always an easy solution to every human problem—neat, plausible and wrong," wrote H. L. Mencken (as quoted, *Baltimore Sun*, February 28,1988). "The human soul is a very complex thing" (George Eliot 1859, p. 172).

Still, we might be helped along in finding answers to these questions in the course of a thorough study and exploration of the essential raw data precisely in those patients who suffer under *severe neurosis* and who show this repetition compulsion in a particularly impressive way.

### Scientific Method and the Autonomy of Psychoanalysis

> Psychoanalysis has proved a fiasco. It is by far the most costly and time-consuming of all psychotherapies, yet it has not been shown to be more curative than a single one of its hundred-plus rivals, even those that require only a few weeks of intervention. Indeed, it appears no better than regimens designed to *withhold* specific treatment factors or ingredients.

This is being proclaimed by Frederick Crews (in the *New Republic* of 1/21/ 1985), a self-touted expert and widely heard pontificator, whose broad literary and polemical skills are uncontaminated by any clinical experience. More recently he devotes even more energy to his debunking effort (worthy of an Ellsworth Toohey):

> In a word, then, Freud had launched a pseudoscience—that is, a nominally scientific enterprise which is so faulty at the core that it cannot afford to submit its

hypotheses for unsparing peer review by the wider community, but must instead resort to provisos that forestall any possibility of refutation. And despite some well-intentioned efforts at reform, a pseudoscience is what psychoanalysis has remained. [Crews 1993, p. 62]

He finds potent succor in the writings of Adolf Grünbaum, a philosopher of science who, summarizing some of his epistemological writings on psychoanalysis, declared in a lecture at Johns Hopkins in the spring of 1986:

It is the *clinical* evidence on which most analysts rest their case. And I conclude that despite the appeal to the latter evidence by these champions of psychoanalysis, the operation of hidden motives in Freud's sense has yet to be cogently tested on an adequate scale. And until it is the widespread belief in psychoanalytic theory in some segments of our culture is hardly well-founded.

And at the end of his book *The Foundations of Psychoanalysis* (1984), he agrees with Karl Popper that "contamination by suggestion does undermine the probative value of clinical data" (p. 285).

With this challenge that, because of its "contamination by suggestion," the theory of unconscious motivation is unproven, the therapeutic value of all analytically reached *insight* and all its claims of being empirically well-founded and justified are being put in question. Grünbaum's challenge to us could be summarized in these words.

You claim that you possess a theory about the causes of the neuroses. All the evidence you have proffered so far is irremediably intermixed with the influence of suggestions and placebo effects. What you assert about causation of neurosis and its specific removal through insight may be right or wrong. Yet you have not presented anything that could stand up under a careful critique. Nothing is proven; everything is at best heuristically of some use, that is, it may serve to find possible connections.

This compels us urgently to inquire into the fundaments of our knowledge as therapists, as teachers, and as theoreticians, especially in that area where alone we may hope to find answers—in direct clinical experience. "For these ideas are not the foundation of science, upon which everything rests: that foundation is observation alone" (Freud 1914b, p. 76).

These questions, which are being asked of psychoanalysis by epistemology, and particularly by Grünbaum (1984), have to be taken seriously, because they force us, whether we want to or not, to examine our *observations* for their strength as proofs (their "probative force," or *Beweiskraft*). They challenge us to delimit with more precision what is to be attributed to unspecific factors, like suggestion, placebo effect, or the effectiveness of the therapist's personality, from that which can be explained by the specific efficacy of certain interventions undertaken in the search of finding inner truth. Which changes are to be ascribed to *suggestion*—the imposition of what the analyst believes, of his system of value and truth? How permanent are these changes? At what price of inner distortion and stifling are they attained? And, on the other side, which of them can be attributed to real self-recognition—*insight*——achieved with the guidance of the analyst? This is the doubleness of our work, the constant dilemma that we can never abolish for good and that we can never escape from either. Each session poses this question anew: Do we have our impact and effect *as a figure of authority* or by *enhancing the patient's autonomous insight?* It is precisely the work with patients suffering under severe neuroses that often forces us to interventions that run counter to the goal of gaining insight.

In searching for an answer to this question it is essential not to be restricted to the study of analytic writings, as the critical philosophers, including Grünbaum, usually are. The written *communication* of the allegedly discovered truth is not necessarily the *whole* truth; many things can only be transmitted with greatest difficulty, and the scarcity of such evidence is not necessarily a testimony for its absence, but rather a sign for the work of transmission yet to be done.

The questions posed to us by a true critique, one which would be proffered rationally, well-founded in knowledge of the entire literature, would be something of this kind: What does what we call insight rely upon? How does the finding of such connections proceed? How do we, in the given case, know whether we are on the right way or have gotten lost?

A work of research like the one presented here, which mostly relies upon case studies, cannot renounce its scientific foundation even with the excuse that it merely deals with statements derived from the immediate context of discovery. Rather one has, albeit with major reservations, to agree with Edelson (1985) that case studies need also to submit to the canon of method and rational conclusion peculiar to science, just as the other forms of research in the natural sciences do. The basic demands of scientific method do not depend upon the subject matter (p. 571), and this entails that the hypotheses should show explanatory power, that they should have been exposed to counterarguments, and they have proven their claim to have greater credibility than the alternative hypotheses (p. 611).

Note that I said, with major reservations. In a radio talk in 1957, the eminent British historian and philosopher Isaiah Berlin said, with regard to the scientific nature of history, and especially the understanding of historical decision making: "There is no natural science of politics any more than a natural science of ethics. Natural science cannot answer all questions." Elsewhere (1996) he comments that the great statesman, like the great novelist, does not require so much the gift or knowledge of abstract generalization, such as be needed in the natural sciences, but a finely tuned discrimination.

> Above all this is an acute sense of what fits with what, what springs from what, what leads to what. . . . It is a sense for what is qualitative rather than quantitative, for what is specific rather than general; it is a species of direct acquaintance, as distinct from a capacity for description or calculation or inference; it is what is variously called natural wisdom, imaginative understanding, insight, perceptiveness, and, more misleadingly, intuition. . . What are we to call this kind of capacity? Practical wisdom, practical reason, perhaps, a sense of what will 'work,' and what will not. It is a capacity, in the first place, for synthesis rather than analysis, for knowledge in the sense in which trainers know their animals, or parents their children, or conductors their orchestras, as opposed to that in which chemists know the contents of their test tubes, or mathematicians know the rules that their symbols obey. . . . Obviously what matters is to understand a particular situation in its full uniqueness. . . . What makes statesmen . . . successful is that they do not think in general terms—that is, they do not primarily ask themselves in what respect a given situation is like or unlike other situations in the long course of human history. . . . Their merit is that they grasp the unique combination of characteristics that constitute this particular situation—this and no other. . . . The arts of life—not least of politics—as well as some among the humane studies turn out to possess their own special methods and techniques, their own criteria of success and failure. Utopianism, lack of realism, bad judgment here consist not in failing to apply the methods of natural science, but, on the contrary, in over-applying them. . . . For, as Tolstoy taught us long ago, the particles are too minute, too heterogeneous, succeed each other too rapidly, occur in combinations of too great complexity, are too much part and parcel of what we are and do, to be capable of submitting to the required degree of abstraction, that minimum of generalization and formalization—idealization—which any science must extract. . . . [Berlin 1996, pp. 40–53]

What Berlin writes about history and political science is also valid for psychoanalysis. It aims at a comprehension of the mind, specifically of the inner life in conflict, a comprehension that places vast amounts of data in a systematic and symbolically presented order, with some predictive power, and that is as such scientific. Yet it connects this with a historical consciousness of the individual life, summarizing an immense quantity of detail, and shares this often in poetic-like form with the patient, or, mutatis mutandis, with the professional public. It involves a consistent application of the understanding of conflict, and of the explanation by conflict of all that occurs incessantly in our thinking, feeling, perceiving, remembering, wanting, and deciding, but in a form that also encompasses the small details—like the great inner connections—pictorially, metaphorically, poetically, sometimes even in dreamlike form, and yet at the same time rationally, logically, clearly. It is therefore a huge complementarity of methods. The theories of the natural sciences or of the humanities are by no means irrelevant, but they do not touch the essence of our kind of science and art. We are reminded of Aristotle's important statement in the *Nichomachean Ethics*:

> It is the mark of an educated mind to expect that amount of exactness (*tosouton t'akribes*) in each kind which the nature of the particular subject admits. It is equally unreasonable to accept merely probable conclusions from a mathematician [more accurately: one who simply wants to persuade: *pithanologous*] and to demand strict demonstration [proofs: *apodeixeis*] from an orator. [p. 9]

Thus we find ourselves in wider and deeper conflict, not only between suggestion and insight, but also between the claim of being *scientific*, as opposed to the necessity of asserting our independence from a methodology essentially reigning in the natural sciences, and insisting upon the *separate dignity and autonomy* of our mode of discovering the truth. This too turns out to be a *dialectic*, moving us incessantly forward.

Inevitably, the psychoanalyst finds himself placed before these challenges: on the one side, the clinically compelling necessity to answer concretely and specifically, in the here and now, the question about the nature of the suffering, and therefore about the truth hidden in symptoms and life problems; and on the other side, the scientific and philosophical obligation to account more generally for his criteria for truth. Continually, he has to ask himself how well-founded his work's claim for truth is, and that means, in a pragmatic understanding of truth, what its *worth* is.

### Categories and Individuality

This question is joined by further problems. "*Aber Lebendige machen alle den Fehler, daß sie zu stark unterscheiden*" (But all living beings make the mistake that they distinguish too sharply [Rilke, "First Duino Elegy"]). No art of treatment and no scientific enterprise can do without order, hence classification. Where one classifies, one has to judge what belongs to what, and as soon as one judges, condemnation is not far away. Categories seduce to categorical judgments. This is a temptation we never entirely escape from.

For a long time I have been concerned about this *spirit of condemnation*, this attitude of *judgmentalness*, so frequently manifest in the talk of analysts, therapists, or psychiatrists—with patients or about them. Many are using the great power given to them by their position to apply, subtly or not so subtly, some pejorative diagnoses and to deal accordingly with those who have been referred to them, who are being evaluated and treated by them. The degradation entailed in this is mostly unintentional, but the patient senses it and proves—with his or her obstinacy, a defiant lack of improvement, or to the contrary, by superficial submissiveness and distance from feelings—that he or she reacts to the shaming in the only way familiar since early times. Thus, *judgment* and *understanding* stand in a dialectical opposition that cannot be abolished. Therapeutic success is the touchstone of every technique, and all dogmatism and judgmentalness must massively curtail such curative value.

## Insight and Emotional Experience, Interpretation and Suggestion

It is often forgotten that psychoanalysis was specifically created by Freud to treat severely ill patients, patients who were crippled by their neurosis and incapable of functioning in wide areas of their existence (often even in their very ability to go on living), and that analysis has not been developed for reasonably well-functioning (though neurotically unhappy) professionals. Psychoanalysis is a *question of life or death*, or at least one of severe invalidity and hoped-for restoration. As Freud (1905) wrote:

> Actually, I have been able to elaborate and to test my therapeutic method only on severe, indeed on the severest cases; at first my material consisted entirely of patients who had tried everything else without success, and had spent long years in sanatoria. . . . Psychoanalytic therapy was created through and for the treatment of patients permanently unfit for existence, and its triumph has been that it has made a satisfactorily large number of these permanently fit for existence. In the face of such an achievement all the effort expended seems trivial. [p. 263]

This view is in agreement with what Thomä and Kächele in their textbook of 1985 said in regard to the ideal of an exclusively interpreting technique. They call this a fiction: "The classical psychoanalytic technique is thus 'one in which interpretation remains the exclusive or leading or prevailing tool' (Eissler 1958, p. 223). This technique exists nowhere in pure form," as Eissler himself conceded (Thomä and Kächele 1985, p. 40). The empirical examination does not support such "a purist method" (*Methodenpurismus*) (p. 41). Rather, the idealization and restrictiveness of this "normative technique" (p. 40) has proven harmful, because it led to a steady narrowing down of the indication for psychoanalysis. Instead they suggest, as a theory of therapy, "a systematic approach to problem solving": "The object of therapy is to master conflicts, under conditions more favorable than those which acted as midwife at the birth of the conflicts concerned" (p. 10). Insight and emotional experience are complementary. One-sided stress on "insight therapy centered on pure interpretation" (p. 263) stands in conflict with the therapeutic aim: "Interpretive purism can prevent a therapeutically favorable atmosphere from developing. . . . in recent years insight has increasingly been contrasted with the curative effect of the therapeutic relationship" (p. 272). With Balint (1968), they see the "new beginning as creative process" in the here-and-now and "the situational and creative elements in the therapeutic situation" as crucial for the mutative effect of therapy (p. 276). "Especially important in this regard is the *spontaneity* of the analyst, as Klauber [1981] emphasizes: '. . . It is this human quality of the relationship which is the antidote to the traumatic quality of transference as much or more than the acceptance of impulses by an analyst who reinforces the benign qualities of the superego.'" (p. 285). With this shift from the intrapsychic to the dyadic concept of therapy, the hitherto neglected "here-and-now—in the sense of new experience as opposed to repetition" (p. 54) assumes new dignity. With Cremerius (1984) they judge that "the limits of analyzability are not the limits of the patients and his psychopathology . . . but the limits of the analyst" (p. 188).[2]

I am in agreement with most of what these authors postulate with regard to their criticism of the rigidity of technical rules and to the criteria of "analyzability." My experience is very much in accordance with that of the Thomä and Kächele team of Ulm: that many more patients, often ostensibly very sick ones, can be analytically treated once relatively minor modifications are flexibly adapted to the exigencies of each case and the postulate of "neutrality" is taken far more relatively (in fact questioned in its value, as these authors as well as some others in Europe [Cremerius (1984) and Haynal (1989)] have courageously done).

In turn, such a restrictive view and redefinition of psychoanalysis has led to the postulate of a type of patient that alone is deemed "analyzable" by most, at least in the United States—"sick enough to need it and healthy enough to stand it," in the felicitous formulation by Waldhorn, quoted by Thomä and Kächele (1985/1987, p. 185). A pristinely defined analytic technique is applied to the "neuroses" of a select club of patients, a club for which essentially the control cases in the training institutes and the candidates themselves are eligible. In contrast to them there exists a vast mass of "borderline cases" who are mostly treated by "confrontation" (i.e., with "reality" and "limitations"), or with intense emotional support (e.g., by stressing above everything else empathy, or, in earlier times, intuition), or with an exploratory-confrontational approach focusing on direct drive interpretations (especially of those of an aggressive content and of "narcissistic entitlement," and of the contradiction between these and their professed wishes)—and of course, in their vast majority, by medication and manipulation, by self-help groups and religious-inspirational suggestion.

In short, it is evident that the patients nowadays being looked at as analyzable are not the same as those treated by the first two or three generations of analysts. Furthermore, there is a discrepancy between the official technique and how in fact most of the patients are being treated, if they are being treated analytically at all anymore (Cremerius 1984).

The detailed exploration of the great and nuanced multiplicity of affects, of the structural conflicts (especially those that involve the superego), and the careful working through of the main forms of defense—and with that the immense richness and genetic multilayeredness of the inner processes—appear to be neglected when it comes to these more severely disturbed (and suffering) patients. Instead of that, a model is being used for these patients that postulates "splitting" as an allegedly basic defense mechanism, employs its interpretation as the major point of leverage, and resorts to a few other so-called "archaic" forms of defense as additional levers: denial, projective identification, introjection, and idealization.

My own experience contrasts with this approach. Most of these severely ill patients are quite accessible to the classic ways of approach and understanding, if this method of treatment is not puristically limited to "insight" but is used in the way it was originally developed—as a method that combines the instrument of recognition (*Erkenntnis*) with the ancillary tools of suggestion, emotional support, and even occasionally medication.

Having said all this, I maintain that the *specific* element of therapeutic influence consists in the careful analysis, moment-to-moment within the therapeutic situation, of the forms of defense, of the conflicts within the superego, of those affects that have a particularly close relationship to the superego, like guilt, shame, depression, and resentment, and, finally and comprehensively, of the entire panorama of affects. The aforementioned *ancillary tools* have their own very important, though *unspecific* efficacy.

I still see the concept of conflict as one of the most fruitful concepts of human science and philosophy and the basic principle for the comprehension of mental processes. I quote from *The Mask of Shame* (1981a, pp. 12–13) about the essence of psychoanalysis: "Psychoanalysis is the natural science of the mind . . . the psychology of the innermost mental processes, of man in conflict" (Kris 1975, pp. 348–349). I believe that everything that lets the eye veer away from this centrality of conflict moves toward the periphery of psychoanalysis. I also postulated there that psychoanalysis is ultimately a field of symbolic forms *sui iuris et sui generis*, of its own lawfulness and its own nature, that cannot be exhaustively formulated through the concepts of its three major neighbors—the physical sciences, the cultural sciences (the so-called humanities), and philosophy. While metaphors from these and other fields may be necessary, indeed basically indispensable, the conceptual structures of psychoanalysis must be formulated cohesively and separately from any other. I hold that the foundation for such an autonomous conceptual framework, its Archimedean point,[3] is simply the reality and operation of inner conflict—observable, central, indubitable. Its a priori premise, still antedating it, is the unprovable principle of psychic determinism, which alone makes any science of inner reality conceivable and possible, just as the principle of causality and orderliness is the precondition for any science of outer reality. Both are necessary to the systematic ordering of experience in general or universal terms ("the conditions for their possibility" [*die Bedingungen ihrer Möglichkeit*], in Kant's terms). Any random occurrence (indeterminacy) would defy both understanding and explanation.

Although I do emphasize this dynamic view, I do not mean that conflict is the only important parameter in understanding the mind. But it is central to psychoanalysis. The study of faculties that develop more or less independently of conflict, "autonomously," ultimately falls into other psychological domains. All these varied perspectives can complement each other in beautiful enrichment of understanding.

## "Classical Neuroses" versus "Borderline" and "Narcissistic" Pathology, and the Question of Diagnostic Inflation

In the discussions about and the treatment of psychopathology and psychodynamics, there has been in the past thirty years a shift toward stressing more and more the similarities with the psychoses and emphasizing the archaic nature of the inner processes.

With that there has come a special regard for both the diagnosis of "borderline pathology" and a radically altered understanding and approach to the severer forms of psychopathology. Simultaneously there has been an increasing reliance and emphasis on the variations of self-image, and the issues of "narcissism" and with that a resorting to the explanatory power of the concepts of "structural defect," "deficiency," "lacunae," and "ego-weakness." This double change has had great implications for the attitude toward patients, and more specifically for the treatment approach, and poses many questions— of validity of claims, of coherence with other lines of research, and of clinical, long-range effectiveness.

As to the former, what had hitherto been counted as part of the core area of neurosis and treated as such was more and more branded as belonging to a borderline land or to schizophrenia and accordingly treated. Moreover, resorting to manic, depressive, paranoid, or autistic positions, states and developmental phases as basic explanatory concepts has become widely accepted. One tries, so it seems, to explain something unknown by something even more shrouded in mystery, about in the same way as the critics of psychoanalysis, like Grünbaum or Crews, foist all insights and the changes wrought by it onto the effect of suggestion. Do we really understand the dynamics and the genesis of the psychoses so well that we should adduce them to the explanation of phenomena in patients who, according to clearly defined psychiatric criteria, do not belong to these nosologic categories? Those who see something psychotic everywhere cannot fail to detect in most neuroses some "borderline condition."

In discussions with students, residents, analytic candidates, and more experienced colleagues, the remark "it is just a borderline case," has become so common that this diagnosis surpasses all others and finally rivals that of narcissism. Both diagnoses, often concomitantly used, are meant to refer to a particularly archaic pathology, one that is very close to that of the psychoses; in it the familiar psychology of the neuroses is replaced by dramatic splits of the personality, the mind is shaken in a mythical back-and-forth of projections and introjections, and driven into a state of confusion near insanity.

Then there is the stress on the devastating loss of mental structure, due to the lack of parental empathy. This lack is supposed to create a completely different pathology, that of narcissism, and to require a very different approach, one that is much more protective than the one needed by the neuroses.

In the "classical neuroses," so it is claimed, it is the sexual and aggressive drives that find themselves in a dramatic but still clearly structured combat with a superego internalized from the parents. In these real neurotics, the superego dictates to an obeisant, analytically compliant, and more or less defectless ego the important task of achieving compromises between defense and instinctual drive, and all this on an oedipal level, pure and simple. This, so it is held by some, is not the case, or at best only with great reservations, in strongly preoedipally damaged patients. In these, namely the narcissists and "borderlines," the ego is rent and riven, always threatened by fragmentation, or suffers in other, easily decipherable ways under lasting structural damages.

There is much in this view that can be agreed to. Yet in this way of argument, what is overlooked is that pretty much all the neurotics have suffered under the same types of lacks, that they have been in other ways severely traumatized to boot, and that clinically, in those cases called narcissistic, the conflicts are more severe, the superego stricter, and the defensive processes more complicated than in those certified as "just neurotics." It is also undeniable that there may be in them lasting and basic disorders of functioning that are very hard to cure, that is, "defects." But we usually are able to ascertain them only in the course of the painstaking conflict analysis over time, not immediately, a priori, in a first interview. Also, the suggestions for empathy and especially for protective interventions are really just as valid for all analysis. It is again a question of a more or less—an issue of complementarity.

Confronting the clinical reality of the patients seen by most of us today forces us to a choice between two options: either we restrict the applicability of psychoanalysis in its supposedly "pure" form to a very small minority of patients, declare everyone else to be unanalyzable, "borderline," or "narcissistic," and turn to a mostly confrontative or supportive, but non-"analytic" technique—or we recognize psychoanalysis as a broad form of treatment that focuses on the centrality of inner conflict, as played out in many variants of resistance and transference in the always unique relationship with a given analyst, a form of treatment that in reality is informed and shaped not only by the very few technical writings of Freud, but also by the infinite exigencies of the clinical reality of severe neuroses and the wide spectrum of patients who can benefit from intensive treatment centered on inner conflict.

## Trauma and Conflict

Within as well as outside the confines of psychoanalysis, the question of psychic trauma has assumed new actuality with the controversies caused by the allegations of retrieved sexual abuse and the opposite view that sees much or all such retrieval as due to suggestion causing the "false memory syndrome." There is no question, however, that the problem of traumatization is central to all understanding of psychopathology.

In regard to the current use of the trauma concept, I refer to the definition in Moore and Fine (1990):

> The disruption or breakdown that occurs when the psychic apparatus is suddenly presented with stimuli, either from within or from without, that are too powerful to be dealt with or assimilated in the usual way. A postulated stimulus bar-

rier or protective shield is breached, and the ego is overwhelmed and loses its mediating capacity. A state of helplessness results, ranging from total apathy and withdrawal to an emotional storm accompanied by disorganized behavior bordering on panic. Signs of autonomic dysfunction are frequently present . . . [p. 199]

A particular version of the judgmentalness inherent in the segregation of diagnostic categories of "unanalyzability" is the quickness with which many leap beyond the understanding of conflict and hastily start talking, already on the basis of phenomenology, about "defects" (e.g., "ego-defects," "super-ego lacunae"). This leads to the opposition between the understanding of genesis and maintenance of neurotic disorders mostly in concepts of defects versus that focused on conflict. I shall come back to this point in Chapter 4.

## Value and Truth

In spite of many commonalities, the inner world obeys laws that are different from those ruling the outer world. It is a questionable endeavor to hold the same scientific strictures applicable to both realms. At the same time, what Fenichel (1941) so poignantly stated is also true: "The subject matter, not the method, of psychoanalysis is irrational" (p. 13). It seems to me that it is especially the laws of *mythical* thinking and the role of *affects*, and therefore the realm of *values*, that determines any rational exploration of the mind. In the course of such inquiry, it becomes evident that facts and valuation, *truth and value*, are not mutually exclusive goals. Rather, *epistemology and value philosophy complement each other in an unexpected cooperation and correspondence.* Here again, qualities that seem irreconcilably divorced belong inseparably together.

## BASIC COORDINATES

*Anxiety and protection, scientific method and autonomy of the search for truth, judgment by categories and understanding of individuality, suggestion and insight, "borderline" pathology and neurosis, trauma and conflict, value and truth*—these *seven polarities, these seven dialectical contradictions* are the coordinates within which the following considerations move. They correspond to seven present challenges: the *demonic force* which often turns the plea for help of many patients and our rendering of help into an issue of life and death; the radical doubt about the value of our main instrument, the *insight into unconscious motivation,* and therefore about our very own, most specific understanding of causality; the necessity of presenting our findings in such a way that they can be *repeated and tested* by others, that is, that they meet certain minimal requirements of scientific method; the destructive power given to *outer authority* if it is allied with the undermining force of *self-condemnation*, particularly in the neurotically severely ill patient; the continuous temptation, again and again, to withdraw from the stringency of thinking in *conflicts* and *polarities*; the temptation either to *blame the outside world* for "the poor child's" suffering or, conversely, to disregard outer trauma and see inner life, solipsistically, as mere reflection of *inner drives* and conflicts; and finally, the quest for truth with the help of *value judgments*.

The tension engendered by these seven polarities goes through all chapters of this book and *Flight from Conscience*. Teasing them out as separate subjects for presentation would fail to do justice to the complexity of these in-depth studies.

The themes chosen for each of the chapters are nodal points where several tension lines cross in ways and forms that are quite specific to the individual described; withal, they ought to illuminate certain *specific* and often unique formations—just as a particular work of art may seem to condense an entire epoch and its dynamic.

## MAIN OBSERVATIONS AND ASSUMPTIONS

*Was gelten soll, muß wirken und muß dienen.*
(What should be valid must be of effect and service.)
—Goethe

Every new book needs justification. In all areas, not least in psychiatry, psychoanalysis, and psychotherapy, the reader is being carried away by such a flood of professional literature that one should raise a claim on his attention only if one intends to submit something original, special, and generally useful. Such a new work should also not simply present a collection of disparate experiences, but rather an ordered whole, an image with focus, perspective, and frame. Yet it ought also neither digress into all-encompassing contemplations and philosophically pious generalities nor spend itself in speculations beyond what can be known by our methods of observation—whether in regard to the experience of early childhood, the biological substrate, or the metaphysics of the soul—nor find its pleasure in concatenations of technical terms.

Its justification must therefore lie in an understandable presentation of new *observations*, thus reminding the clinician of some of his own cases and hinting, in a fascinating way, at the possible solution of old riddles. With this it should propose new *treatment strategies* and *tactics* and also describe in detail how they have opened up access to otherwise intractable cases, while stating how generally used ways of understanding and methods have failed with these cases. On the basis of such experience it should become possible to sketch the most helpful *concepts* and *models*, and thus to come closer to some scientific truth. Such approximation always brings up questions concerning the inevitable *philosophical* presuppositions that underlie how we comprehend and act.

As far as this is possible, I have tried to let the phenomena appear and speak to me with a new freshness and not to allow theoretical prejudices to obstruct the view. Observing over hundreds of hours the immense richness of the mind, we may recognize and understand ever fresh forms, renewed transformations, and, with them, new, often unexpected theoretical connections.

One image symbolizing this particular intent emerged in a session: we search for the pieces of a jigsaw puzzle hidden in a sandpile. But it is not enough to dig out piece for piece; we have to find the right order in which they fit together. We may not force them together and break them. A priori, we never know how the picture in the riddle really looks. This applies to every case.

One of my teachers told me: "I usually understand the dynamics of a case in the first session." Really? It is neither false modesty nor incompetence if I would respond today: "Lucky you! I am often not so sure after five hundred hours."

At the beginning of this work, there was no obvious center around which everything effortlessly gathered, as had been the case in the previous two works, the treatment of the subject of shame (1981a), and the psychology of compulsive drug use ( *The Hidden Dimension* [1978]). Instead, there lay in front of me a vast amount of experience chock-full of interesting and promising connections and possibilities and that even gave the impression of some inner unity, but one that could not be easily joined together without its being bent, twisted, and broken. Much of it seemed very familiar psychoanalytic knowledge. However, when I allowed this material to speak to me, as much without prejudice as was feasible under these circumstances, slowly certain new configurations began to appear, complex images of connections that repeated themselves. Certain dilemmas, sequences, and equations kept emerging that had been present in the therapeutic work, yet which I had not been aware of with such clarity nor had known from the literature. Eventually, it was the power and importance of "repetition compulsion" that proved a kind of red thread through everything—but as problem, not as answer.

The following considerations took their issue from several simple observations:

## Approach

A number of *severely sick* patients were treated by me with psychoanalysis although they would have been, according to the usual recommendations, viewed as unanalyzable and sometimes actually were explicitly warned of the dangerousness of such an approach by representatives of other psychiatric orientations, by physicians in other specialties, or by "experts" claiming prerogatives for their special area of symptomatology. Though the treatment often proved very difficult and complicated and required certain modifications of the customary method, it could, all in all, retain the paradigm of the analysis of resistance and transference and the search for unconscious motivation. However, it proved necessary in most of the cases, and always in those most difficult, to *combine* psychoanalysis with other methods of treatment. Such simultaneous combination surpassed by far in efficacy every single method, and is comparable to the usual treatment today in somatic medicine (e.g., batteries of convergent medication in the treatment of tuberculosis, leukemia, and AIDS). Although these cases would under the ordinary criteria have been viewed as *unanalyzable*, they could be treated this way effectively and with lasting success.

The question is asked: How is this possible? How can we use suggestion and other modifications of technique and still claim that we *analyze* the transference, that is, that we interpret it in its original meaning as *distortion* and thus resolve it? If we become a *real* figure in the life of the patient, how could it still be possible to examine the as-if character of transference? Do we not here replace true analysis with the ill-reputed "corrective emotional experience"? Do we not violate left and right the basic rules of abstinence and neutrality by inadmissible gratifications of the patient's neurotic demands?

Certainly, these are difficult issues, hard questions that must be taken very seriously. As already briefly mentioned, I believe that analytic neutrality, the endeavor not to become a real figure in the life of the patient, is a utopian ideal, a "regulative idea" in the Kantian sense. In severe psychopathology, silence and extreme emotional restraint are often just as much being experienced as a real, non-neutral intervention as a more active participation of the analyst (cf. Thomä 1993).

I ask myself whether the actual question in each case should not rather be what the focus of our activity should be if we want to attain an *optimal, long-term change*. This optimal form of focusing has to be individually specific. This means that there exists not just *one* analytic technique but that *every patient requires his own optimal technique,* a technique comprising a wide spectrum of interventions. These have to be set up so that they permit, facilitate and protect both the *rational alliance* and the *reexperiencing of irrationality.*

This implies that these patients who suffer from severe neuroses pose far greater demands on specific analytic know-how. They require both a more differentiated technique and a more precise discernment of dynamics and diagnostics than the usual group of "analyzable" patients (cf. Thomä 1993). They need more, not less understanding, tact and respect, more attention to conflicts, more awareness of the oppression by conscience and ideals, and more sophistication in the analysis of complex ego-functions—especially defenses—not less!

In the light of the research of the last twenty years, the traditional theories about the mental processes in earliest childhood, which are still very often being used to justify many present-day approaches with these more severely ill patients, have been shown to be largely ill-founded, wrong, or skewed. Interventions with these patients based on splitting, confrontation, and direct drive interpretation are not so much erroneous as less useful than expected; in and by themselves they are valuable tactics suited to bring about mainly short-term behavioral alterations, but for greater efficacy they need to be complemented with other ways of understanding and treating. Here again it is not so much a question of either-or, as a matter of as-well-as, that is, it is an issue of *complementarity.*

The literature pretty much lacks thorough descriptions of cases and treatments of such difficult cases. Therefore, a presentation of their successful analyses which aspires, at least in spirit, to a certain inner unity, may claim some interest.

## The Therapeutic Atmosphere

Approach and understanding diverge, therefore, in decisive aspects from those that are being recommended today for these cases by most psychiatrists, analysts, and therapists. Instead of declaring them "borderline states" and treating them under this diagnosis as if it were a unitary category, I see them as many different forms of neurosis which, though uniformly severe, are clearly differentiated from each other and require an equally differentiated understanding. Most importantly, they can be made *accessible to the classic psychoanalytic method,* provided that as much as possible we *avoid being put into the role of an authority, induced to take on the functions of an "external superego, "* and that we take care not to become a *real figure of conscience* for them and thus not to anchor the sadomasochistic transference in a subtly *real relationship of sadomasochism.* In that, the therapeutic atmosphere, particularly its affective tone, is decisive. Confrontations are the exception, not the rule. It is this fundamental attitude of forbearance (*Schonung*), of tact and friendliness, and of avoiding condemning words or behaviors that shapes certain technical guidelines. These "rules" are, therefore, only means to an end and are themselves already expressions of the basic attitude; they should never turn into a demand of *l'art pour l'art*, as has often been suggested, especially here in the United States.

## Moments of Rightness

Certain sessions and certain therapeutic episodes stand out from the entire course of treatment like high peaks jutting out from a mountain chain. The lower hills and mountains lead up to these summits, yet it is just from these peaks that we can gain new clarity and overview. These "*good analytic hours*" (Kris 1956, p. 255) are not only breakthroughs in the treatment itself, but, if rendered in detail, might permit the reader, following the words of the therapeutic dialogue, to let himself be persuaded by the relevance of the connections, and thus to grasp for himself the core dynamics of representative cases. Such "going along and being with it" might make it possible for many to apply these insights in other instances. Although everything is individual, it is also general: "It would be the highest thing: to comprehend that everything factual is already theory. . . . One should not look behind the phenomena; they are already in themselves theory" (Goethe).[4]

Moreover, these detailed presentations of "good hours" might also make it easier to deal with the difficult problem of how to distinguish between specifically effective factors and those of an unspecific nature. Such *moments of rightness* may permit us a glimpse of something that is the essence of the psychoanalytic process, that is, a look into the tightly interwoven texture of interpretation, insight, and clinical change. And with that they might begin to give an answer to the radical doubts of the epistemologists (at least as far as their critique is itself rational, which, alas, it rarely is).

I do not mean by this to slight the relevance of what we all know so well: how much of the work is slowly inching forward, groping, and yet cumulative in its effect. Progress is made not only in sudden illuminations, but in small, plodding steps. And then, there are of course also stagnation and deterioration. The former—alleged slowness—may also hide the latter: failure.

## Role of the Superego

As already alluded to, the *superego*, with its manifold functions, plays during the therapy of all these difficult patients a dominant and especially important role, far more than it is commonly credited with in the professional discussions and writings. With all these patients there are episodes during which they rebel in one way or the other against part of this inner authority, when they try to overthrow it altogether or to flee from it. While this dynamic aspect of the *defense against the superego* is only one part of the therapeutic work, although a very important one, it is significant enough to form one of the major perspectives of this entire book (and gave the book its original German title: *Flight from Conscience*). Thus the book should be a novel contribution to the *defense and superego analysis of the severe neuroses*.

During the in-depth examination of the case material, it also becomes more and more evident to us that impulsive actions are not simply attempts to defy momentarily the harsh despotism of conscience, because we can also distinguish quick sequences of conflict solution in which also all the prohibiting and restraining processes partake. Conscience, ideals, and values themselves stand in contradiction, *the superego is split*. Thus, during the compulsively occurring repetitions and the observable identity splits, observing the conflict between opposite superego aspects is crucial and, in fact, of the greatest practical significance.

## The Spirit of Resentment

A particular form of such *flight from conscience* can be detected in *resentment* (*Ressentiment*).[5] Nietzsche and Scheler detected and stressed this affect's great role in the structure of traditional morality. Put into our own terminology, it has to do with how the superego and its value structure are rooted in the drive for power and the aggression derived from it. Something we can observe in many patients is to what extent the "inner judge" is filled with this spirit of *ressentiment*. This is one version of it. An even more virulent form occurs when intense self-condemnation, especially deep shame, leads to burning resentment, which in turn then justifies a radical revolt against all human bonds and obligations. It consists in the self-righteous identification with one's own categorically judging conscience (a merging of the ego into the archaic superego). The accusation is being turned around: the self changes from being the victim of self-accusation to being the brutal judge and avenger; the other becomes the one who is radically blamed and rejected and who ultimately must be exterminated.

Some patients show this episodically. The resentment may break through with demonic drivenness, or it may be disguised by self-righteous justifications. In a few instances, and usually in historically prominent or literary figures, this sequence can be studied almost in pure culture, as for example in world literature in Shakespeare's *Richard III* or *Othello*, in Balzac's *Cousin Bette*, in *Canetti's Auto-da-Fé*, and in particular in Lagerkvist's *Dvärgen* (*The Dwarf*). It is a *ressentiment* reaching for naked power, and it behaves as if it were a "new conscience" and a revolutionary ideal system, namely a conscience whose highest commandment and aim would be to pull out the roots of envy, vengefulness, and jealousy by exterminating their objects. How should it "succeed" in that? Very simply: by countering the sense of deepest helplessness and overwhelming anxiety, of paralyzing shame and impotence with an equally total ideal of omnipotence. *Conscience thus becomes itself the carrier of malignant narcissism: this is the nature of evil.* The outward sadism and totalitarianism is a turning outward of the cruelty and absoluteness of the superego's demands toward the self (cf. also Berliner's term "countermasochism" [1940, 1947]). It is a peculiar form of superego pathology and already as such a kind of defense against overwhelming feelings—and principally treatable.

More generally speaking, the clinical phenomena of masochism, narcissism, and compulsive drug use are central ways of dealing with such superego conflicts and thus, indirectly, with chronic traumatization.

Yet there are a few more considerations to this concept of *ressentiment*. It is described by Scheler (1915) as a "mental self-poisoning" (*seelische Selbstvergiftung*), "caused by the systematic pushing aside [repression] in the discharging of certain emotions and affects" (p. 38).[6] While it is "vengefulness, envy, jealousy, scornfulness, pleasure about the other's suffering and malice" (p. 41) that underlie resentment (*Rachegefühl, Neid, Scheelsucht, Hämischkeit, Schadenfreude und Bosheit*), these only lead to the formation of resentment if "a yet more pronounced sense of powerlessness impedes such action or expression" (p. 41) [*wenn*] (*ein noch ausgeprägteres Bewußtsein der Ohnmacht ein solches Handeln oder einen solchen Ausdruck hemmt*) (p. 41). What is left out in Scheler's description though is the relationship to the sense of justice that is inherent in the affect of resentment, and that is to be found in the definition of the French root word: "le fait de se souvenir avec animosité des torts qu'on a subis (comme si on les ressentait, ou les 'sentait' encore)" (as the *Micro Robert en Poche* put it) (the remembrance with animosity of suffered instances of injustice as if one still or again felt them). However, such an injured sense of justice can only occur once the value of justice itself, in whatever version, has already been accepted. *Ressentiment* has to be viewed therefore against the background of *loyalty*, and loyalty is more than some ordinary "object relation": it is the bond toward somebody who is being seen as a binding authority, as a source of obligation and commitment. Loyalty entails the expectation of reward—lastly, in the form of acceptance, respect, and love—as service rendered for the faith kept. It is the violation of this expectation that engenders *ressentiment.*

Loyalty is one form of superego bond, and loyalty conflicts are among the most important and most burdensome conflicts in the dynamics of the severe neuroses.

## Secrets, Denial, and Double Conscience

When opposing superego figures within struggle with each other, *denial* is needed as a crucial defense. Many patients are haunted by a *secret* throughout their life.

Such a blockage of entire areas of perception always leads to a *split* of their inner and outer reality. Without their being clearly conscious of it, these patients feel forced to lead a double life and to assume a *double identity*. Most of the cases to be described here fall therefore under the diagnoses of *multiple personality* and *dissociative disorder*, categories that today are, again, used more often and with a broader meaning than for most of this century.

What underlies such double identity is a kind of *double conscience*, and, corresponding to it, radical value conflicts and contradictions in the formation of ideals. The temporary realization of one identity dictates the denial of its antagonist.

Such a doubleness of both the outer world and of one's own identity must be reflected in behavior and affects. Something similar can be observed in most dreams: one's own identity is typically split up into several figures. Yet, these partial identities are not final elements either, but themselves represent attempts at resolving inner conflicts. Moreover, there is a conflict between the patient's everyday existence and the one or several regressive forms of identity. The exploration of the dynamics of such split identity is not only a very important part of any understanding of the neuroses in general and especially of the "impulsive action sequences" (Lansky 1984) in them, but also might contribute something to the comprehension of the finding and maintaining of identity (M. Stern 1986). Thus, the phenomenon of double identity is not merely of great clinical interest, and not only a lead symptom of pathology, but it also engenders fascinating literary and cultural-philosophical considerations.

## Vicious Circles in Ego States

Strikingly, long-term intensive work gradually discovers characteristic *circular sequences* of ego states—of compromise formations of conflicts—that can be reconstructed for the current inner life, and for the current transactions in transference and the immediate environment, but also for the past. Such *reconstructions of ego states* took on, in my experience, greater relevance than the restoration of narrative continuity by reconstruction of repressed trauma. These vicious circles also assume a certain specific regularity for different pictures of pathology.

## The Realm of Affects

Particular and independent significance must be ascribed to the realm of *affects*. Affect theory has in the last few years reclaimed an existence and dignity independent of drive theory. Only the accurate grasping of the great variety and richness of experienced and veiled feelings, moment by moment in the session, permits optimal empathy and understanding of the patient.

In psychoanalytic theory, the role of affects has for a long time been much underrated. Their attentive examination has to lead to a great enrichment and deepening of clinical and theoretical acumen. On the one side, affect psychology points toward *value philosophy*. On the other, affect psychology is also always part of *conflict psychology*, affective discord perhaps being the most accessible manifestation of inner conflict, as affects very typically can enter into conflict with each other. They stand in the service of what we psychoanalytically understand as the ego, but whether they can so simply be viewed as ego-functions seems nowadays quite questionable. Their independence accounts for the fact that they can be observed in surprising multiplicity from the very earliest time, even shortly after birth on (Tomkins 1962, Nathanson 1992). There are simple as well as highly complicated affects.

## The Centrality of Metaphor

The analyst's work has to be largely *metaphorical*. Primary process thinking underlying both neurosis and dream follows the logical laws of mythical thinking. Because metaphors work with images, and because they overstep the lines between perceptual categories, they appeal to mythical thinking. The etymology of the word *metaphora* already indicates the close relationship to one of the basic concepts of psychoanalysis: it means "transference" (Grassi 1979, Wurmser 1977a).

One of the most fascinating discoveries in the research on early infancy is the newborn's and infant's striking "capacity to transfer perceptual experience from one sensory modality to another" (D. Stern 1985, p. 47). Such "yoking of the tactile and visual experiences is brought about by way of the innate design of the perceptual system, not by way of repeated world experience. No learning is needed initially . . ." (p. 48). This implies "that the infant, from the earliest days of life, forms and acts upon abstract representations of qualities of perception" (p. 51). In other words, *abstraction*, that is, the ability to transfer formal qualities between different modalities, exists from the very beginning, independent from all experience, and thus is an immediate given—an a priori. Metaphorical thought is only a special case of this fundamental characteristic of our mind.

What Aristotle (*Poetics*, 22.16/17—1459 a) saw as the "token of genius" (εὐφυίας τε σημεῖον) in the poet, that is, the use of metaphor—(πολὺ δὲ μέγιστον τὸ μεταφορικὸν εἶναι)—can by rights also be claimed for the analyst: "Seeing what is similar." Similes and figures of speech are an important road that may lead very directly to what is unconscious. Philosophically, it also means a great deal that the analytic models of insight and of ordering the data are themselves of metaphorical nature.

In addition, this philosophical attitude does greater justice to the complexity of inner life than a closed and dogmatic system of theories could do. Theoretical models as metaphorical renderings that allow approximation to "the truth" but are not absolute; models that are more useful for this purpose than others; models of all the different schools being attempts to order smaller or larger segments of observations, some handier than others; based on such models and the technical guidelines being more or less effective, short or long term, helpfully and yet unfortunately also often harmfully—these are the *pragmatic* foundations upon which, in my own psychoanalytic work, the concept of truth is built.

## Complementarity of Experience

Many have arrived at the conclusion that in this type of work it becomes philosophically imperative to turn away from a naïve and positivistic knowledge of reality. The *philosophy of complementarity* appears to be most helpful: to reunite again and again the seemingly contradictory viewpoints, and to see them as mutual conditions of each other—as for example in the understanding of intrapsychic processes versus those of interpersonal communication, and thus of a broadly understood "self-psychology" versus an equally broadly conceived "object relations psychology"; or, derived from this, the significance of transference versus the significance of genetic construction; or, what is experiential in the therapeutic relationship versus the value of cognition as decisive therapeutic factors; or finally the exploration of the psychoanalytic situation itself versus that of experience and action without.

> Thinking and doing, doing and thinking, this is the sum of all wisdom, acknowledged from time immemorial, implemented at all times, not recognized by everybody. Both must, like breathing out and breathing in, eternally move back and forth in life; like question and answer, one should not take place without the other. Who sets it as a law for himself what the genius of human reason secretly whispers in the ear of every newborn: to test doing by thinking, thinking by doing, cannot err, and if he does err he will soon find back to the right way. [Goethe][7]

The following is inscribed on the sarcophagus in the "Hall of the Past" (*Saale der Vergangenheit*): "Think to live!;[8] it seems to be the intention of the "secret powers of the Tower" (*geheimnisvollen Mächte des Turms*) "to separate what is connected and to connect what is separate,"[9] and thus engage alternatively in analysis and synthesis.

A similar complementarity exists, in my view, between great literature and clinical experience. They are like two rows of mirrors. Both rows reflect in manifold images and refractions the essence of the soul, yet alone are unable to grasp it completely: "Never can you find the boundaries of a soul, even if you went down every path; thus deep is its ground, Logos" (Heraclitus).

It is a questionable procedure to use psychoanalytic categories in order to fathom literary works; and, in turn, literary concepts and symbols do not suffice to comprehend the essence of the unconscious. However, both together aim at a third entity, one that is *partly* understandable and explainable, and yet, in its individual uniqueness, encompasses a world in itself and can never be *completely* comprehensible. Such skepticism in regard to the reach of our knowledge does not mean that we would have to appeal to some religious faith.

Therefore, it is evident that the insights of psychoanalysis (and of the clinical work altogether) stand in dialogue both with the world of culture and with biology—and yet, they are ultimately independent from both: *sui generis et sui iuris.*

## The New Concept of Causality

The new concept of causality, emerging from the observations mentioned, is also a subject of philosophy. The causes and reasons (the latter understood as inner causality) that are being adduced for the understanding of neurotic symptoms and character problems, and that can be submitted to analytic treatment, cannot be found in single events,[10] —whether these be internal or external. Rather, it is a matter of many layers of outer and inner conflicts that constitute the *new causality* only in their playing together. This form of research into causality, which in psychoanalysis is being carried out individually,[11] is as much in need of a scientific canon as the other realms of science; but this canon presupposes different methods from those used, for example, in the natural sciences or in the scientifically proceeding humanities (*Geisteswissenschaften*).

In this context it proved always very helpful not to be snared by clichés, to question again and again traditional wisdom and generally accepted dicta— those seemingly self-evident truths that Ibsen (1882) called "old inherited popular lies";[12] "they are like putrid, spoiled, but freshly salted bacon."[13] Of special interest for us will be the precipitous *leap from description to explanation* that has been a favorite stunt in our field from its inception; it has not lost its popularity. That too found a wonderful critic in Goethe: "When one examines the problems of Aristotle one is amazed about the gift of observation and about all that the Greeks had eyes for. Only they commit the mistake of hastiness because they immediately step from phenomenon to explanation, which brings to light totally insufficient theoretical pronouncements. This however is the universal error that is still being made today."[14]

## METHOD OF PRESENTATION

"*Was man nicht versteht, besitzt man nicht.*"
(What you do not understand, you do not possess.)
—Goethe, *Maxims and Reflections*

### Understanding the Individual World

In the Grünbaum debate, the philosopher of science Peter Caws (1986) remarked,

> psychoanalysis is a natural science all right, but the natural domain of which it is the science is *the idiosyncratic world of the individual patient*, not the class of human beings over which the natural science of psychology applies. In other words, I think that clinical findings *cannot reliably be extrapolated beyond the case from which they are drawn*. Every new patient who walks into the analyst's office is a new world to be explored . . . [p. 230, original italics]

It seems to me, too, that it is essential to find the lawfulness in what is singular and particular; in other words, what is generally valid (or rather, what is frequently valid) can often be better grasped if we present what is particular and special than if we proceed mainly with the help of abstract terminology.

It also strikes me that many descriptions in the psychoanalytic literature lead to misunderstandings because they stake out claims for either—or distinctions that prove ill-founded, as with self-psychology versus conflict psychology, intrapsychic versus object relations, transference versus past experience, trauma versus inner conflict, defense versus drive, and so on. Because of that, valuable new observations and therapeutic recommendations run the danger of not being taken as seriously as they merit—and the bigger danger that they cause less experienced therapists to lose their way. The same may hold true for some groups with other orientations where the rich and full unfolding of therapeutic work and efficacy seems curtailed by theoretical writings that give the impression of one-sidedness. Precisely because of this, I consider it crucial *not to be restricted to cursory case descriptions*, but to present directly, as far as this is feasible, what *really* happens—not only to *say* what has happened—and to give it as a *whole form.*

One way of elaborating the observations and conclusions might be to go schematically from one illness to the other, or to study one dynamic problem after the other, such as certain forms of defense or of superego pathology. However, in the course of many years I have become more and more skeptical about excessive schematization and generalization. Although we cannot get by without certain categories with whose help we sort out our experiences, we have to acknowledge their limited validity.

Instead of such a procedure I have decided to let the cases themselves speak to us, as it were, immediately, the way it occurs in the analytic situation. In these detailed excerpts the reader may rediscover his own concrete experiences, and that may permit him to come to his own abstractions that might or might not be at variance from the author's.

Of course, such a presentation also remains a matter of selection, which is determined by the underlying principles of ordering. We cannot get around such prejudgment, a kind of a priori. Still, at least such an approach should not succumb to the danger of overcategorization and thus of losing the individual reality.

In what follows I shall select mostly treatments which, in spite of often desperate difficulties, ended with a good outcome and where we get in retrospect the impression that there were specific groups of interventions and insights which, at times very dramatically, made the breakthrough possible.

For that I employ a kind of presentation that to my knowledge has only seldom been used: the concentration upon characteristic excerpts from the treatment, given in a pretty detailed form. Usually, these are quite faithful reproductions of the therapeutic dialogue during the sessions that both patient and analyst valued in looking back as high points of the entire treatment. In that way I shall try to avoid the excessive abstraction and the technical jargon marking most clinical case descriptions, without, however, falling into the opposite mistake of the excessively detailed way of quoting from direct transcriptions (I mean mistake only for the purposes of this work). Even so, many of the methodological problems raised by epistemology remain unresolved.

Therefore, it is advisable at first not to worry too much about the philosophical contentions and instead to propose and describe at this point a method of developing and confirming theory that I hope is at least *practically sufficient*. This method, chosen for the clinical chapters, differs from the more usual ones.

## *Kairós*: The Right Time

In Sophocles' *Electra* we read: "The right time is the greatest teacher in every work of man" (καιρὸς γὰρ ὅσπερ ἀνδράσιν μέγιστος ἔργου παντός ἐστ᾽ ἐπιστάτης 75/76). I have already mentioned that not infrequently the great inner connections show up in single sessions and sequences of sessions. The exact study of such representative episodes, "the right time" (*kairós*), will form the basis of this work. Moreover, this method might also be a contribution to the present epistemological debate about the justification of psychoanalytic claims.

With the type of research used here I mean that the concentration upon certain critical hours permits the *investigation of specific interventions and specific connections*, as far as they can be correlated with subjective and objective changes—even the question of whether this is not the case. (This includes the examination of the possible fallacy *post hoc propter hoc*.) What such a focusing pushes toward the periphery are the less specific cumulative effects of the therapeutic work—experiencing trust and acceptance, restoring narrative and introspective continuity and coherence (cf. Loch 1976, Spence 1982, 1983), and sensing the therapist's empathy or the tension of discovery or uncertainty (Friedman 1985; Lichtenberg 1983, 1985).

A clear disadvantage of this concentration of research upon the "high points" of work lies in the fact that in such sessions there are far more interpretative comments and conjectures by me than are being expressed in the "lowlands." This form of condensation evokes the appearance of far greater activity on my side than is in reality the case.

One presupposition for such a selection of the material is that there are real differences in quality between certain hours and periods of analysis (Kris 1956, 1975). The checking up on this premise is itself a question that should be investigated separately from the careful study of the selections themselves. One form of inquiry does not make the other redundant. Here I will restrict myself to the latter.

It would of course be very helpful if a serious epistemologist were himself to compare the tapes or the more or less verbatim notes of such a good hour with those of a banal or bad hour, or of series of hours over longer periods, and if he were to examine what impact the interventions of an experienced analyst or therapist have: how they showed to be *very effective* only in very specific forms and quite rarely, in a proportion perhaps of 1:100, if not less, how they could be noxious or at least interfering in others, or without any influence, or moderately but cumulatively effective in the rest.

The questions raised in this type of research would be these: What distinguishes the good from the bad sessions, the good from the bad therapists? What does change, and how is such change manifested? Short or long term? Does it regularly occur after certain kinds of interventions? How would he—this ideal, critical inquirer—understand the so often prevailing insecurity and confusion? How would he evaluate the sudden feeling of clarity that often happens in patient and therapist?

Being the objective observer, how would he judge the generalizations arrived at by an experienced therapist on the basis of dozens of patients whom he has intensively worked with, insights that he now carries over into other cases he knows only from supervision or in short focal therapy? Or the theoretical developments in his writings based on these experiences?

## Controls

Then the question raised by Grünbaum (1984) would become relevant: What would be truly representative control studies? Since double-blind controls or comparisons of groups are either impossible or irrelevant, new forms of objective control would be required. Good hours or interventions compared with bad ones? Observation of the same patient or therapist as his own control in the form of "single subject research" (Edelson 1984)? Or the comparison of effective treatments or mutative interpretations with ineffective ones in different therapists, maybe even with those from different schools? How far do selective tape recordings or stenograms suffice for this purpose?

## The Value Conflict of Reliability versus Relevance

A particularly daunting practical problem seems to me to consist in how we can deal with the enormous surfeit of information that has piled up over hundreds of hours. I believe it is this problem above all that has defied all the attempts to objectify the findings in a satisfactory way, and that has left the inquiry for the most part to those persons who are directly engaged in this shared investigation—namely the duo of patient and therapist. As regrettable it is, it cannot be denied that this kind of exclusively clinical and directly participatory investigation suffers from all those shortcomings Grünbaum (1984) scathingly expatiates upon—all the dangers of distortion, the deception due to suggestion and to inevitable memory alterations—and that these infringements of observation and investigation may be corrected only unsatisfactorily by supervision and group processes. Not least, such critique is supported by the often sharply contradictory claims.

With that we have to ask how we may combine the method of sufficient *reliablity* with the method of sufficient *relevance.* That is, what are the primary data which should be selected and used? This has proven so difficult because most of the insight does not occur in sudden revelations but in something that proceeds step by step, with the help of accumulating evidence, a kind of accretion.

Furthermore, the process notes taken down after the sessions are indeed far too "contaminated" as such to satisfy in any way today's research requirement for more valid proofs. I trust my own memory much less than many colleagues trust theirs. Moreover, I noticed, at least in myself, to what extent the need to remember as faithfully as possible mightily interferes with the unbiased, "evenly hovering" attention required for the work itself.

On the other side, taped material can, already by its sheer quantity, become so overpowering if used for the purposes mentioned that its volume simply inundates what would be relevant; it is the problem of the noise factor. Quantity alone and the exactitude of what has been boundlessly accumulated cannot supplant the response to questions about quality that I consider crucial for judging scientific truth. Many of these problems are currently being studied with great seriousness (cf. e.g., Edelson 1984, Luborsky and Auerbach 1969, Thomä, 1993, Thomä and Kächele 1973, 1985, 1987, Weiss and Sampson 1986).[15]

"Much is true that cannot be calculated, and much that cannot be brought to the decisive experiment."[16]

In the following inquiry I have therefore decided upon a middle course as one that is practically most satisfactory: Since the beginning of my work with patients, about forty years ago, I have found that the *stenographic* notes, made during all sessions with all my patients and kept in systematic order, were an extremely valuable research tool. Thanks to this procedure it is possible to review and quickly sift within one hour the material of about a hundred hours of therapy or analysis; even a more careful study and transcription of what appears most relevant from such material is a matter of only a few hours. In addition, everything that needs to be examined precisely and in its depth dimension, often including my weighing of theoretical reformulations and of countertransference reactions, stands at my disposal, although typically in somewhat simplified and condensed form. In this way it seems possible to *combine the advantages of sufficient reliability with sufficient relevance.* With such an approach it should also be possible to apply *quantitative* means in order to find evidence for those *qualitative* factors (and their value) that assume such centrality in the therapeutic work, instead of engaging in the vain attempt to prove causality by some kind of *pars pro toto* thinking, hence by inadmissible simplification. In fact, an investigation of this kind is nothing else than an elaboration and systematization of what is anyway an integral part of the entire psychoanalytic enterprise, that is, the process of supervision.

In short, the important epistemological question is not so much: Are these or those theories correct? but: How can we explain that severe and complicated neuroses are getting resolved after certain, often very precise and deliberate interventions, or at least let themselves be strongly modified by them, whereas they prove refractory at other times and vis-à-vis other interventions? What is the satisfactory explanation, very concretely, for success and failure in every single case?

These are hard, but nonetheless empirically solvable questions. No philosophy is able to respond to them. But systematic, objectivating clinical investigations (*process research*) have a good chance to hit upon answers that have greater evidentiary power than those found in the clinical situation alone (cf. Thomä and Kächele 1985, p. 369 f., 1987).

In the following chapters (and *Flight from Conscience*) I shall make use of this method to the extent as it is feasible for me as an individual investigator. The treatment notes of the cases are, at least in principle, available for an independent reexamination. In accord with what I stated earlier I select out of the enormous mass of available material single hours (and series of them) that are particularly remarkable and decisive for the entire course of treatment. They could be taken as analogous to very precisely chosen biopsies whose essential segments can then be studied microscopically. Although this approach too can be subjected to scientific criticism I still believe that in this way we approximate the "probative evidence" properly demanded by Grünbaum (1984) more than is possible when cases are only presented in global descriptions or as anecdotal vignettes.

## SELECTION OF CASES

It is evident that psychoanalysis goes through a process of revolution. Higher requirements for its scientific quality and accountability as well as the impact of new results of research in many neighboring fields have gradually led to a greater readiness to pay more closely focused attention to clinical experience, to the "raw data," so to speak, than to the theoretical presuppositions and to treat the latter as metaphors that should be used pragmatically, not in a doctrinaire way.

I believe that it is part of such a reorientation to open up new clinical areas with the precious instrument of the psychoanalytic method. As mentioned earlier, it has been for many years one of my intentions to investigate how one may psychoanalytically treat severely ill patients—those commonly regarded as *unanalyzable*—and, in doing so, to find which minimal modifications of technique one can get by with in order to combine long-term therapeutic effectiveness with maximal insight into the dynamics. I am very much convinced that the treatment of these severe forms of neuroses is not something peripheral, but that it does belong to the very essence and main task of psychoanalysis. It is just this work with severely disturbed patients that can serve as a touchstone for the theoretical conceptions. It soon shows which assumptions prove themselves, hour by hour, case by case, and which ones may give a short-range explanation, but in the long run do not help further. Other ways of expressing this would be: Which types of interpretations seem to have more of an authoritatively imposed effect as suggestions, hence are short-lived in their efficacy, and which types lead to ever-widening circles of spontaneous self-observation on the side of the patient? Which interventions are more supportive, and which are more illuminating to the patient, not just to the therapist? Which approaches cause "resistance," and which actually resolve resistance? (cf. Gray 1994). Such an application of psychoanalysis would enable us to return to why it has originally been created.

### Characteristics of Severe Neurosis

In accordance with the scientific requirement to identify precisely the matter of inquiry (Edelson 1985, p. 597), I present now the characteristics that I have used to designate cases as severe neuroses:

1. Repeated periods of inability to work, or severe work inhibition, due to overwhelming affective states of restless tension, anxiety, self-disparagement, depression, or anger;

2. States of altered consciousness that are decribed by the patients as such and are not merely inferred from without;

3. Rapidly corrected (not persisting) disturbances of perception in the form of hallucinations or semihallucinations;

4. Experiences of more or less extensive and severe depersonalization and derealization (especially the former);

5. Life endangering actions of self-destructiveness and self-sabotage, usually of an impulsive nature, with admitted knowledge of the dangers involved;

6. Those phenomena that are today often called splitting: extreme valuations of the own person and of others (totally good and totally bad, pure and dirty, holy and demonic),that is, an absoluteness of judgments, as well as the experience of inner doubleness (feeling split);

7. The manifest "repetition compulsion": a sequence of symptomatic actions and experiences that keep repeating themselves in pretty stereotypical fashion with the feeling of inner drivenness, and that affect the entire existence;

8. More generally, the prevailing feeling of a lack of inner freedom, and with that the dominant sense of compulsiveness of behavior and experiencing;

9. The addictive or emotionally dependent use of alcohol and drugs;

10. Striking manifestations of one form of neurosis, usually with admixture of the symptoms of other forms;

11. The repetitive, apparently irresistible tendency to react to tension and anxiety with impulsive actions that endanger the patients themselves or others or break the law;

12. Severe disruption of relationships with others: extreme ambivalence (like the 'splitting' described under Item 6), usually with a hostile dependency, or an almost complete lack of interrelationships entailing deeper feelings of closeness and intimacy.

For the classification as "severe neurosis" more than just one or two of those signs are necessary; at least six out of those twelve should be there without great doubt. One may also note that I have avoided the use of psychoanalytic terms in this enumeration. I am of the opinion that relevant factors like intensity of transference or individual characteristics of the transference, the nature of the main defense constellations and sequences, and the real nature of the underlying conflicts and main traumata can be ascertained with some reliability only in the course of extended and careful treatment. It has struck me how precisely overschematization and hastily assigned diagnostic claims as to severity and main dynamic factors in patients have led to the current one-sidedness in setting up indication and technical rules and thus have strongly contributed to the spirit of judgmentalness.

It will also be noted that hospitalization is not one of the mentioned characteristics. Only three of the major cases described in these books have been hospitalized for psychiatric reasons (all for withdrawal from drug addiction) although several had to spend time in jail or were entangled in legal proceedings. This mark appears to me to be too superficial and almost accidental. In a whole series of cases it was just the treatment regime described here that was tried *instead* of the hospitalization that would otherwise have seemed inevitable. Moreover, there were during the treatment of most cases recurrent times where the question of inpatient treatment had to be seriously entertained.

I also do not claim to have dealt with *all* forms of severe neurosis. The (by necessity) narrow compass of my own experience means the exclusion of other types of patients that I have either not yet treated myself with the required length and intensity, or that I do not yet sufficiently understand. On the other hand, such narrowness has the advantage of depth and of seizing the actual complexity of the inner world.

**Main Treatment Hypotheses**

Hence, the main hypotheses underlying this work are the following:

1. What have just been circumscribed as "severe neuroses," and which correspond more or less to the "borderline" category (cf. e.g., Kernberg 1984, pp. 10–15)[17], can very well and with great gain be approached by the analytic method, provided certain confinements and exclusions of technique that have been installed in the last decades are given less weight.
2. The consistent technical concentration on inner and outer conflicts, particularly from the side of the defenses and the superego, extends the efficacy of the analytic method to cases that otherwise are easily seen as unanalyzable. In other words, the analysis of inner conflict remains the central (albeit not the exclusive) interest of psychoanalysis.
3. In this work, the examination and working through of the transference of defense and superego aspect is of special clinical value.

4. For the understanding and treatment of these cases it is not necessary to resort to a clinical reorientation to Kleinian concepts or to the
   practical recommendations founded on them, if one wants to attain
   lasting changes. Most of the concepts of Freud's clinical theory (above
   all, the structural theory and the central, although not exclusive, role
   of oedipal conflict in the pathogenesis of the neuroses) as well as Anna
   Freud's and Fenichel's recommendations for the treatment are very
   well applicable to these patients.

5. In all cases, oedipal and preoedipal conflicts are so interwoven that it
   does not appear advisable to try to understand these severe neuroses
   as predominantly preoedipal. Much that in them seems to be preoedipal serves the defense by regression, or results from the temporary collapse of certain ego functions because of the severity of inner
   conflict and affective storm; and the other way around, the oedipal
   conflicts are also in less severe cases inherited from preoedipal times,
   from earlier disturbances, especially of an affective kind (disturbances
   of affect regulation), or result from oral and anal-sadistic elements in
   the superego.

6. On the other side, some basic assumptions of metapsychology are in
   dire need of a radical and urgent reformulation, in particular as result of infant observations; for example, those concerning the nature
   of the repetition compulsion and of the drives, the theoretical position of the affects and many aspects of the development and structure
   of the superego, and, all in all, the entire theoretical comprehension
   of the first two years of life (Lichtenberg 1983, 1989, Stern, 1985).

7. Severe neurosis means particularly intensive conflicts and hence particularly strong anxiety. What Freud (1926) said still holds: "anxiety
   would be the fundamental phenomenon and main problem of neurosis" (p. 144).

8. These cases often and at certain times require a combination of psychoanalysis with other forms of treatment, like medication, behavior
   therapy, and family interventions, yet in such a way that the analytic
   situation is not too strongly compromised.

The rival hypotheses can be deduced by negation of these eight postulates, and can be brought to the simple common denominator that these
patients are said to be either not analyzable at all, or, if analytically dealt
with, only treatable by understanding splitting as the basic process, by focusing on a few other defensive processes that are seen as equally archaic,
by seeing narcissism as an independent drive either to be gratified or re-

nounced, or by treating aggression/destructiveness as an instinctual drive
of biologically founded peremptoriness requiring obligatory discharge (in
Mitchell's [1993] formulations with which I concur: "the endogenous, spontaneous, propulsive origins of aggression" [p. 355], and in contrast to "regarding aggression as a biologically based response to subjectively perceived
endangerment" [p. 372]. Sometimes they entail the view that the structural
model and the role of oedipal conflicts are not essential.

   This book, together with its companion *Flight from Conscience*, continues
the work of *The Hidden Dimension* (1978) and *The Mask of Shame* (1981a) and
builds on the insights presented there. Like those earlier books, it is a kind
of accounting by an analyst of his successes and failures, in particular concerning those interventions and attempts at comprehension that were experienced as decisive in a given treatment, as well as what went wrong in
the same treatment. The examples given are from patients seen in the last
years prior to the initial writing of this work. It was even for me surprising to
recognize how many of the patients here presented could be successfully
treated with this approach of intensive, conflict-centered treatment, usually
four to five times a week, although even in this regard flexibility mattered a
lot. I estimate that the success rate has been over eighty percent, in the sense
of an outcome that has been desired by both partners in the endeavor, not
counting those who dropped out after the first few sessions. Of course, and
yet unfortunately, this statement cannot live up to a strict methodological
criticism. Still, it seems to me that it nonetheless speaks for the value of such
a broadly applied psychoanalytic treatment that the large *majority* of patients
showed excellent results, also catamnestically confirmed, after having pre-
viously tried out many other methods and having seen their individual neurotic symptoms and their neurotic character constellation as a whole remain
unchanged. This does not mean that other methods are ineffective, but only
that in severe cases the flexible approach shown here has been by and large
successful. All rigidity of frame needs to be especially shunned. Many treatments were wrecked by such authority-driven insistence. The superego transference was being used instead of being analyzed (Gray 1994).

   Moreover, the comparison of my experiences with less intensive psychotherapy, on the basis of a psychoanalytic orientation, is interesting. I still
see about double the number of patients in such nonintensive treatment
(at this moment fifteen), as those intensively seen (seven). They are not
unsuccessful, but the goals of treatment are far more delimited. Sometimes
the great investment of energy and money would not seem justified in view
of the goal desired; not rarely, though, such limitation in goal and method
evokes in the patient and me a slowly rising chagrin. The patient's treat-

ment goals frequently appear larger than nonintensive therapy could achieve, and the discrepancy between these as compared with their life goals becomes much wider and therefore far more painful (Ticho 1972) than is the case in psychoanalysis proper, even with severely neurotic patients.

Although it is true that (in the latter instance) a great amount of time is being invested in the individual patient, no treatment, or insufficient or incompetent treatment costs far more. This becomes especially clear in the case of the drug addicts. The right investment of time and energy at the right moment and in the right way can be lifesaving or may save other immense expenditures. Some time (one decade) ago it was reported to me (by Dr. Jack Matteson, of Charleston, West Virgina) that the average cost of a successful suicide attempt comes to $45,000: fire department, ambulance, emergency service, intensive care unit, funeral, care for the surviving next of kin, not to mention the long-term consequences for the latter. The costs of serious but unsuccessful suicide attempts and of their consequences might be no less. In comparison, the costs of a successful psychoanalysis of such severe cases, as presented here amounted at the same time to about $50,000 to $75,000 (at present rates, all these numbers may be roughly twenty to twenty-five percent higher).

## MAIN THEMES AND ORDER OF TOPICS

The order of topics will be the following:

At first I shall present the presuppositions on which the work with the patients was founded. They can be located in the (repeatedly mentioned) constant tension between insight and suggestion. Within this problematic, I shall describe those technical directives which I have found most useful and their application to two microscopic samples illustrating sequences of certain defensive processes.

The successful analysis of a case—Vera—with severe masochistic-depressive illness and a deep split of personality represents in a dramatic way some of the dynamic connections that can regularly be observed in the severe neuroses. Furthermore, her treatment led to a particularly interesting modification of technique, one which can be fruitful for many other cases. Her very marked denial, accompanying the split in identity, and the severe superego disturbances causing this split lend themselves to a discussion of some more general considerations of the main themes of the book.

The study of a case with a severe phobic narrowing down of the personality—Jacob—will give us the opportunity to study the process of change and large-scale cure during the therapy. In the forthcoming parallel work (*Flight from Conscience: The Psychodynamic Treatment of Trauma, Conflict, and Repetition Compulsion*) the following case studies ensue:

A series of patients who had been diagnosed as showing "pathological narcissism" ("narcissistic characters") permit first a clinical probe into the manifold and fascinating dynamics that are covered over rather than illuminated by this diagnosis. The presentation should show both the central position of superego conflicts precisely in the case of narcissistic character issues and the relation of absolutistic claims by the superego and of split identity to the underlying traumatization.

This will be followed by the description of a case—Dilecta—where the defense analysis of acting out and denial, and of the "defiance against conscience," eventually led to an uncovering of the original rupture in the experience of reality and the nature of the denied secret, especially of the masochistic beating fantasy. At brief moments in the analysis of this patient, her deep resentment against her mother shines up as she reveals the way the mother had used her power over the child to raise her resolute condemnation of the child's individuality to an absolute kind of validity, thus convincing the child that she was completely unacceptable and shame-laden, and evoking in her rage and vengefulness. The sexualization of such suffering was repeated in the core phantasy of masochism, but had to be covered over by its seeming opposite, her triumphantly beating a rival, a process that was inevitably followed by renewed humiliation. Quietly, this sequence was the main motive for her impulsive actions.

Subsequently, several sections are devoted to the flight from conscience observed in drug addicts and to the treatment built upon these insights. Among the severe neuroses, those of compulsive drug users play a particularly important role because they show attempted solutions and compromise formations of neurotic conflicts that deviate considerably from those we commonly encounter in more mainstream neuroses. The same is true for the perversions, which will find separate representation.

Particularly with these patients who so powerfully provoke countertransference reactions it is crucially important to watch out for the judgments and condemnations implicitly at work in psychiatry and psychoanalysis. Diagnostic categories ("borderline" and "narcissism," "hysteria" and "masochism") and some dynamic concepts ("splitting," "ego weakness," "superego lacunae," "manipulative") offer themselves as pejorative and rejecting designations. As useful as many of these categories may be, they express a power that can be deployed both for good and for harm. Decades of experience in psychiatry have taught me that the latter is not rare, particularly when these terms are excessively used. Yet, countertendencies also keep cropping up, and at times these have assumed an accusatory, even paranoid tone (as in the movements of antipsychiatry, like those connected with Alcoholics Anonymous or with methadone programs). These have also regarded it as their sovereign duty to declare the judge's chair to be their permanent throne. I will here carefully avoid their claim and title.

Not each of the patients I treat can be called a "severe neurosis" (alias "borderline" or "narcissistic neurosis"). Occasionally, I will also adduce illustrative material from lighter forms of neurosis that could be treated with psychoanalysis alone. Yet I will especially draw attention to this fact and not simply smuggle in such material, which could skew the conclusions in the direction of confirming the hypotheses.

The temptation to use grand designs and spectacular attempts at creating order is always present. Whether they are precious or often rather misleading and do violence to the individual case is a question threading itself through many of these chapters. In spite of this caution, I shall try in two final chapters to draw some more general conclusions, as a contribution to the theory of neurosis and the treatment of these severely ill patients.

The second volume of *Broken Reality, Blindness and Tragic Truth* (Wurmser 1989a) is built upon this same body of clinical work. In literary examples, the clinically often observable sequence of shame, resentment, and the subsequent usurpation of conscience can advance to a manifest main motive. These are reflections of political reality, namely, the character images of leaders of political terror who succeed in making themselves mouthpieces and strategists of the general resentment. Tragic character and tragic worldview have many profound connections with the problems of superego analysis developed here.

The more philosophical, and especially epistemological, third work, *Conflict and Complementarity* (1989a) takes its starting point in the newer criticism of psychoanalysis, especially by Grünbaum, and counters it more thoroughly, to reach a more comprehensive philosophical view.[18] The tragic worldview of the ancient Greeks, the role of shame in Greek culture, the Talmud, and Chinese tradition, the issue of conflict and complementarity in Confucius and Lao-Tzu, and other fundamental polarities, accompanied by specific denials, as met with in the Jewish, the Chinese, and the modern American-European culture provide an opportunity to establish some connections between the clinical insight into human nature and the more general human experience. This reference to what is universal should give us the framework for the direct experience and its methodology.

*The Riddle of Masochism* (1993), weaves together the problems of moral masochism with those of the perversions, the external victim position and the façade of narcissism and sadism. Discussions of the work of three great writers—Ibsen, Nietzsche, and Thomas Mann—are interspersed between extensive case studies.

## THE BATTLE WITH THE DEMON

I revert to the starting point, and to our major task.

> I had a terrible anxiety dream last night, Vera reported. It was in an old Victorian house. A woman was lying on an iron bedstead. Then I went to the bathroom and sat on the toilet. There was an uncanny mood; some threat was hanging in the air, as if I was going crazy. Suddenly I was noticing a spider crawling on the floor toward me. I felt compelled to make spiderlike movements with my hand. I sensed something demonic within me—that I was insane. It was dark, and I saw the shadows of spiders climbing up on the door. Then I heard a muffled sound as if somebody were being stomped in the stomach. I went back through the bedroom. The woman was not lying there anymore. I went down the stair. The beige carpet was wet from blood. As I was turning around a body fell over the bannister, to the end of the stair, and I heard demonic laughter from the top floor. Then a face fell to the ground, not a body, but an evulsed face, a child's face. It was lying on the ground, expressionless and very sticky with blood. It looked more like the face of my sister than that of my brother. Then I woke up in a cold sweat.

That what is felt to be "demonic" is something aggressive is of course true and almost self-evident; it tells us, however, nearly nothing about the real dynamic meanings that sought expression in this and countless other of Vera's just as frightening dreams and hallucinations, in which overwhelming feelings and wishes created for themselves symbols of often compelling expressive power. More specifically, the demonic is the resentment haunting her from within, and in two ways: a resentment filled with envy and jealousy toward others who seem to have gotten more than she or who have allegedly cheated her, and a resentment speaking in the pitiless voice of her conscience that poisons every joy and seems to spoil every one of her (great) accomplishments with malicious scorn. The torn-off face is not only her burning jealousy at her (younger) siblings, but also reflects her own searing shame that lets her again and again "lose her face" and that she tries to deal with by turning it around: that she would like to humiliate others just as much as she feels ashamed herself, without usually admitting this wish of reversal to herself.

Yet, what is this demonic force that forces her entirely under its power, compels her to devastating actions, the consequences of which she regrets and dreads and yet is unable to avoid? And in particular: How is it possible to break the irresistible force of this will to repetition and to help the counterforce, the wish and the consciousness of a deeper freedom, to assert itself?

I now address this double question.

## ENDNOTES

1. A bracketed number refers to the number of the session.

2. I have modified some of the translations.

3. Δός μοι ποῦ στῶ καὶ κόσμον κινήσω (Give me a firm point and I shall move the world).

4. (*Das Höchste wäre, zu begreifen, daß alles Faktische schon Theorie ist. . . Man suche nur nicht hinter den Phänomenen; sie selbst sind die Lehre.*) (from *Wilhelm Meister's Wanderjahre*, "Betrachtungen im Sinne der Wanderer," [end of Book 2], vol. 18, p. 57).

5. I prefer the French word because it is far stronger than its English derivative and took on special importance in modern philosophy, especially in Nietzsche's and Scheler's writings. I deal with it extensively in *Broken Reality*.

6. (Die durch die systematisch geübte Zurückdrängung von Entladungen gewisser Gemütsbewegungen und Affekte entsteht.) [Scheler 1915, p. 38]

7. (*Denken und Tun, Tun und Denken, das ist die Summe aller Weisheit, von jeher anerkannt, von jeher geübt, nicht eingesehen von einem jeden. Beides muß wie Aus-und Einatmen sich im Leben ewig fort hin und wider bewegen; wie Frage und Antwort sollte eins ohne das andere nicht stattfinden. Wer sich zum Gesetz macht, was einem jeden Neugebornen der Genius des Menschenverstandes heimlich ins Ohr flüstert, das Tun am Denken, das Denken am Tun zu prüfen, der kann nicht irren, und irrt er, so wird er sich bald auf den rechten Weg zurückfinden.*) (Goethe, *Wilhelm Meister's Wanderjahre*, Book 2.9; vol. 18, p. 22.)

8. (*Gedenke zu leben!*) (*Wilhelm Meister's Lehrjahre*, Book 8.5; vol. 16, p. 239 f.)

9. (*Das Verbundene zu trennen und das Getrennte zu verbinden*), ibid., p. 246.

10. The red herring assiduously angled for by some of our epistemological critics.

11. And it *is* a *research into causality*, as correctly posited by Grünbaum, in opposition to the hermeneuticians.

12. In the singular, "*en gammal arvtatt folkeløgn*," from Henrik Ibsen, *An Enemy of the People*, p. 201.

13. (*De er liksom harske, ulne, grønnsaltede skinker*), ibid., p. 199.

14. (*Wenn man die Probleme des Aristoteles ansieht, so erstaunt man über die Gabe des Bemerkens and für was alles die Griechen Augen gehabt haben. Nur begehen sie den Fehler der Übereilung, da sie von dem Phänomen unmittelbar zur Erklärung schreiten, wodurch denn ganz unzulängliche theoretische Aussprüche zum Vorschein kommen. Dieses ist jedoch der allgemeine Fehler, der noch heutzutage begangen wird.*) (Goethe, *Wilhelm Meister's Wanderjahre*, Book 2, vol. 18, p. 58.)

15. Cf. also my work, *Broken Reality* (1989a) about the philosophical implications. All my books deal with these questions in praxi.

16. (*Es ist vieles wahr, was sich nicht berechnen läßt, sowie sehr vieles, was sich nicht bis zum entscheidenden Experiment bringen läßt.*) Goethe, *Wilhelm Meister's Wanderjahre*, "Aus Makariens Archiv," vol. 18, p. 210.

17. "Borderline: Identity diffusion: contradictory aspects of self and others are poorly integrated and kept apart. Defensive operations: Mainly splitting and low-level defenses: primitive idealization, projective identification, denial, omnipotence, devaluation. Reality testing: Alterations occur in relationship with reality and in feelings of reality" (1984, p. 20).

18. Both volumes were joined in one in the German edition, as *Die zerbrochene Wirklichkeit* (1989a).

# 2

## Defense and
## Superego Analysis

A crown's worth of good interpretation.
—Shakespeare, *Henry IV*, *Part II*, II, ii

Before starting the presentation of cases it is fitting to deal more in detail with the method of treatment that has led to the findings and conclusions.

The analyst is also in many ways a wanderer between two worlds—an ambassador representing the inner world against the impetuous and often unreasonable demands for adaptation, but also an ambassador of reason facing the equally pressing demands of irrationality. At this point, however, I would like to talk about a particular form of doubleness, a dilemma which, as mentioned, we can never quite avoid and that we cannot solve once and for all either.

## THE PRELIMINARY DECISION

If we speak about the technique of psychoanalysis and psychotherapy, a value judgment inescapably resonates: What would best serve the aim of bringing about, in a given case, such a deep inner change that, *in the long run*, would allow the patient to become happier and more fulfilled? What would interfere with such an endeavor, and would support it? That means: What is good, and what is bad? And thus: What are the interventions and the more general treatment strategies that would be most useful for certain patients, when and in which form, with which therapists? What is in the given case the specific treatment goal?

However simple and banal these questions seem, their discussion becomes complicated, may turn emotional or even polemical, and opens important problems for the epistemology of psychoanalysis. I have dealt elsewhere (Wurmser 1989a,b) with Grünbaum's (1984) philosophical criticism of the foundations of psychoanalysis. Above all, these questions require the systematic, empirical investigation of the psychoanalytic process, something often demanded yet rather infrequently undertaken. Here I shall restrict myself to the practical question of which treatment approach has proven itself most suited in the long-term treatment of cases with severe neurosis, as certain

49

rules gradually emerged that showed themselves particularly helpful for that purpose and the avoidance of certain "mistakes" was found particularly necessary.

The decision one must make, based on an implicit value judgment, and one that has to precede everything else, is this: Which treatment strategy is more apt to help this patient, in the short or in the long run? Is it to be directed at helping him or her to *solve inner, mostly unconscious conflicts*, conflicts above all that stunt inner growth and force relationships and the ability to find gratification of many kinds into stereotypical, rigid behavior patterns? Or should it rather consist in helping him or her directly to master tasks on the outside better, to change the behavior, to make up for inner deficits, to question faulty judgments, to diminish or increase self-condemnation—whatever may be of need? The first is a *vertical* approach, the second a *horizontal* one. If we choose the former, we basically decide for psychoanalysis; with the latter, the choice is for a more educating, advising kind of psychotherapy, one more interested in behavior. Aim and result are drastically different in the two paradigms. I shall return later on in this chapter in more detail to this basic differentiation and complementarity of methods.

Therefore, the value judgment, addressed by questions of technique, can only have the form: Which of the two principal methods (or rather: groups of methods) is better suited to a certain situation and pathology? It is not: Is one method in itself better and of greater dignity than the other? In many situations, the insistence on a rigorously psychoanalytic procedure is inappropriate and may even be very damaging; the reverse is just as valid.

Especially fascinating is the gradually accruing experience that in the severe forms of neurosis, as with drug addicts, and severely phobic and masochistic-depressive personality disorders, only a *combination of methods* may lead to real improvement, and that specifically and only the simultaneous application of vertical and horizontal approaches leads to improvement and lasting success. Of course, it is well known that preferably such a combination is not carried out by the same therapist. I shall speak in detail about this in the context of the treatment of compulsive drug users.

In what follows now, I restrict myself at first to the psychoanalytic aim, that is, to the question: What is the technique allowing us to solve unconscious inner conflicts? In other words, What is the approach we decide upon when we not only wish for a short-term change of behavior, but consider deep inner change possible and desirable—a change that is durable in regard to the problems at hand (the neurotic difficulties) and accompanied by the patient's deepened self-respect and self-fulfillment? What are the guiding principles for such a technique?

In answering this question I rely entirely on my own clinical experiences. In the course of the past twenty-five years, I have found the defense analytic model I have learned with my two main supervisors, Jenny Waelder-Hall and Paul Gray, far more useful than those techniques offered by others, or those I myself had followed at other times in my work.

It should be added however that the severity of these cases dictated modifications of a more interactive kind that will require special reconsideration, especially also in light of the vivid and fascinating discussion over the past few years about the complementarity of the interpretative and the interactive approaches.

## TECHNICAL GUIDELINES FOR DEFENSE ANALYSIS

An indispensable precondition for the psychoanalytic treatment of these severe neuroses is the fundamental decision on the side of the patient to be honest and open. Sometimes I state at the inception: "You have asked me for help with problems the origin and nature of which are unknown to you— as it were, veiled by a curtain. In order for me to help you to look behind this curtain it is necessary to avoid pulling a second curtain in front—in the form of drugs or lies or conscious concealment. With the first curtain I may very well be of help, for the second one you would rather need a detective than an analyst. We cannot fulfill both tasks at the same time."

Modifications of the following guidelines that are required with the special problems of severe neuroses will become clearer in the next chapters in the presentation of single cases.

### Beginning at the Surface

The first and perhaps most important guideline consists in the suggestion, particularly stressed by Fenichel (1941), *to go out from the surface of the moment*—that is, always to observe what is for the patient of greatest emotional importance. This does not necessarily mean that he speaks about it at that very moment, but rather that we sense in how he behaves and talks that something that distresses and frightens him is omitted, circumvented, or only peripherally addressed. "Surface" does not by necessity refer to what the words of the hour are concerned with, but what he wants to talk about but is too scared to do.

Often dreams, external preoccupations, or childhood memories serve to divert from this "battle in his soul." Therefore it is the main task of the ana-

lyst to ask himself: *What is the conflict right now?* What does the patient right
now avoid? Hence: What is he afraid of right now?

In this it is generally accepted that *contiguity* is a main guide in the search
for such deeper connections. The deeper context of meaning is found in a
regular *sequence*, the repetitive occurrence of certain images, fantasy wishes,
fragments of memory, feelings, and thoughts, rather than in the logical
surface threads. Hence the insistent inner questions have to be: Why now?
Why in this context? As Arlow often stressed (e.g., 1979), such contiguity in
form of sequences allows us to surmise the deeper, hidden meaning that is
just now crucial. It is such sequence that is above all meant with the term
"surface."

The interpretative process is mostly a shared search for answers, and at
that a very difficult investigation aiming most of all at *tying together again the
connections that have been torn*, as Anna Freud (1936 p. 15) stated, and much
more than the dramatic discovery of some hidden repressed memories (of
special, that is, traumatic, events). A great part of my own work consists in
reconnecting broken threads of meaning and in reencountering hidden
inner sequences and fantasies, "at the border of perception," as one of my
patients once called it. Such concealed sequences of feelings and images,
hiding in the shadows of the superficial themes in the more or less uninter-
rupted talking of the patient, may become relatively easily visible, in the form
specific for that moment, if we draw the patient's attention to the main
contents of a period of twenty or thirty minutes in one session, or also of a
series of sessions, if we review and summarize them in his or her own words
and submit them to the patient's own "evaluation": "What do you make of
this? What may this mean? How may we understand this?" Of course this
"close process monitoring" (Gray) is just one way of gaining access to what
is sought and should not become something done by rote.

Dreams may easily tempt us to go too deeply. Whenever a dream comes
up we have to ask ourselves above everything else: Why does this dream come
just now?—in the context of this hour (Gray 1994), but also in the current
context of his or her life, that is, Why has it been dreamt last night (or just
the other night)? What does it have to do with the immediate present? Only
when its meaning is safely anchored in the felt and experienced present does
it become possible to approach the deeper meanings. I do not dismiss the
importance of dreams, for example, in favor of the analysis of transference,
as often happens now. I still see again and again how the dream indeed is
the *via regia* to what is unconscious and that it can be of very great help,
precisely in the comprehension and treatment of defense and superego
processes within and outside the transference. Still, I often find its greatest

value in showing us where the "point of urgency" lies, meaning, which conflict is of pressing actuality.

## Defense Analysis Precedes Drive Analysis

The second well-proven technical principle is that "defense analysis precedes drive analysis." Sometimes this is misunderstood as if the former is done for the first years and only then do we turn to the latter. A more appropriate formulation therefore is that it is mostly preferable to present the interpretation of the inner conflict *from the side of the defense*: "I fear that . . . ," "I do not want that . . . ," "I cannot allow myself the thought . . . ," "I avoid thinking of it . . . ," "It would be particularly dangerous to deal with this, to wish that, or just now to feel such and such . . ."

Such indirect interpretations replace direct drive interpretations like: "You want (or wanted at that time) to kill your brother," "You hate me like your father and really want to take revenge on me by doing this or that . . . ," "You want to take me within yourself, to devour me, in order never to lose me," "You love me or are bound to the other in a masochistic bondage as you wanted to behave toward your father," "You find gratification in suffering," "You forbid yourself that greedy demand . . ." All these ways of directly bringing up the drive side are experienced as reproaches by the patient. Thus I am particularly cautious about directly commenting on aggressive or narcissistic wishes; such statements are viewed as superego interventions, namely as reproach, as blaming, or at least as criticism, and are fought off with increasing resistance. More and more this leads to a battle of wills and to stalemate.

This indirect approach to aggressive feelings, wishes, and fantasies represents in fact a main criterion of the defense analytic method and stands in sharpest contrast to treatment forms influenced by Melanie Klein (1952a), Wilhelm Reich (1933) or Ferenczi (1932). *The clinical consequences of this difference in methods can in my view not be overestimated,* as can be seen in supervision. It has repeatedly happened during supervision in Europe that such a change of approach led to a dramatic unfreezing of a "transference clinch," a breaking up of what had seemed like fatal resistance.

At the beginning of our analytic practice we are often so impressed when we gain meaning with the aide of such *magical drive interpretations* in what had seemed meaningless, and understanding in what had appeared bizarre and nonsensical, that the temptation may be irresistible to employ this newly found wonderful instrument. Dreams show such endless fascination especially because they seem to bring wishes that otherwise are deeply hidden and of a very archaic and secret nature suddenly to the light of day and at once to explain so much. However satisfying this may be in the short run and however much we may find in the patient a consenting player, such a drive-conscious honeymoon does end before long. Resistance will suddenly be the greater, and now we feel called upon to "overcome" it, to argue or command it away with a stance of authority: "You don't want to hear this, you refuse to accept this. You feel injured in your self-respect that I tell you this . . . ," and so on. We fall into teaching, lecturing, explaining, into adhortation and admonishment—in short, we camouflage suggestion by analytic jargon—but quite obviously we have run off the road we had chosen as treatment strategy.

In my experience, defense analysis does help us very much by protecting us against missing the path, and even if we have landed in the ditch it is mostly not too late to ask ourselves: Which form of anxiety (or more generally: painful affect) and, with that, what form of defense have I overlooked? What did I fail to grasp? Where did I go too deeply and thus have mobilized forces of self-condemnation that are too strong, excessively interfering influences of unconscious guilt or shame? In Fenichel's words: "How could I have interpreted more superficially?" (1941 p. 44).

## Affect Defenses

An especially important kind of such defense analysis, one also stressed by Anna Freud (1936), yet one often overlooked in literature and supervision, is noticing and interpreting *affect defense*: anger instead of anxiety or mourning, happy excitement instead of sadness or wrath; pain and sadness in the place of rage, and, especially well known, anxiety in the place of sexual exitement, or the reverse: sexualization as cover for painful affect, especially traumatic terror. Generally, it has become clear that the affects are of the greatest importance for the understanding of psychodynamics and have to be treated independently from the drives (or, if we follow Lichtenberg [1989, Lichtenberg et al. 1996], the motivational systems).[1] They are very much a kind of Ariadne's thread, guiding us into the darkness both of inner depth and of early childhood, if we only observe that they too have become highly structured, multiple layered, and that they too are, like symptoms, compromise formations. The thread of Ariadne has many knots! Still, problems and disturbances of affect regulation between mother and child, and between other family members and the child flow into the later conflict-centered psychology that is, in essence, the rightful realm of psychoanalysis. Both forms of approach and understanding—regulation versus inner conflict—

are, as stated by Lichtenberg (1986), in a complementary relation to each other. Efforts at regulating affects partly change, with the increasing ability to symbolize, into defensive processes against affects. In the severer forms of neurosis such transformation succeeds to a much lesser degree than in the lighter forms; the affect defenses fail. For the rest, in light of the research into early childhood, affect theory has to be separated from drive theory (see Chapter 6).

## Transference of Defense

A further refinement of the first two principles lies in something first described by Anna Freud (1936) and studied with particular care and depth in the past three decades by Gray (1982): the interpretation of the *transference of defense*, and thus the dealing with "negative" transference from the side of defense. We are all well aware that transference interpretations are preferred as more effective. Yet, as supervision shows, it is very often overlooked that this preference refers particularly to the *defense analysis within the analytic situation*: "I notice how you have avoided at that moment to continue talking about it . . ." Commonly it is a sign of anxiety of being ridiculed, condemned, attacked by the analyst—with special poignancy the transference of shame or guilt feelings. The analyst appears as a threatening superego figure who stands in hostile opposition to affects and drive derivatives and their reflections in wishes, fantasies, memories, and present-day concerns. "You are afraid to approach this topic here, in my presence . . ." is the general meaning, although there are many other and often apter formulations to draw the patient's attention to it. In the first line, we need to ascertain what the nature of the actual anxiety is, in the second, with which kind of self-defense the patient deals with this danger, and only in the third line, which earlier conflicts he or she is reminded of—which earlier threat and danger, which earlier form of defense, and finally, which earlier wish. Almost always in the neurosis, the superego appears as the most imminent source of anxiety.

Yet, it is obvious that with this approach neither the past nor elements outside of the transference nor the drive side are neglected. It is merely the question: From whence is it best to gain access to the anxiety that is at this moment strongest, and yet hidden—and other affects of unpleasure like pain, shame, guilt, depression—and hence to the resistance as well, without our still adding to them or our sliding into what is removed from conflict, unessential, away from "surface" and "point of urgency"?

Perhaps this can be formulated even better, so that the main concern is basically not the analysis of defense in the transference, but the *analysis of the kind of anxiety and danger*, at this moment, within the analytic situation. If this is moved into focus and loses its present justification (shows itself as distortion)—if we do good analytic work—everything else gradually falls into place. For, without my needing to state this, I really do not ridicule my patient, I do not judge him, I do not deprive him of his self, his identity, his creativity, and of his own judgment, nor do I burden him with guilt, nor do I shame him. *Tact* is therefore absolutely indispensable, in fact of such paramount importance that, if we truly tactfully proceed, we find more and more in the patient an indispensable co-worker and co-investigator if we lead him to confront ever new inner experiences of unpleasure. But it also means that it is just such an approach that renders many severely ill patients again analyzable who otherwise would have to remain inaccessible to this kind of treatment.

The right interpretation cannot be a *confrontative*, that is, really quite aggressive intervention (a scornful or sarcastic remark, or one which otherwise could be taken as critical), as long as we decide to proceed in a stricter sense analytically and not in a more guiding, suggestive, pedagogical manner, and even in this latter instance, we would have strong reservations against such confrontative interventions.

It is often very helpful to treat the transference and conflictual meanings of experiences or actions as additional to their significance in everyday life, not as supplanting them, as in Gray's frequent expression: "in addition, not instead."

It is also evident how centrally important with this approach the various layers of shame and guilt feelings are, as revived within the analytic situation. As Fenichel (1941) remarked, "The superego . . . is in essence itself a defense structure" (p. 62), but it is, as we shall see, more than that (Brenner 1982).[2] In this connection it has also been a very valuable strategy in dealing with particularly severe forms of self-destructiveness and self-condemnation to *drive a wedge between the superego and the rest of the self*: to help create a therapeutic split between the "inner judge," "inner demon," or "executioner" and the rest of the personality, by asking, "How can we understand the cruelty, the resentment, the envy of this inner figure that wants you destroyed?" In other words, we try to make the judgmental part of the person the problem, instead of the value of the self as the patient has hitherto done.

My experience is in accordance with that of Anna Freud and Joseph Sandler that it is better not to "*force it* [the material] *into the transference.*" Often it seemed to me preferable only gradually to refer to the transference aspects. Sandler (1985) states:

I think that sometimes one has to go along with the patient for quite a long time, showing him the mechanisms he has been using, leaving oneself out until the patient is well and truly in analysis. My experience is that taking up all the material in terms of transference early in the analysis may put certain patients into resistance and may lead to a breakdown of the analysis. [p. 89]

And Anna Freud replies: "Because it extends the transference to a phenomenon that the patient has no need to feel. The original idea about transference is that it is something the patient feels that is going on in him, not something that is dragged in by the analyst" (p. 89).

Especially with more severely ill patients it may at times be advisable, even while maintaining the psychoanalytic model, to move away from the transference, instead of bringing it into consciousness by interpretations. In such cases the *defense by intellectualization* may be useful, by its deployment rather than by its interpretation, specifically when the transference is too intense and too close to be put into action. This is true in particular for patients who suffer flooding with affects, hence with disturbances of affect regulation, usually of a very early origin, or patients with pronounced paranoid tendencies. Thus an interpretation, like: "This does not refer to me, but to this or that earlier figure," that is, an *interpretation downward*, may lead to a therapeutically needed calming. I mean with this that in such cases it may be better, even in the long run, during times of such affective storms not to dwell on the transference fantasies and to work through them, but to move rapidly away from them to the more distant past. This may seem to be "bad" analytic technique; but is is "good" psychotherapeutic technique: away from the conflict solution, toward a more pedagogical approach, a sort of teaching warranted by authority, carried by intellectualization, leading away from the otherwise unbearable anxiety or from forms of paranoid shame and injury, with the rage entailed by this. Again, this is meant as a (time-) limited pull-back during overwhelming affect, not as a continuous stance.

Thus, however harmful intellectualization as resistance in obsessive-compulsive patients may be, we may often count ourselves fortunate to be able to resort to it when the regression becomes too threatening, or to use it as a temporary expedient or even as a lasting help if it can be gradually transformed into sublimation.

## Defense Against Superego Functions

There is one aspect of defense analysis, however, that is particularly important, delicate, and hard: that of the *defense against superego functions*, both within and without the transference. Occasionally I use a short explanation here that at times conscience and ideals are being treated as if they were the main enemy one has to seek protection against, just as, in other connections, it is certain feelings or wishes that seem the menace. *Defiance* above all expresses such a defense against the necessity of submitting to a hated inner or outer authority; defiance is a strongly censored and yet exceedingly important affect frequently serving essential self-defense. I often add that such resistance and spiteful rebellion is a weapon of despair, an indispensable self-protection at a time of weakness and humiliation, and that it deserves to be taken equally seriously, treated with the same respect, and understood as all the other feelings and wishes.

The *rebel against conscience* is a frequent and not easily treatable character type, yet not one always inaccessible to analysis. We have to place into the same context the problems of addiction, a good part of which has to be understood as flight from conscience, as a defense against various superego aspects.

Gray (1987) emphasizes the possibility and necessity of analyzing the superego, instead of using the superego transference for the purposes of treatment: "I take the position that optimal analysis of the superego, as of resistance generally, is best achieved by perceiving and interpreting superego manifestations primarily as part of the ego's hierarchical defensive activities, mobilized *during the analytic situation*" (p. 145). As he says, "This technical approach aims at providing an opportunity for a *maximum* of new, conscious ego solutions to conflict and a *minimum* of solutions involving new internalizations" [i.e., of an external authority] (p. 149, original emphases).

**Values, Outer Reality, and Acting Out**

Sometimes, outer reality and questions of values and conscience are being viewed as lying outside good analytic work and are being neglected or approached by turning to psychotherapeutic measures, like confrontation, instruction, and setting limits. Especially with more severely ill patients it may indeed become inevitable to resort at times to such means. Yet even with them it often remains very possible to stay with conflict analysis and thus to avoid compromising the transference by massive imposition of authority and influencing.

In particular, we find ourselves again and again faced by the problem of what to do with patients who, although being in analysis, seriously imperil themselves or the treatment. Repeatedly then we have to ask the question whether the analysis can simply go on that way and whether we should patiently watch, or whether we have to intercede as superego figures, thus compromising the further course of treatment from an analytic point of view. The answer usually is clear in extreme cases, but there is a broad range where this is difficult to determine.

This brings me to the very important point of *acting out*.[3] Because, since Freud's essay of 1914(a), acting out has been treated as an important form of resistance, the tendency has been in general to call it that way and to let the patient know that it would be hard, if not impossible, to analyze a conflict as long as part of it, that is, the drive, is being put into action, hence gratified and discharged, and that analysis needs to be carried through in abstinence. I myself have been insistently taught this and have dutifully relayed it to my patients at one time or another.

More and more it has struck me, however, that such enactments may not only contain crucially important material for the analytic work, but that in certain cases the latter may depend upon observing the repetition of such dangerous actions in order to attain decisive progress. In other words, what is not being experienced in action may remain intellectual and thus cannot be effectively interpreted. In these instances *enactment, or acting out, is both resistance against insight and vehicle for insight.* With this I do not of course mean to imply that acting out should be promoted, but it also should not be treated as if it were an enemy. Rather, it should be valued as salient communication and as matter for exploration, just as any other form of defense.

A brief distinction in definition: Rangell (1968) calls acting out a special type of neurotic acting that is specifically directed against the attainment of effective insight, especially in the analysis, but not necessarily restricted to it. This is contrasted to neurotic actions outside of the analysis. Acting out and neurotic actions relate to each other like resistances and defenses, or like transference in analysis and transference-like displacements of a more general nature.

Brenner (1976) postulates that when the analyst sees himself faced by analytically unmanageable actions this means that he has failed to interpret an essential aspect of the transference in time. I believe that with such a claim the possibility is overlooked that at times we may not be able to understand correctly the transference phenomena before they have presented themselves in the form of actions, however risky these actions may then turn out to be. I shall often have occasion throughout these books to refer to such problems.

Much severe and dangerous acting out can be understood as turning the tables: "Instead of being lied to and shortchanged and instead of feeling wounded and shamed I inflict this now on everyone else if only I have come close enough to them." It is the prominent defense of *reversal,* especially from the *passive to the active* form, and *role reversal*, accompanied by *archaic iden-tification*, that makes much acting out understandable and analytically treatable.

Often the defense by *denial* of reality is in a very dramatic way connected with this. Many therapists might therefore point, by interpreting or confront-ing, to the lived-out "grandiosity" and to "deep narcissistic disturbances," perhaps somewhat in this sense: "Nothing is going to happen to me, I am immune against dangers and invulnerable because I am so special and can lay claim to such entitlement." Yet such interventions easily slide into self-righteous moralization on the analyst's side and lend themselves to the as-sumption of a superego role by the analyst, which harms further analytic cooperation. Instead of this I usually find it far better to regard and treat these narcissistic premises as protective fantasies that are used to fight off the underlying anxieties and various forms of helplessness, especially pain, shame, and severe loss, with the help of the prevailing denials. This array of defenses may show up, for example, in the following (reconstructed) se-quence: "I behave in such a dangerous—or ruthless, defiant, lawbreaking, or obnoxious—fashion because I can ignore important parts of reality, and I may even decree them to be inoperative. This is so because I have special rights and see myself as invulnerable and invincible. These claims rely upon my profound conviction that only in this way I can protect myself against feeling once again my deepest helplessness or loneliness, my sense of utter unlovability and sinfulness." Such a dynamic sequence can again be found especially in the transference as seemingly antianalytic acts of defiance and in behaviors endangering the analysis. (Much of this defensive stance is taken up in *Das Rätsel des Masochismus* [*The Riddle of Masochism*] [1993] as "counter-masochism," and in Wurmser [1981a] as "shamelessness").

### Constructions and the Repressed Past

What is to be said about the *repressed past?* Both extremes are there, its un-der- and its overvaluation. What counts is what helps in the long run and can turn into a lastingly effective insight. Here too the detailed defensive measures may be at least as important, if not more so, than what is defended against; this is particularly true for the recollections observable and experi-enced within the sessions themselves. *Constructions* have in no way lost their value as therapeutic means. Microscopic analyses of sequences, of the innu-merable variants and complex series of anxiety → form of defense → wish or affect, allow macroscopic interpretations and genetic reconstructions of the original main conflicts and of their layering. I still consider these genetic constructions an integral part of all *lege artis* carried out analytic work, yet in connection with the viewpoints spelled out here. Only if such a *synopsis of the original conflicts* grows from careful conflict analysis in the present, especially in the transference, can it attain its hoped-for psychoanalytic value.

Gray (1994) draws attention to a special form of construction first mentioned by Anna Freud: the construction of the defensive activity of the ego *then*, as it inadvertently repeats itself *now*. It is to be noted, he says, to be mindful of what Freud himself called "the resistance against uncovering resistances" (1937, p. 239). As the second case example later on in this chapter will demonstrate, such a form of construction permits us to show to the patient the correct sequence, the fitting together of layers of defensive endeavors, with the help of the current material. In general, such *series* of defenses open up especially valuable insights into inner life.

## Drive Interpretations

At times, direct *drive interpretations* are also fruitful. On the one hand, anxiety and defense may have been already so successfully analyzed that the patient could almost have said it himself. In that case, though, it would be better not to express it oneself but to leave it up to the patient. On the other hand— and this is the much more important case—drive derivatives themselves serve as a defense against far more threatening affects or wishes (see also Brenner 1982). The uncovering of this dynamic is a particularly important and frequent example for prominence and priority of defense analysis.

What I mean with this is the following: On the surface, sadistic fantasies may protect against more dangerous masochistic tendencies, and these in turn may do so against up to now inaccessible, deeply repressed, original aggressive wishes from childhood, which in turn are ways of trying to deal with traumatic states. Superficial exhibitionism may protect against much deeper shame or against its opposite, the wish to look, curiosity, as a more dangerous drive. All this has been outlined by Fenichel (1945) with the well-known concept of "threefold stratification." Necessarily we would have to focus on this meaning of defense, not on the seeming drive gratification, which at once would be taken as condemnation.

## The Nontechnical, Personal Relationship

I concur with Leo Stone (1984) and Samuel Lipton (1977a,b) that it is not possible to reduce the entire analytic relationship to technical aspects (philosophically, in fact, an absurd proposition anyway). There is a *nontechnical, personal relationship* between analyst and analysand, in analogy to the one existing between physician and patient; it can be understood best from the aspect of the personal interest in the well-being of the other, and may be meant with "professional tact." Within this, the shared task of how best to resolve unconscious conflicts is being tackled. Since for this task the analysis of defense *in the transference* is of cardinal importance, the encompassing relationship should not be such that it stands in the way of this task (historically, much stress in various schools on relating and interacting has in fact done just that). For this, what Anna Freud (1936) has postulated may still be valid much of the time as the viewpoint of the analyst in general: to take "his stand at a point equidistant from the id, the ego, and the superego" (p. 28). Analytic "neutrality" and "abstinence" should not go over into unfeelingness, indifference, or unfriendliness. *The concept of neutrality refers to inner conflict, not the person of the patient* (cf. Hoffer, 1985).

I agree with Thomä and Kächele's (1985) pleading for a flexible and warm therapeutic attitude. As they state, to a large extent therapy consists in "how the therapist *is*," not only in how he is being seen in the light of the past. The realistic perceptions of the patient have to be acknowledged, not merely interpreted genetically. With that the ideal of the resolution of the transference at the end of therapy turns out to be utopian; it "was part of a monadically conceived treatment process" (p. 65).

I consider these authors' critique of the "rule of abstinence" particularly important: it

> had clearly unfavorable effects on the development of psychoanalytic technique. . . . The conception that necessary frustration constitutes the motive force for change has become more than questionable and has above all distracted attention from the unfavorable consequences which exaggerated neutrality on the part of the analyst has on the therapeutic process. [Thomä and Kächele 1985, p. 220]

In their view, the rule of abstinence in its radical form has been practically as well as theoretically more harmful than useful.

Thomä and Kächele (1985) also criticize the authoritarian formulation of the fundamental rule and the stereotypical refusal to respond to any questions, which is experienced as rebuff and humiliation. All such rigidity increases the danger of malignant regression. Part and parcel of this caveat is that

> in view of the practical necessity to be just as prudent in using silence as the spoken word, the fact that a stereotype is made of silence is a real cause of con-

cern. . . . Hand in hand with the highly stylized view that interpretation should be the analyst's only form of verbal communication, a high, even mystical, value has been attached to silence. [p. 294]

Instead, "all technical steps should be directed at creating the most favorable conditions for the ego" (p. 305).

I find that *the emotional responsiveness,* the *affective resonance* of the analyst just with these patients has a very strong therapeutic effect, because they usually come from a milieu in which most feelings had to be banished, ignored, skewed, or suppressed—where "one could not be oneself" and the world of feelings was most strongly put under the pall of shame. This is more than empathy, more than support (and it is not suggestion or insight), but it is of cardinal importance (see also Owen Renik's [1995, 1996] recent papers on self-disclosure).

What always proves a failure and needs to be rejected out of hand is a basic attitude on the side of the analyst that is cold and impersonal—a kind of personified "No." This drives those seeking help out of analysis or harms them by establishing a sadomasochistic relationship in fact, not just in fantasy. Who would be able to approach what is most embarrassing and what deeply terrifies him in his fate if no atmosphere of trust is offered and when a rational and emotional alliance is missing?

Not only do I believe that, depending on the situation, considerable latitude exists within what is still compatible with good analysis, in accord with Fenichel's (1941) dictum, "Everything is permissible if only one knows why" (p. 24), but also that the more severe neuroses are only analytically treatable if tact, friendliness, and active *interest* for what is *very particular, very individual, in every single patient* are allowed to have a central part in the therapeutic relationship.

## Timing and the Specific

I have already pointed to the importance of choosing the right form and the right time—what the Greeks called the *kairós.* I now stress how significant specificity always is. At its core, *psychoanalysis is the art of the specific.* Vague, general remarks about aggressions, anxieties, wishes for dependency, or sexual feelings are not yet effective interpretations but at best prepare for them. In fact, *the more specific, the more effective,* and the right moment should not be missed. Too much passivity and reticence is just as damaging as intrusive overinterpreting. The form should be brief and poignant, not longwinded and intellectual, but also should not turn into being the sign of an authoritarian know-it-all. Much of the time I find it advisable to formulate the interpretations cautiously as questions: "Isn't it so . . . ?" or "Would it be too far-fetched to see in it . . . ?" or "I wonder if . . . ," or "We might ask ourselves . . . ." or I may complete a statement of the patient by "so that you felt this and this?" As mentioned before, I very often repeat also the main points of the associations of the hour up to that moment, or some major remarks of the patient from the previous sessions, with the intention of submitting possibly meaningful sequences and then allowing the analysand him- or herself to bring forth the interpretation. The more the patients interpret on their own, the more they develop their abilities for analytic self-observation and thus the readiness later on to continue the therapy on their own.

**Education in Self-Observation**

This last point leads on to the postulate that psychoanalysis should ultimately be an *education in self-observation* (Gray 1973), that its lasting gain lies in the continuation of the analytic work by the patient, and that therefore all those measures that enhance the observing ego are of particular help and significance. Often I remark (with Jenny Waelder-Hall) to the patient: "This is a very good (or important) point (or idea); what do you think about it?" Or "This is an excellent question; how might we answer it?" Frequently, I summarize, as mentioned, the main associations of the patient and ask directly: "How would you interpret this yourself?" or "What meaning may this have? or "What meaning could you give to this?" or "Do you have an idea what this aims at?" This is usually done with the clear understanding that I may myself not know precisely where this leads to nor what the meaning is of what has already been given. Often, the thinking in historical connections can be encouraged: "This must have a long history. Can we hear more about it?"—again a specific suggestion by Jenny Waelder-Hall. Also her simile: "We, you and I, are like customer and bank employee who want to open a bank safe. You have a key, and I have one, but only you and I together are able to unlock it."

Thus what counts in the interpretations is the learning of self-observation, and with this the capability of arriving at the insights oneself. The content of the interpretation is the less important part; more important is the other part of insight: one's own experiencing of inner connections and of the feelings accompanying them.

## PROMINENT FORMS OF DEFENSE

Here several specific forms of defense are examined whose consideration and deeper understanding has often been very useful for me, but aspects of which may not always be given the respect they deserve.

### Repression, Denial, and Ego-Split

First, I would like to mention briefly how I understand the following terms: *Repression* means the unconscious "No" toward certain *wishes* (drive derivatives) and the *memories* connected with them; the corresponding form of rejection in conscious experience is *renunciation*. *Denial* is the unconscious "No" toward certain *perceptions*—either, as Freud (1927, 1940) originally meant it, toward perceptions of certain external facts, or, as much more usually meant today, toward the perception of the *meaning* of such facts, of their affectively charged importance (Basch 1974, 1983). The conscious correspondence to denial in the first sense—that of facts—would be lying, the outright rejection of truth, but also the conscious avoidance of painful truths, with the meaning "I simply cannot think of that." What corresponds to denial in the second sense, that of affective relevance, is what Freud (1925) has described as *negation*: the conscious, intellectual form of "No" against the importance of a perception. The *blocking of affects*, often equated with repression, is the unconscious "No" toward certain *feelings*; its conscious correlation is the *suppression* of certain emotions. *Isolation* is the unconscious "No" toward the *connections* of affects and thoughts, of wishes and images of memory and imagination; their correlation in consciousness, as presented by Eissler (1959), is the conscious splitting off of everything that intrudes in *concentration*.

Because of the significance of denial for the rest of this book I deal with it somewhat more in detail. It was defined by Trunnell and Holt (1974) as "a failure to fully appreciate the significance or implications of what is perceived" (p. 771). In other words, it is a defense mechanism making unconscious the *emotional significance of perceptions*.

As it is noticeable how very close this stands to repression, their separation may be questioned. Freud (1927) discriminates between them only with reservation: "If we wanted to differentiate more sharply between the vicissitude of the *idea* as distinct from that of the *affect*, and reserve the word '*Verdrängung*' [repression] for the affect, then the correct German word for the vicissitude of the idea would be '*Verleugnung*' [disavowal]" (p. 153). (This differs from the distinction made earlier by me, one that more closely reflects, I believe, the development of psychoanalytic thought since.)

We then have to ask ourselves: What do we really mean with the significance that gets lost, especially in such marked ways in the states of depersonalization? Clearly, it is not a matter of logical or semantic significance, but of the *value* these perceptions (or ideas) possess for us. It should therefore not come as a big surprise that the inner evaluating and value giving agency, that is, the superego, plays a decisive role when such states of massive denial and voided meaning occur. This is not just the case for external perception, but also for that of the self: for example, we can clearly distinguish between feelings we fully experience and others we register but cannot fully "feel." The reason for this distinction seems to me to lie in the presence or absence of a kind of inner warrant, an acceptance and testimony, which our conscience gives to these perceptions. It is a kind of sanction from above: "You are permitted to, or you ought not, accept meaning and value of this for yourself." Nothing else is blocked with this, neither the affect nor the perception themselves, but solely their personal valuation.

Denial as defense is accompanied by an *ego split.* Since this term is nowadays being vastly overused, I would like to delimit it.

Freud described it both at the very beginning and at the end of the wide span of his psychoanalytic creativity.

In his (1895) case description of Miss Lucy R., he mentions how the result of repression is "a splitting of consciousness" which is "a deliberate and intentional one. At least it is often introduced by an act of volition" (p. 123). He notes later that "it was a peculiar state of knowing and at the same time not knowing—a state, that is, in which a psychical group was cut off" (p. 165).

Freud (1940a) also wrote:

> He [the child] replies to the conflict with two contrary reactions, both of which are valid and effective. On the one hand, with the help of certain mechanisms he rejects reality and refuses to accept any prohibition; on the other hand, in the same breath he recognizes the danger of reality, takes over the fear of that danger as a pathological symptom and tries subsequently to divest himself of the fear . . . this success is achieved at the price of a rift in the ego which never heals but which increases as time goes on. The two contrary reactions to the conflict persist as the centre-point of a splitting of the ego. [p. 275f.]

He described (1936) this doubleness also in regard to depersonalization.

Such "disavowals of perceptions," which "occur very often and not only with fetishists" (1940b, p. 204) lead to half-measures, incomplete attempts at detachment from reality: "The disavowal is always supplemented by an acknowl-edgment; two contrary and independent attitudes always arise and result in the situation of there being a splitting of the ego" (Freud 1940b, p. 204).

The doubleness of self- and world experience as described by this con-cept of "splitting" or "ego-split" has often been remarked upon as a crucial event in the severe neuroses; it has recently served, under the heading of "borderline-pathology" with changed meaning and used as an explanatory term, to demarcate both the technique and theory of a very vast area of psychopathology. Much of what follows tries to present an alternate model.

## Reversal

There is an array of drive reversals that are, as forms of defense, of much greater significance than what we often would conclude from the literature about these severely ill patients, including turning from active to passive, turning from passive to active, and turning against the self. The latter, turn-ing against the own person, is of course of special importance in the depres-sions. We shall see a good example of this later on in this chapter in the excerpt from the analysis of Anne, a depressive woman with strongly mas-ochistic character. The first, the turning from active to passive, is typical for the masochistic character. The phobic patient Jacob, described in Chapter 5, shows this defense in steadily new variants.

However, it seems to me more and more helpful to see in the middle kind of reversal, the *turning of passive into active*, the cardinal type of defense in severe psychopathology, and very specially as a defense against aggression suffered from the outside. It is therefore a form of defense that is decidedly interpersonal in nature (against what is experienced as attack or as threat from the outside), in addition to being of intrapsychic character (against the simultaneous, intolerable anxiety). Thus it is, in spite of the parallel-ism, not quite in the same sense a defense against aggression, in the way that repression is directed above all against libido. In contrast to repression, turning passive into active is mostly an *interpersonal* form of defense.

The severer the psychopathology, the more valuable I have found this type of defense for my understanding and my interpretive work. This is es-pecially so in my work with compulsive drug users as well as with severely "narcissistic" and even many masochistic-depressive patients. Most acting out consists at least to a considerable degree of such turning passive into active. In a general formulation, this defense means: "Instead of suffering it pas-sively what I am constantly afraid of, I am now the one who actively inflicts it on the other." Or: "Instead of permitting myself to be suddenly surprised by a calamity, I prefer to bring it about myself." It is an attempt to reenact the traumatic situation under the stage management of the ego, instead of the helplessness of the original state. Thus, much of revenge, of deception and lying, of self-righteous indignation can be traced back to this defense by *turning the tables*, and becomes treatable only if understood in that way. Its comprehension also usually effects a strong reduction in countertransference.

## Identification

Hand in glove with such reversal there usually is identification as defense, *identification with the aggressor* above all, where the aggressor is an accuser, a reproachful, judging, shaming authority. Now it is the patient who becomes prosecutor and lets the therapist or the environment at large feel guilty or ashamed. Everything is now so set up that the other sees himself profoundly in the wrong. The patient has become the voice of the accusing conscience. Especially depressive-masochistic patients develop consummate skill in treating the other reproachfully, to turn him, explicitly or implicitly, to a sinner burdened by inexcusable guilt. This occurs by combining these two defensive processes (reversal, and identification with the accusing aggressor) and is clinically very frequent. The "negative therapeutic reaction" can be understood to a good extent in this way.

I find little use for the concept of *projective identification*. Does it mean that one *provokes* in the other what one fears most intensely within? In that case I would rather see in it again a special form of that turning of passive into active, and easily and elegantly interpretable in this way: "Instead of suddenly suffering punishment, unexpectedly and without control—or the humiliation, or injury, or abandonment—I bring it about on my own; I am at least the one who determines the point in time." As Abend and colleagues (1983) have put it, the expression "projective identification" is often used when we simply deal with projections (see also the valuable review study by Grefe and Reich [1996]).

In the analysis of masochistic pathology, the defense of *identification with the victim*, the mirror image to identification with the aggressor, and with it the *turning against the self* (or turning active to passive), stand in the foreground. Their lives seem to put those afflicted always anew into situations where they find themselves as victims. They are tormented human beings who have sacrificed more to family and civilization than is compatible with competence and efficacy, and thus live a life deeply inimical to any pleasure, joy, and happiness (see Novick and Novick 1996). What lurks beneath this as an especially shameful secret is the intertwining of almost all sexual feelings with suffering (and vice versa!). Thus it is, as will be illustrated later in this chapter in the case of Anne, as if they begrudged themselves any joy, any present, unless they have paid an exorbitant price in form of physical and emotional torment and disgrace. They are commonly people who as children had been exposed to great brutality or other severe traumata and who now, in the form of that identification with the victim and with the help of manifold *affect reversals*, seem to state: "I am not afraid anymore of suffering, I even seek it out. I don't suffer anymore under violence, I even enjoy it as victim. I am not debased anymore as a helpless creature, on the contrary, I am a martyr of God's grace, of higher worth than my tormentors. I am not helpless anymore, but now I am in control, because it is I who brings the calamity about" (see also the case of Elazar, in parallel book).

Therapeutically, it is not only the reversal of affect, but also in particular the reversal of aggressive wishes that assumes crucial importance: every desire to attack, to take revenge, to inflict pain and to kill is turned by the weak and impotent against the self. This turning against the own person is often the Archimedean point from which the masochistic fantasy system may be lifted out of its hinges.

### Regression, Polarization, and Exaggeration

As far as I know, one special form of defense has so far not received any systematic attention: the *defense by exaggeration*, by amplification or hyperbole. The analysis of dreamwork, with its attendant use of condensation or compression (Freud [1900]: "The intensity of a whole train of thought may eventually be concentrated in a single ideational element," p. 595), may then endow its interpretations with such extra force. Anger at once turns into murder and killing rage, disappointment into desperate frenzy, injured self-esteem into overwhelming shame and its compensation by delusional grandiosity, gracefulness and gentility into obsequiousness and submissiveness. While in fact such exaggeration may frequently reflect what is in the background and repressed, it also might quite likely serve directly defensive purposes: by exaggeration, the actual feeling is being devalued; moreover, the listener is secretly being ridiculed. In some school traditions it may often be much simpler to talk of murderous rage against the analyst—"it is after all expected of me"—than merely to confess: "You have offended me yesterday by your approach (by your silence, by your intrusive interpreting and overinterpreting, by your tactlessness); you have annoyed me." The "interpretation upward" is here, as often, a more effective measure, one closer to the surface of the mind. In turn, if it is mainly the analyst who, mostly on the basis of dreams, introduces such intensification—"You want to kill your wife" or "You want to sleep with me"—he (or she) runs the risk of increasing anxiety and hence resistance a great deal, exacerbating the current conflict *ad absurdum* and thus debasing it, not to speak of the questionableness of the direct drive interpretation. Such a caveat is of course much more in order for the earlier than the later phases of analysis.

It stands to reason that this defense by exaggeration is a variant of the defense by *regression*. Another manifestation of it would be the defense by *polarization*, or as preferred by many, by *splitting*. All in all, I believe, however, that it is here less a matter of a particular defense mechanism, let alone one that excels by its archaic and elementary nature, than that it is, as we will observe in most cases presented in this volume, the phenomenologically very important result of a number of defensive processes: regression, condensation, displacement, repression, reaction formation. The more severe the neurosis, the more extensive this phenomenon.

"In order to solve the problem of ambivalence she displaced outward one side of her ambivalent feeling. Her mother continued to be a love object, but, from that time on, there was always in the girl's life a second important person of the female sex, whom she hated violently."

"My emotional life has always insisted that I should have an intimate friend and a hated enemy. I have always been able to provide myself afresh with both . . ."

Borderline and splitting? The first quote is from one of the classic cases described by Anna Freud (1936, p. 45), the second is one of the untold autobiographical elements in Freud's (1900) *Interpretation of Dreams* (p. 483).

As I shall detail in Chapter 6, I consider splitting (or for that matter polarization) *a descriptive, not an explanatory concept*. In this regard, one difference of my way of understanding from that of Melanie Klein or Kernberg lies in that, for them, such polarization represents a basic element, irreducible rock bottom, whereas for me there the work of exploration and interpretation only begins. Another issue is its specifically pathognomonic significance, namely for a special category of patients, the "borderlines," a significance not existing for me—except that these phenomena of polarization, when very prominent, hint merely at a severer version of the neurotic disturbance at issue; in and by themselves, they do not as yet call for a change in the technique.

By the way, it seems to me that all kinds of splitting and dissociation are particularly typical for hysteria. All repression is itself nothing other than such a kind of "split," phenomenologically understood, as stated by Fingarette in his book *Self-Deception* (1969).

## Externalization

This defense mechanism is in my view just as much a counterpart to denial as Waelder (1951) suggested for projection (which is anyway often not clearly delimited from externalization). With its help, "the whole internal battleground is changed into an external one" (A. Freud 1965, p. 223; the specific reference is to displacement and externalization in infantile phobias), that is, *the inner conflict is being reenacted on the outside whereby others are being treated as if they were disavowed parts of the self.* In other words, externalization is that kind of defensive activity whereby *external actions, things, and human beings* are being used in order to deny an inner conflict; an inner conflict is transformed (back) into an external one.

Novick and Novick (1996) differentiate very neatly between the specific use of the term as "externalization of aspects of the self representation" (p. 126) and projection proper as a "defense against a specific drive derivative directed toward an object" (p. 115). The former is "aimed at avoiding the narcissistic pain consequent upon accepting devalued aspects of the self" (p. 114); the latter is "motivated by the sequence of fantasied dangers consequent upon drive expression" (p. 115).

Under the influence of externalization, the actions on the outside and especially their retelling and reliving in the sessions stand in the way of observing inner conflicts. The outside events reflect inner conflicts as they occur *now* in the therapeutic situation and specifically in the transference and serve the transference of defense.

As an example, aggressions suffered within, under the lashings by the conscience, like derision, rebuff, and chastisement, are now not only expected, dreaded, and suspected, as with projection, nor simply "given back" to the others, as with the turning from passive to active, but they are being provoked and enacted anew on life's stage. Or limit-setting from the outside is being evoked and invited, as incessantly demanded by one's own conscience, yet this is then being ferociously fought off. Or acceptance and approval and support are ostensibly being sought, very concretely in form of "oral" or "narcissistic" supplies; but then these are, with seeming disdain, rebuffed, while they are at bottom actually shunned as being undeserved. At the same time and as counterpart of the same conflict, every restriction of those gifts evokes intense envy and rage.

Much "acting out," many impulsive sequences serve such defense by externalization; the actions aim at establishing magical, omnipotent control over what is not controllable. One braves extreme danger, dares the risks of separation, humiliation, and physical injury, in order to prove, counterphobically, that the fear of those threats is unfounded. Of course, there is in this again much of "turning passive in active," but what essentially distinguishes this defense is this: "Instead of inner danger, instead of drive anxiety, superego anxiety, and unconscious, archaic castration anxiety, I now have to deal with reality anxiety, with bare knuckles and out there. I vanquish those hidden inner dangers by triumphing over these dangers in outer reality."

I believe that what the concept of "projective identification" of Kleinian coinage aspires to explain are the phenomena resulting from the defenses of externalization, projection, displacement, and role exchange, working together in complex ways.

## EXAMPLES FOR SEQUENCES AND RECONSTRUCTIONS OF EGO PROCESSES

### A Case of Pseudostupidity

One of the symptoms that brings this 35-year-old physician, Thomas, into treatment consists in very dangerous actions involving astonishing misjudgments—like going snorkling in the sea with only part of his gear and thus nearly drowning, trusting people with his money who have deceived him before, overlooking in peculiar ways obvious medical signs of severe dangers in patients, and so on. Such episodes are followed by hours and days of self-castigation and rumination on how to undo the damage done, days of bitterly raging at himself, and of profound sadness. With all this he is a deeply conscientious and honest man.

It is interesting that these dangerous episodes characteristically begin with some perceived humiliation and slight followed by a transitory, usually very brief state of rage about this offense.

This sequence has to be seen against a severely traumatic history. The mother appears to be a phobic and obsessive-compulsive woman who clearly dominated the household with her temper tantrums. After having given up a successful career as a civil service employee to take care of her children, she showed to the world a chronically depressive, angry scowl. The father, a weak and meek man entirely under her thumb, suffered from a congenital severe impediment of vision that left him legally blind and only able to fulfill subordinate types of work. Especially during the later childhood of Thomas, and with the advent of more and more children, he too became very irascible and abused the children physically.

Both parents evinced a terrifying blindness toward the individuality of their five children. In an entirely one-sided and obstinate, ruthless way they forced Thomas and his three brothers from early childhood on to direct all their activities toward a single goal: to become physicians, with the outspoken demand that he or they would cure father's blindness. For example, one refrain was: "Don't waste time with those toys. They won't help you to become a physician later on. You don't need to write [school-]compositions; that is not important for a doctor. Why are you not more observant [e.g., in regard to passers-by]? As a future physician you have to be that. Why are you interested in math? What good will that do you later? You will have anyway your own tax accountant, and much money in addition . . ." The fixity and violence with which this choice of career and other prejudices were imposed on the children had a nearly delusional quality and had for some of them catastrophic consequences.

The family was quite poor and lived in extremely cramped conditions: five children to one bedroom, under constant terrible noise, "seven people on three different tables in three different rooms craning their necks to look at two different television sets."

In a more detailed analysis of the sequence:

> I find myself caught between rage and guilt. Every time when I refused something at home or was not in agreement with them, my mother started screaming and crying; "After all I have done for you, this is now the gratitude I get! You nothing, you pile of crap, you bad person!" And then my father joined in yelling: "You are killing your mother. You will be standing at her grave and say the prayer for the dead! You want to be religious, don't you, you hypocrite!"

A similar mixture of rage and self-condemnation overwhelms him today when he feels exposed and helpless. Then all evil thoughts and wishes vanish. He can think of nothing anymore; his mind is now only blank and empty. Such an altered state of consciousness, entailing emptiness and constriction of the ability to hear, understand, think, and remember, may increase to the extent of his being all confused and dumb. Everything around him becomes meaningless and incomprehensible; conversations turn into senseless noise.

In less intensive states of this kind there may be only severed feelings of anxiety, anger, and especially sadness, or weird ideas that appear to him ridiculous and absurd, such as that during intercouse he would cut off the leg of his wife with his own, or that during a lecture or a theater performance he would, by cocking his finger, shoot the person standing at the center of attention.

Yet all this is a minor matter compared with the impulsive action itself which turns into a fateful peril. He describes it so:

> When I was playing chess with my father or my brother it kept happening that I planned ahead and foresaw very precisely everything and pondered every one of my draws, everything I would do in order not to be overpowered, but I planned it in a very repetitive, stereotypical manner, leaving fully out of account what *his* next draw would be, and suddenly I would find myself beaten.

The same would happen when they tickled him or fought with him, at play or seriously. Unexpectedly he was overwhelmed because the others took advantage of his vulnerablity: "I was unable to anticipate the catastrophe." It is a narrowing of his consciousness that keeps befalling him in such competitive or fighting situations. This *narrowing of consciousness* and *isolation of affects* is accompanied by a radical form of *denial of perceptions*. In particular, whenever he feels helpless and degraded, everything appears suddenly without meaning; it loses all its affective significance. It is in this state that the most stupid decisions are made, which implement at the same time his aggressions against others and the self-punishment bound up with it. This state of foolish action is then followed by sadness and crying.

The first time we are speaking about this so precisely he remembers his crying when his mother used to leave in the evening for her work and his father brought him to bed. After such memories of separation anxiety and separation grief, there occur to him recollections of wishes and games in which dolls were thrown—it is unclear whether by him or friends—into the fire; he describes an uncanny incinerator in their apartment building. Again the clear references to babies are easily evoked, but without emotions, except for some amusement. These emotionless images of memory veil the murderous wishes. The screen affect of sadness serves as defense against the unacceptable feelings of jealousy, rage, guilt, and shame. Images as well as affects are displaced.

The *sequence* appears therefore in the following, pretty regular form: (1) the feeling of loss, humiliation, or threat → (2) anger or helpless rage → (3) guilt or shame about such evil feelings and wishes → (4) attempts to undo them and make them harmless—by severance (isolation) and displacement, and especially by "emptiness and confusion," an altered state of consciousness → (5) as a part thereof or as accompaniment to it, a narrowing of consciousness, with massive exclusion and blocking of perceptions, that is, denial → (6) decisions and actions of pseudostupidity → and, finally, (7) return of the original affects, but in altered form, mostly as sadness, feeling ashamed, and anger at himself, or return of the original aggressions in pale, unfelt form. However, what is specially characteristic in this sequence is the *denial of external dangers*: either they are not perceived at all or simply insufficiently taken into account, and thus punishment is eventually brought about from within or from without. How this basically masochistic sequence could be understood in deeper ways and eventually resolved will be shown in the detailed examination of the entire course of his analysis (in Wurmser [1993], Chapter 6).

This first case shows something else which is theoretically of great significance: Several authors have mentioned that the *splitting of the ego* typical for denial—the parallelism of rejection and acceptance of perception—often does not remain restricted to this, but becomes far more comprehensive and, as both Lichtenberg and Slap (1973) and Wangh (1985) have described, opposes entire complexes of id, ego, and superego parts in stable combinations. It is always newly impressive to observe this strange oscillation between two opposite *part identities*. Such a doubleness thus always occurs when there are extensive processes of denial at play, especially as reflected in states of depersonalization. The *acknowledgment of one part-identity* includes necessarily the *denial of the other part-identity*, and with that a more or less radical falsification or at least narrowing down of perception. It is not only essential in this that the two part-identities are in conflict with each other, but that the superego plays a central role in this event. Thus, and crucially, we find in Thomas a kind of "*false*"—that is, *depersonalized*—*part-identity*, an imposed submissiveness, docility, and goodness, an obsequious acceptance of all the dictates from parents and profession, regardless of how unreasonable these might be. Opposed to this stands the *bad, rebellious child*. In a dream these two self-figures appear without too much disguise; on the one side, there is an innocent child who plays, but who also shoots at people in cars and hits them, and on the other side, there is the dream-ego that watches, forces the child to the ground and ties it down. Or there appear howling lions, tigers, wild hounds, and snakes that hunt him as prey and chase him out of his sleep. Or he plays in an interesting reversal some practical jokes, like hiding in the closet and suddenly leaping forth at his wife—I mean with reversal that he redirects his aggressive wishes originally meant against his pregnant mother; probably the same is true in his shooting (in the dream) at the cars. This second part-identity comes very much to the foreground in temper tantrums in which he resembles a 3-year-old screaming and crying child.

Corresponding to his own double life there is the split reality in the family of his childhood; hidden behind a façade of joviality and friendliness are strife, violence, and unhappiness. In a still different formulation, the children either took over the stereotypical role assigned to them, that is, the role of the physician, and joined in with the parents in the massive denial of their own identity, wishes, and feelings, or they rose up in brief but unsuccessful revolts, in desperate anger and defiance, only to succumb soon again to their sense of guilt and revert to their docility. It is interesting to note how this entire sequence proceeds now in the main unconsciously and entails that dangerously severe denial of the *meaning* of facts—of their risks— which leads to the most stupid judgments.

The very strong split in his personality experienced by Thomas does not have to be seen however as "borderline pathology." It should also be added that the analysis, which was unusually difficult and long, could successfully be terminated after nine and a half years and 1,550 hours. The complex psychopathology of a severe masochistic character pathology with depression, tendency to passivity and "blaming," as well as the here briefly outlined symptoms of pseudostupidity, depersonalization, and outbursts of rage had gradually yielded to our analytic work, although with many setbacks, mostly in form of "negative therapeutic reactions." A very detailed study of the evolution of the dynamics in the analysis is given in the book *Das Rätzel des Masochismus* (1993).

### Reconstruction of the Sequence of Defenses in a Case of Neurotic Depression and Masochistic Character

The second patient from whose analysis I present some excerpts is Anne, a married woman in her thirties, whom I described more in detail in my book *The Mask of Shame* (1981a). Her analysis was successfully concluded after five and a half years or 971 hours; six years later she returned for a period of reanalysis (70 hours). She had come to treatment because of chronically depressive, but also anxious or rageful moods, generalized social anxiety, and painful inhibition, self-sabotage, and unhappiness. She was the oldest of four; her next brother, Paul, had been born when she was 5 years old. Her mother was herself depressive, shy, and withdrawn, her father a brutally explosive, highly paranoid man. Thus he penalized Anne and the entire family for some smaller mischief of hers by being silent for several months and let her in that way feel that she was the cause of the whole family's unhappiness. Anne idealized her mother, but unconsciously she was very bitter about her because she had not been able to protect the children against the father's terrible outbursts of rage. Her jealousy toward her siblings and hence also a strong rivalry with my other patients and tasks and with my family was an important theme in the analysis.

Here I bring only a microscopic excerpt, which should nevertheless show certain sequences and their interpretation partly worked out by the patient herself.

She opens the 618th hour: "As I came in I was angry. I'm not certain if it was because of you, but I hadn't been before. I had the fantasy over the weekend: I wanted to go with my sister-in-law and her baby to the zoo—, and the fantasy was that I would see you there, and you would have your wife and your grandchildren with you, and you would be very proud of them and show them much love. And when I would see you, my reaction would be that I would be very hurt and would cry and wouldn't come to the next hour. I know this is so unreasonable—that you cared for somebody else, and that is for little children, and that I would feel like an outsider—because I'm not related to you, and you could never care so much for me like for your family. I tell myself: 'You stupid idiot! How could he have such feelings for you, how could he care for you more than for his family?'"

"So that you assume it would have another origin, that it means much more than it says?"

"Yes, I guess so. I'm reminded of father's favorite sentence that 'the world doesn't owe anybody anything'—probably because I acted as if the world owed me something. Or it was simply something for him to scream about." She comments about the expression of her longing to be accepted and her resentment at being excluded and shortchanged as repetition, as identification with her hated father, and as a transference phenomenon, without pointing as yet to its unconscious root.

"Or is it not rather so that you had it [the feeling of belonging] and lost it?"

"That is true."

"And that it is this losing that you painfully reexperience with me?" In my comment I shift the focus from one type of affect—resentment and jealousy, both being aggressively tinged and strongly tabooed feelings—to the affects of pain and sadness that were in the past eminently important and are being reactualized right now in the transference, that is, to a kind of affect that in this context has to be assigned traumatic significance and thus causal efficacy. Implicitly, the predominantly aggressive affects are treated as resulting from defense and attributed to *affect reversal.*

Thereupon she describes her mother's temporary absence during her later childhood because of an operation and mentions how nobody cared for the child's feelings. I remind her that, at the time when her mother was hospitalized for the delivery of Paul, she refused to take her lunch at the neighbor's. She adds how important it had been for her to get the food from her mother herself. "It was an act of love, of tenderness. If I had switched my lunch for that of my girlfriend it would have been like dishonoring my mother, rejecting her love. I had this feeling that my mother was better than everybody's mother and that she prepared perfect lunches. That lunch was her presence; [through it] I was in touch with her when I was in school. How could anybody be a good mother who didn't do this? Well, my mother-in-law!" Here both her identification with the victim (the mother) as well as again her conscious and expressed jealousy (against mother-in-law and sister-in-law) resonate, both being elements of the "surface," namely continuing the theme raised at the beginning of the hour.

"And you were very afraid to get away from your mother."

"I was just thinking that the making of the lunches would be a big thing, and that I would like to be like my mother." (The patient is at the time of this therapy excerpt still childless.)

"That you wish to undo the separation from your mother by identifying with her." Anxiety, wish, and defense are here interpreted together.

She continues complaining about her feeling left out by mother, but then interrupts herself: "The fantasy that began all this was about you and your grandchildren. Why would I punish myself with such thoughts, or indulge in them?" (She notices the self-tormenting, i.e., masochistic character of these thoughts.)

"Yes, what about it?"

"You mentioned it as reenactment of earlier loss. Why would I want to do that? Reenacting alone would not solve it, but understanding would." Here she expresses the basic expectation accompanying the analytic process: the Socratic faith that insight heals.[4]

"But the reenactment may also have deeper meanings," I counter; "for one, the outcome could now be different, and second, it would give you reason to feel sorry for yourself, and we know how important this is for you." Although not meant in this way, this comment is a direct drive interpretation of her masochism and clearly has an undertone of condemnation or criticism that she at once picks up, in accordance with the very content of the interpretation that refers to her masochistic attitude: "That seems important, the enjoyment about it [the suffering] although it has no value." It is noteworthy how she arrives at her own self-critical drive interpretation stimulated by the one I had given. I chose at this point, instead of the defense and superego analysis, the affirmation of the interpretation, probably standing under the assumption that this aspect of the dynamics by and large is already known, although by far not yet fully worked through: "That it says masochistically: 'Look, I'm again the ugly duckling'—and the secret pleasure in it." (Today I would presumably rather throw light on the same aspect from the side of the self-criticism within the transference, as for example, "What I just have been saying did have a critical sound which immediately was taken up by that side of you that criticizes you, saying: 'Now you again connect suffering with pleasure . . .'.")

At once, however, she concurs with my drive interpretation: "I understand what you say, and I agree with it. I wish I could change it, but in *that* regard I have not changed. This is not completely true though. I remember times of disagreement with my husband when I do not 'enjoy' it so much. I'm not sure whether I will ever eliminate this—this masochistic enjoyment."

"Or rather: whether you ever *want* to eliminate it entirely. But we see also something else: that this masochistic pleasure is the last step in a sequence."

"I don't see that."

"The fantasy has several stations; that you are sorry for yourself is only the end station."

"I think that this is too hard for me to figure out. As if I thought: How do you expect me to understand this?"

"That this kind of pseudostupidity would keep the fantasy intact?" (An indirect, but emphatic defense interpretation: turning of the aggression against herself, a questioning of her implacable self-condemnation, that is, of the tyrannical power she assigns to her conscience.)

"I don't think that this is pseudostupidity."

"That it would be the real thing."

"Right."

"You turn it against yourself—because the fantasy says simply—"

"Now I turn the aggression against you, that you know it, and I don't."

At this point, instead of responding with an interpretation, I recounted the fantasy she had told at the beginning of the session and then added: "You want love and attention from me and are angry and hurt for not getting it in that form, and then you direct that anger against yourself: I'm so dumb and cannot understand anything. How can we understand your not-understanding?" I don't take this for an interpretation but only for a clearer, more explicit presentation (a clarification) of the wish sequence she has hinted at herself; but I'm quickly taught better:

"Part of it was," she says, "that I didn't want the fantasy to be torn apart by your analyzing. And now I think that *you are angry at me and that I want this.*" Each of my comments and especially those referring to her wishes consistently are being experienced as reproaches, regardless of how much she already had expressed them herself. The masochistic basic attitude is being repeated in the transference, and this specifically, as it is ubiquitous for her, in form of the *superego transference*, mostly using shame feelings.

"That it would confirm the masochistic position, and this, including the pseudostupidity, the not-understanding, and being sorry for yourself, as a *protection against the anger at me and against the jealousy*. It keeps the jealous memories away, repressed, the jealousy directed against little children."

"I was just thinking that also: I feel so much shame about my jealousy in the fantasy."

"That *shame* is the motor for why you want to *repress* it."

"Now I can see where I repress it. But I still do experience anger and jealousy before I change them in feeling sorry for myself. Why would it be only partly?"

Today I would here rather respond with a counter-question, like: "What do you think?" or "What is really repressed are the memories—of what?" Yet I answered then with a direct defense interpretation: "The feelings are *displaced* onto *my* children. What is really repressed are the memories of the jealousy at the children in *your* family." Today I look critically at my usage of technical terms, like "repress," "displace." There probably would have been expressions that would be nearer to feeling and experience, less technical, and hence preferable. I continued: "It is probably also not without significance that this happened in the zoo." She does not get the allusion, and I resume after a while: "I was thinking of your play in childhood with animals." I am referring to her fantasy plays in which she tortured and killed human dolls and animal toys and also to current fantasies about me that involve torture and concentration camps. "It is as if it meant: 'Throw those rascals to the beasts!' And we shouldn't forget that you had great fear of an animal attacking you." I hint here at the murderous wishes against her siblings, but now still from the side of the anxiety (punishment) and the defense (repression, reversal of drive, projection, displacement).

She reacts: "It is the *wish* that the animal would kidnap them (the siblings) and we would never see them anymore." She gives the drive interpretation although still in the form of an externalization.

I reply: "So that what is repressed is the specific content of those jealous memories—that animals would take them [the other children] away."

To the following session she comes in "one of my worst moods ever," for a number of reasons: disagreements and strife at home and a rotten day at work (as secretary). Then she adds that her husband has asked her for fellatio. At first she refused him but felt then she could not rebuff him. Now he is annoyed at her because he is sensing that she is accusing him of having forced her into it. But this is completely ridiculous, she adds. He is complaining that she keeps attacking him with reproach; he wouldn't take that much longer. He makes her feel very guilty. At one point he has told her that she is very difficult to live with, and she would like to throw this back in his face. But she is afraid she would never hear the end of it. She then starts crying about his financial messiness and his accusations of her. She laments how at work too she has to pay for something her boss had cooked up. I connect both situations by the common feeling of humiliation. Immediately she starts talking (again) about her jealousy toward her husband's sister and mother; that he pays them more attention, gives them more time and flowers than her. He does not have any regard for her feelings. He lets her feel poorly about herself, that she is a sissy in his eyes, and she has to agree with him in that. So that the end is always, I say, that she would spare him the criticism and attack and humiliate herself, turning it again against herself. She counters that she probably is giving me a one-sided view: "Am I not really attacking him as he claims?"

"You probably do—but mostly to invite punishment from him."

In the following hour she feels much better without understanding the sudden change in mood.

"One thing that bothers me: we spoke earlier this week about my masochistic tendency—"

"—as a defense—"

"Right. But I look at it as something in itself: that I seem to enjoy it so much that I don't have the motivation to change it. In a sick way I also enjoyed [the suffering] yesterday." The interpretation of her masochistic attitude as a defense is being made by her into a cause for self-reproach by transforming it consciously into a drive interpretation, one that actually is also a correct insight into the secondary gain of her masochistic orientation. I question this by referring back to the original sequence: "But what was it related to? When did this masochistic form of sexual pleasure occur?"

"My mind began to wander. I have a new dress. I wonder whether you have noticed. I have feelings, I would like to look attractive for you." It is a direct love offering, but one in a triangle with her husband, with strong undertones of revenge against him, and all embedded in the overall masochistic transference.

"And that masochistic 'orgy' happened as we followed the zoo fantasy into the depth, and that had to do with wanting to be attractive for me."

"That made me think about the fantasy of seeing you with your grand-children, and then, that we were talking about my feelings toward my siblings, and my feeling that I cannot change the past, and I don't know how to deal with that feeling."

"But there was something much more specific that we had not heard before."

"I don't know what you're talking about, except about throwing them to the animals or having the animals taking them away."

"Yes; what about it?"

"I have a thought right now. It is hard to understand what this has to do with the [bad] feeling yesterday. Namely that I have to trust you. I don't believe this is an important connection."

"You left something out that is a bridge to it."

"I don't remember it. At the end it was only about the animals taking them away."

"It was that *you turned it against yourself in the animal fantasy,* already then."

The defense is not only observable in the present sequence, within the hour, but can also be inferred in the recent memories as well as in those from her childhood.

"I don't understand. I don't remember what that was about."

"Your phobia; that an animal was attacking you and eating you."

After a longer silence she enlarges and deepens the interpretation in a significant way: "I remember something. When I was young, various friends of my parents used to take me to the zoo. Very few of them had their own children then. They would borrow me. This time I was swinging so long that I could not walk afterwards. I was about 3. So they put me in a stroller and took me to the zoo. I was indignant about it. Otherwise I don't remember anything about that visit. But something else that I realize just now: they had a child the same year as Paul was born. I lost their attention too."

"You mention this in the context of . . ." and I repeat my last two remarks. Again a longer silence.

"I thought about the dream I had as a child, about the *bear chasing me.* I think of a house close to my grandparents' house in the mountains of Appalachia where my grandparents were living. It was isolated. An old lady was living there, the mother of that couple I was just talking about. It was a mountain cabin. She had a picture in the living room of an Indian family—an Indian brave and his wife and his child. And they were in these mountains, and they were pursued by a bear and trapped on a ledge. The brave tried to protect his family with bow and arrow alone. Now I also remember that dream: it was in the yard of that house, and I was walking around, and everyone else was in the house. And suddenly I saw this bear, and I started running. And now I just have the thought—I was running away from the house instead of toward the house and security. He caught me and bit me in the shoulder. I thought it would be painful, but it felt very warm, almost in a sexual way."

"So that the bridge is complete."

"I can see the similarity."

"*First the aggression: that the animal would take away the siblings, the family; then, secondly, that you turn it against yourself and experience this with anxiety; and thirdly that you feel this anxiety and this attack against you as something sexual.*" This is the *reconstruction* of the *sequence of defenses* which interprets in summary form both the observations made in the session itself and what she had dreamt at age 8. But, as will become clear shortly, this interpretation is not yet complete.

"I understand all that. I try to understand what that has to do with yesterday."

"The ball is in your court. It is a good question."

"I take it literally—to get rid of the siblings, of the family—and yesterday the wish to get rid of my husband."

"That bear that you could not bear—" She laughs about the wordplay. "—and then, to complete the explanation—"

"—how I turned it against myself."

"You felt persecuted by him."

"Right."

"And you enjoyed it."

"Right. One thing that gets in the way; over and over again, all the things that he has done wrong, the things that I don't like: I ask myself: Am I being persecuted by him? I don't want to admit that I'm all wrong, that this suspicion is invalid." She recognizes and interprets herself the projection contained in her fears. "That doesn't mean that I don't also have legitimate complaints, and I was also wrong in certain regards, and he has legitimate complaints against me."

I try to deepen this insight: "You say: 'Am I being persecuted by him?' meaning, that all aggression is turned against you—when the bear catches you."

"Yes, I was also thinking of it. That I was *ashamed* how I behaved yesterday, that I feel that this sense of persecution doesn't help my credibility with my husband."

The facet of the masochistic transference is here also conspicuous, specifically the consistent superego transference; it could have been interpreted in this connection without difficulty, and it probably should have been. Instead, I say: "Your reality now is being shaped in the mold of that dream. The bear is now there, newly created and maintained in reality."

"I just think how strong my feelings were yesterday, of being persecuted, as if a switch had been turned on, and I couldn't turn it off. And when he told me it was my foul mood I used it as more persecution. I cannot get out of it when I am in it."

"It had been stirred up here, in the hour." Here too it might have been advantageous also to remark on the specific transference meaning; I do not mean that of the jealousy but that of the condemnation: the bear biting her from behind. "Then you presumably had a dream in the night referring to those three steps [jealous aggression, turning against the self, and sexualization], and when you woke up in a bad mood, you were stuck because the beginning was unconscious. It was like a broken record. And everything during the day fit to this persecutory fantasy and the masochistic attitude."

"I'm reminded that this week his sister has been calling my husband every night and how jealous that makes me."

"So that the bear fantasy is linked to the sister-in-law and then displaced onto me in the zoo."

After longer silence: "I feel very ashamed about these feelings, and how I behaved yesterday."

"I believe this is a very important feeling also here: that *you are afraid I would ridicule and shame you for these masochistic feelings.* We can add this as a *fourth step* in this whole sequence, and assume it even for then: that you felt ridiculed and were ashamed. When was the dream?"

"Between 6 and 8."

"What is so important in this: that the same sequence that is still so troubling today was already present then in the same form."

"That reminds me of something else: I was 10 or 12. Every summer I went with two girlfriends to the swimming pool. Sometimes my feelings were hurt. I would begin to go under water and I would cry. I was very sad. It was like a game. And when I came out of the water I would pretend as if nothing was bothering me."

"Like the masochistic part of the fantasy now and the shame about it."

"This is true. I compare it with when I was crying so much that I was almost sick. That too I did in secret after having gone to bed."

"And I assume that there also was a lot of pleasure with it."

"This is true. I remember: when I was crying so much I had the fantasy that my parents would find me half dead, and that they were sorry for all the wrongs they had done against me. And last night I had the fantasy that I would be so upset and traumatized that I would walk around like a zombie, with no emotion and no response, and would be very ill, and you would have to take me to a doctor. It reminds me of my father's silences. My father got a lot of enjoyment out of it—he let us know that he could speak but did not. In my fantasy I would not be able to speak."

"This is an important additional piece. If this too is part of the *turning against yourself*, how would it sound—I mean the translation back into aggression?"

"To do to my father what he had done to me."

"This also. But more: Couldn't being silent mean: to be dead? In the fantasy you play the corpse: *you turn the death wish against yourself*."

Critically I would like to make two comments here: For one, that I have here missed the opportunity to take the transference meaning she has expressed into the defense interpretation: that she would like to force me by her suffering to step in vigorously as a forgiving power, that is, as a good superego figure, to protect her in spite of her killing fantasies, and to heal and love her. The second addition would be something that got much clearer to me only much later, namely when I was reading the work of J. and K. K. Novick (1987, 1991): how she was here transforming her overwhelming helplessness into magical power, the "delusion of omnipotence," as the Novicks call it: *her suffering should magically bring about forgiveness and redemption*, and how this is being repeated with me.

She stays silent, then says: "I'm just thinking how much better I feel today; and I wonder how I got out of that masochistic orgy. I can only guess that it was the dream that has solved the conflict."

"When you allow yourself here to be angry in thought, feeling, fantasy, or dream, without turning it against yourself, then the break in the record is jumped over." The first item missed just before is here, at least indirectly, made up.

"That reminds me of the last thing just before falling asleep. My husband said I cannot make any compromise. I always want to be right. I responded: 'Only if you do something *you* don't want to do. Then we shall meet halfway.' It was the first rational comment that I made."

"You put him in his place and were not cornered by the bear, not driven by him into the masochistic position. And that may be the answer to your question."

I have chosen these two vignettes mostly to describe the multilayeredness of the defenses as they manifest themselves in relation to the current outer reality, to the transference, and in newly emerging memories from childhood. It was also to present how this kind of combined reconstruction of ego and superego processes may be dramatically successful, both on the small scale and all in all. In Anne's case, the crucial dynamics were, as presented in *The Mask of Shame* (Wurmser 1981a) and, in spite of the noted omissions, worked through to the extent that gradually a lasting and deep character change occurred.

## SUGGESTIVE PSYCHOTHERAPY AND PSYCHOANALYTIC TECHNIQUE

It may well happen that many of the things I presented earlier in this chapter in the section on the eleven technical guidelines for defense analysis may prove not to be feasible and that their opposite is desirable. With that we return to our first dilemma, that is, to the choice of treatment strategy.

In some situations, behaviorally oriented psychotherapeutic interventions might be preferable to psychoanalytic ones.

As mentioned in the introduction to this chapter, it is an issue of two fundamental paradigms, one psychoanalytic, one pedagogical. The former frees inner growth, the latter guides, leads, steers. Both complement each other. Where conflict is the prevailing problem, psychoanalysis is the better model. Where something, on whatever level, seems to be lacking, where there may be a deficit or defect, the psychotherapeutic-psychagogic approach—ultimately some form of education—may be preferable. This *complementarity*, however, reaches more deeply. There is probably no psychoanalytic treatment in which such educational elements, such psychagogical admixtures are entirely missing: "and even with the majority, occasions now and then arise in which the physician is bound to take up the position of teacher and mentor" (Freud 1918, p. 165). But characteristically Freud immediately adds: "But it must always be done with great caution, and the patient should be educated to liberate and fulfil his own nature, not to resemble ourselves" (p. 165). Shortly afterward, he makes the often quoted comment that we may feel compelled "to alloy the pure gold of analysis freely with the copper of direct suggestion" (p. 168).

In turn, there is probably no effective education in that deep and encompassing sense of "erudition," *Bildung, paideia*—in psychotherapeutic or any other form—which could entirely do without truly psychoanalytic admixtures and could go on without deeper insight into the conflicts incessantly arising during development.

This requires a more careful examination of the contrast between these two basic types. What is essential in these two counterpoised and yet almost indissolubly interwoven paradigms? Suppose we say, "Break the ice of your doubts; overcome yourself; all of this is only imagination, habit, self-indulgence; everything is a matter of will power. Experience will teach you to get rid of the unreason that dwells in your neurosis. Reward and punishment rule the world, and if you follow me in everything things will turn out all right. What I give you is good and will cure you; what reality tells you will help you. Follow these two taskmasters." This is, in a somewhat parodistic and exaggerated form, pedagogic; it is suggestion, a more or less subtle leading of the soul and guidance, more or less naive or wise psychagogy.

But how far is this different from the specifically psychoanalytic approach that works through and resolves conflict? After all, we deal here (in the psychoanalytic approach) also with transference—which is, after all, the vehicle of suggestion. We also overcome resistance and thus use our authority, and in some ways we even appeal, at least implicitly, to some faith in the method. And in order to be even more modern: Isn't ego-analysis ultimately nothing other than a method of demonstrating the discrepancy between the actual and the past anxiety situation, and don't we therefore reduce the entire linkage to "imagination," and isn't the procedure an appeal also ultimately based on the suggestion to recognize that the anxiety has become without basis? Isn't therefore the analytic approach nothing less than a special case of the other, the suggestive-educational paradigm, a kind of learning? Or, to follow our hardest critics, Grünbaum (1984) and Crews (1993), nothing but placebo and suggestion?

The answer is not easy. Is it, after all, not well known, almost a cliché, that in analysis transference and resistance are used as means for imparting insight and not for influencing? Yes, but what does that mean? Is it correct when Gill (1994a) states that

> the *decisive* criterion of psychoanalysis, one intrinsic to that therapy as against its extrinsic features, is that transference—the patient's experience of the interaction—is analyzed as much as is possible, whereas in psychotherapy it is to a greater or lesser degree *wittingly* left unanalyzed. [p. 62, quoted in Miller 1997, p. 37]

This is certainly one criterion, even a necessary one, but it is not sufficient.

The psychoanalytic modality means above all that the forms of defense and anxiety situations are taken seriously, that they are studied from the continually changing surface, and that they are traced back to their origins and creatively relived in the regression (Loewald 1980), not dismissed as more or less absurd. It is a technique of tact and intuition. It is "permitting the autonomy," not persuasion. Here, the anchor lies in the inner experience, and the focus dwells on *the inner conflict* and not on the goal of how it would be resolved. The interpretations serve the purpose of sharpening this focal inner attention, to free up self-reflection, not to submit or impose a solution. Parallel to this, transference is not used to break resistances but serves as a microscopic lens through which to study those forms of anxiety and defense. The metaphors are telling: here it is a matter of exploring, looking, searching, there it is a matter of overcoming, conquest, power, mastery. Both are thoroughly valid, valuable, and noble forms of providing help.

Admitted! But is not this approach of educating self-observation something quite intellectual, something that vanishes into the thin atmosphere of high rationality?

Indeed, it may well come to that, as a caricature, just as the other approach may degenerate into brutal overpowering.

In both, a kind of conversion is aimed at, a form of deeply felt transformation. It is *in what way*, however, that such a radical change is to be attained that makes the difference. It comes down to shifting the focus *from the belief in a directing authority* to the *autonomous*, reiterative, *and self-convincing insight*.

What is the decisive difference in this? It lies in the fact that what has been *torn asunder* by the defensive processes, especially by *repression*, and has been made unconscious in its *connectedness*, is being brought together again. It resembles very much what Goethe asked from art: "It is the [human] spirit that has to *detect connections* and thus to bring forth works of art . . . [The young artist] learns to think, *to bind properly together what fits* [together] . . ."[5]

To state it somewhat exaggeratedly, authority *forces* together what insight into inner experience *brings* together and lets *grow* together. What the belief in the authority binds together stays so only so long as that belief remains standing. Certainly, such a belief is also not to be disdained, but what the always repeatable insight joins together grows more and more into a unity. In other words, *the synthesis* is *striven for*, it is *not made*. The connection changes from one that has not been known before to one that is more and more familiar from within, and that is not dependent on persuasion from without. What such psychoanalytic insight accomplishes, in a strict sense, which should be truly effective and mutative in a lasting way, will be presented in detail in the following chapters.

In contrast, perhaps the most valuable aspect of the psychotherapeutic-psychagogic approach is to be a *good superego figure* and to tactfully assist the patient in acting within the bounds of reality. Intellectualization may be welcomed, interpretations of transference may often be less than judicious. Still, it seems to me that a good knowledge of defensive processes is also indispensable for good psychotherapy. The focus lies here more on the achievement of the *goal*, that is, the taking over of certain values and the adaptation to outer reality.

We have seen what gaining of insight that is in the true sense psychoanalytic, and that should be deeply mutative over time, consists of. It can be summarized in the following watchwords: (1) going out from the momentary surface, with the special relevance of contiguity: "Why now? Why in this context?"; (2) the precedence of defense analysis over drive analysis; the detailed, complex recognition of defense processes, moment by moment; (3) the often neglected and difficult interpretation of the transference of defense; (4) the careful, cautious, yet decisively important use of reconstructions; (5) the role of the nontechnical, personal relationship, with maintenance of neutrality and abstinence (though even this requires rethinking); and (6) the principle: "The more specific, the more effective"—and with that, the significance of the right moment, the *kairós*.

I turn now concretely to the suggestive-psychotherapeutic measures that sometimes also prove necessary in the psychoanalytic treatment of difficult cases:

The past may serve as a protection against a present that is too conflict-laden and cannot be mastered, and against unmanageable transference aspects; it may, as content for interpretations, be preferable. "Premature" genetic interpretations may be capable of bringing order into chaos and thus of mediating at least a sense of reestablished mastery and control—be this illusory or not. In that way they may also strengthen the trust in the knowledge of the therapist at a time of helplessness and despair.

As already mentioned and as stressed by Anna Freud (1936) and Gray (1986), intellectualization may be a strong and bitterly needed defense against acute inner and outer dangers. Transference interpretations may often be premature, unsuitable, or comprehensible to the analyst, but not to the patient. Thus, obsessive-compulsive and other strongly narcissistic character forms may have a too strong defense against the recognition of the transference aspects. "Why are you so interested in yourself?" the patient may reply. In other severely ill patients the tendency toward regression would be deepened by them.

Comments about the outside world often show a superego quality and are received either as critical or as advisory and protective. The sicker the patient or the more entangled the situation, the more necessary such an abandonment of the equidistance, but also the farther one usually moves away from the model of psychoanalysis. With increasing urgency the question then becomes whether or not one should resort to the initially mentioned combination of vertical and horizontal approaches. If such of the analyst's behavior as a protective, warning, or even condemning authority oversteps a certain measure, it becomes ever harder to find the way back to the analytic procedure. What Freud (1937) said about the mistaken setting of a deadline is generally true for interventions that are seen (like those) as "blackmail" or as "threats": "A miscalculation cannot be rectified" (p. 219).[6]

Of course, beyond a certain limit, authority and suggestion make not even for good education, and, in contrast to the psychoanalytic model, good psychotherapy follows, in its essence, the educational paradigm. It aims at the taking in of a better, more benevolent and more reasonable superego and therewith the learning of better outer adaptation. When we deal with disturbances of affect regulation and consequently with impulse problems often such external measures are indispensable, measures aiming at affect control, for example, drugs, or setting limits, like the conjoint setting up of additional therapeutic structures (e.g., Alcoholics Anonymous, Antabuse, marital counseling, etc.). These horizontal types of intervention do not have to be principally opposed to the analytic method, provided they are applied in very tactful, careful and nonauthoritarian ways; in fact, they may be synergistic with it.

It seems to me, by the way, that analytically oriented psychotherapy is all in all technically even more difficult and demanding than analysis.

So far we have spoken of the concrete-empirical side of these two paradigms. They complement each other and stand, case by case, in a variable equilibrium during the treatment; both possess the same dignity, and require, if well used, the greatest skill and thoughtfulness.

## THEORY AND TECHNIQUE

Now a few concluding remarks to this section. "Technique" stems from *téchne*—"art, skillfulness, artfulness." Usually, it is assumed that it is largely theory that determines technique. This is certainly partly correct. But the countervailing statement may have at least as much validity: that *technique must lead to specific theoretical consequences*. Because in my view psychoanalytic technique is extraordinarily difficult and because we are often guided in the development of such a style by implicit, perhaps even unconscious factors—

above all the idealization of one or more teachers or of one's own analyst, but also its opposite, the assumption of a counter identity—it often turns out so that the technical limitations and skewings bring along the same effects for theory. *Faulty technique leads to faulty theory, which then, in a circular turn, confirms the former.* Both are then viewed with great affect and presented with dogmatic conviction as good and as the only salvation.

Obviously, not every technique handled with great conviction is good. In this regard a critic of psychoanalysis like Grünbaum (1984) is justified when he emphasizes the influence of unspecific factors like suggestion and placebo effect on the formation of theory, as well as on therapeutic efficacy. The decisive questions concerning the scientific nature of psychoanalysis and the *specific* efficacy of certain interpretations relate to this problem of the quality of technique; they can only be answered if we discover what distinguishes a "good" intervention, a "good" hour, a "good" therapy from a "bad" one. It is quite likely that from case to case, from moment to moment, only very few interventions by the analyst or therapist are optimal, with many others harmful in the short run and still others in the long run.

Much in today's theoretical Babel might be traceable to such technical unclarities and could be resolved once they were cleared up. Since commonly case presentations are limited to highly condensed and abstractly held summaries, it is really impossible to examine the soundness of the theoretical and practical claims and often very hard to apply them to one's own cases. The hasty and abrupt leap from clinical observation to generalization and metapsychological formulation contradicts elementary requirements of scientific etiquette (see Brody 1982, Slap and Levine 1978).[7]

Although it is no simple task to render by description and explanation the essence of the therapeutic endeavor, such investigative work is indispensable if the enterprise of psychoanalysis and its training is to be placed on a scientific foundation. Philosophical criticism and our own epistemological conscience compel us to separate out the effects of suggestion and of other unspecific factors from the specific efficacy attributed to *true insight*. This can occur best by exact observation of the interaction in analysis, whether by tape recordings and their detailed study, or on the basis of stenographic notes *during* the sessions and critical considerations and reexamination afterward, as I try to do here.

In that I shall begin from the initially mentioned assumption that there are so-called "good" hours that show certain processes with particular clarity, bring about deepened insight in both participants, and are followed by a noticeable clinical improvement, sequences that could illustrate what Grünbaum (1984) called "Freud's tally argument": that those interpretations that correspond to an inner truth in the patient are being retained because of their efficacy and power of illumination whereas all those lacking these attributes fall away.

In all this, it is important not to be restricted in the clinical work. A patient presented later on (Dilecta, in the parallel volume) stated late in her analysis: "I was afraid that analysts have their little theories into which they fit their patients. I did not feel that with you. You did not try to force me into a model. I would not have survived all these years with you if you had been an inflexible analyst. I would have rebelled and left the analysis long ago."

Each patient is a new riddle. What I have suggested here are merely road signs pointing into the unknown. Often they may help us some part of the way, but at some other time they may lead us into what is impassable or pathless. If we then still hold onto them we stay lost.

How the analytic attitude I have sketched up to now shows itself practically in the treatment of the severe neuroses and to which findings and results it leads I would like now to demonstrate with the help of a series of thoroughly portrayed cases.

I conclude with two quotations: "Receptiveness is a rare and massive power, like fortitude," we read in George Eliot's *Daniel Deronda* (1876, p. 553). The following wonderful words about the novelist we find in Henry James' "The Art of Fiction," quoted by Leston Havens (1997) in the discussion about Friedman's plenary lecture; "We work in the dark. We do what we can—we give what we have. Our doubt is our passion, and our passion is our task" (p. 49).

## ENDNOTES

1. Cf. also Lichtenberg and colleagues (1996) in their recent book *The Clinical Exchange*: "From both self psychology and infant studies, we derived our emphasis on emotions as a principal guide for appreciating self-experience and the desires, wishes, goals, aims, and values that come to be elaborated in symbolic forms" (p. 9).

2. My book (1981a) examining the feelings of shame is therefore ultimately a treatise on a special form of defense analysis.

3. The term itself precedes its psychoanalytic use: "Only your brother's passionate nature drove him to act out what other men write and talk about," says Tito Melema in George Eliot's *Romola* (1862–63) about the transformation of Neoplatonic "theosophy" into the fervent mystical faith of Savonarola's followers (p. 171).

4. Clearly, this is an a priori presupposition that is being deprecated by Grünbaum (1984) as a placebo factor. (How happy we all would be if all placebo factors had indeed such a drastic impact!)

5. *"Der Geist ist es, der Verknüpfungen zu entdecken und dadurch Kunstwerke hervorzubringen hat. . . Er lernt denken, das Passende gehörig zusammenbinden . . ."* ("Betrachtungen im Sinne der Wanderer" DTV, vol. 18, p. 41, emphasis added).

6. The German version sounds to me much stronger: *"Ein Mißgriff is nicht mehr gutzumachen"*—A misstep is irreparable.

7. Rubinstein (1983) documents similar premature or insufficiently founded generalizations in Freud's work.

# 3

# Reconstruction Made Possible by "Acting Out"

*Ach wehe, meine Mutter reißt mich ein.*
*Da hab ich Stein auf Stein zu mir gelegt,*
*und stand schon wie ein kleines Haus, um das sich groß*
   *der Tag bewegt,*
*sogar allein.*
*Nun kommt die Mutter, kommt und reißt mich ein.*

*Sie reißt mich ein, indem sie kommt und schaut.*
*Sie sieht es nicht, daß einer baut.*
*Sie geht mir mitten durch die Wand von Stein.*
*Ach wehe, meine Mutter reißt mich ein.*

*Die Vögel fliegen leichter um mich her.*
*Die fremden Hunde wissen: das ist DER.*
*Nur einzig meine Mutter kennt es nicht,*
*mein langsam mehr gewordenes Gesicht.*

*Von ihr zu mir war nie ein warmer Wind.*
*Sie lebt nicht dorten, wo die Lüfte sind.*
*Sie liegt in einem hohen Herz-Verschlag*
*und Christus kommt und wäscht sie jeden Tag.*

R. M. Rilke[1]

## SOME TECHNICAL ISSUES RAISED
## BY ACTING OUT AND NEUROTIC ACTION

Before I enter into the very detailed case study that takes up much of Chapters 3 and 4, I will give a few preliminary remarks setting out the problem that stands at the center of the material presented in Chapter 3.

Moved by the serious clinical and social problems that acting out posed in a number of cases as well as by an increasing awareness of the detrimental impact that the therapist's or the analyst's interventions may have when he tries to stop such dangerous actions, I was trying to find ways between the Scylla of tolerating acts of unimpeded self-destructiveness and the Charybdis of the analyst's acting as superego—both being deemed incompatible with good analytic technique.

This is not going to be a thorough theoretical and bibliographic study of the topic, but an attempt at formulating some of my observations and my experiences in dealing with a clinical problem that I find particularly daunt-ing. I do not offer it as an example for good technique, but rather as a pre-sentation of how I tried to retain a psychoanalytic stance in circumstances that appeared inimical to it.

The question posed by those situations is: How can we reconcile the *cen-tral psychoanalytic task* of bringing about *long-range* change through making conscious what has been warded off, and help to experience it convincingly, with the *need for psychotherapeutic help in the present situation* when the actions (or the passivity) of the patient seem to present an immediate danger to her (or his) future, to safety and life, or to the continuation of therapy? The dilemma can be phrased this way: How can patient and analysis be protected against sabotage by the neurotic process without the interventions in the service of such protection irreparably compromising the analytic process itself?

Or, turned into a positive statement: How can the resistance by severe acting out be made into a tool for insight—from something interfering into something mutative?

The original description of acting out is in Freud's (1914a) paper "Re-membering, Repeating, and Working Through": "The patient does not *re-member* anything of what he has forgotten and repressed, but *acts* it out. He reproduces it not as a memory but as an action; he *repeats* it, without, of course, knowing that he is repeating it" (p. 150). It is specifically related to the analytic process and, as Boesky (1982) notes, so defined "that the en-tire transference was an acting out" (p. 40). And it is the result of resistance: "The greater the resistance the more extensively will acting out (repetition) replace remembering" (Freud 1914a, p. 151).

With his characteristic incisiveness and clarity of thought, Rangell (1968) similarly restricts the term to acts of resistance against insight (mostly, though not exclusively in analysis) which, like all resistance, can offer valuable clues as to the dynamics:

> Acting out is thus a specific type of neurotic action, directed towards interrupt-ing the process of achieving effective insight, thereby seen mostly in the course of psychoanalysis but also elsewhere. . . . While defenses occur in psychic life in general, resistances are the defenses against insight which are specifically un-covered during the analytic process. Acting out is to extra-analytic defensive actions as resistances are to defenses, or as analytic transference is to extra-ana-lytic transference-like displacements. [p. 197]

As to its technical handling, Rangell (1968) reflects and strongly advo-cates "a more permissive and understanding view":

The persistence of a critical and even moralistic attitude towards this specific type of defense stems, it seems to me, from the persistence of an older technical manoeuvre which is the residue of an earlier historical period, i.e., the use by Freud [1915, 1919] and other early analysts of the rule of abstinence . . . . Counter-acting-out, like countertransference, promotes acting out, whether by an authoritarian or an excessively permissive deviation from the analytic position. . . . I have seen a wrongly moralistic, anti-action attitude which creeps into some analyses fortify the patient's own phobic avoidance of action. . . . [pp. 199–200]

I shall not present a thorough review of the entire, especially also more recent literature, this having been done competently by Erard (1983). I present instead a concise summary of its conclusions and then proceed to the detailed case presentation. He states that a number of authors recognized the difficulties of regarding acting out purely as either resistance or communication, and suggested that acting out may serve both purposes. He refers to Boesky (1982), who has gone so far as to propose that acting out and the transference neurosis are inseparable. Erard continues:

The conceptual vagueness behind the term acting out rests on its simultaneous use to denote, on the one hand, a resistance against remembering, transference feelings, or insight, and, on the other hand, a pre-verbal or performative means of communicating with the analyst and promoting the transference. . . . Since resistant behavior in treatment may itself in principle be a form of repetition, acting out is best understood not in contrast to transference resistances but rather as a specific type of transference resistance the function of which is to undermine the requisite treatment conditions in which a transference neurosis can be established and maintained. Specifically, I am proposing that the term "acting out" be used to denote behavior threatening the professional relationship, the health or safety of analyst or patient, or the treatment alliance, insofar as it is used as a defense against affects or fantasies attending the development of the transference neurosis. In contrast to resistance against remembering or insight in general, on the one hand, and simple impulsive behavior on the other, acting out requires interpretation not only in terms of the specific fantasy or affect against which it defends but also in terms of its function of undermining the specific conditions in which effective treatment can occur. [pp. 69–72]

Very concretely, as to its handling, and in a way that is very pertinent to our discussion of this issue in the work with the severe neuroses, Brenner (1976) suggests:

If an analyst is confronted by transference manifestations that are analytically unmanageable, e.g., so-called acting out, one of the questions he should ask

himself is whether he has failed to interpret an important aspect of the transference to his patient in good time. . . . Persuasion and suggestion are not analysis.
They may produce welcome symptomatic improvement, but they cannot serve
the purposes of analysis as we understand analysis today. The actions of an analytic patient are one source of analytic material and are to be analyzed like any
other when it is useful and possible to do so. . . . One will do better to call transference analytically manageable or unmanageable rather than analyzable or
unanalyzable . . . A common reason for transference behavior that is analytically
unmanageable is undue delay in interpreting to a patient his transference wishes
and conflicts." [pp. 124–125]

This is undoubtedly true as far as it goes, but, as we shall see very shortly
in the extremely difficult cases to be studied here, the practical problems
appear with a complexity and severity of regression that would require omniscience and omnipotence on our (the analysts') side, were we to be expected
to prevent them—unless, of course, we were to lay down our arms and
betimes call the case unanalyzable.

Yet, once we are faced with this problem, it seems to me that even patients whose transference is, on the face of it, particularly difficult to manage—be it because of their overall impulsiveness, or because of their masochistic needs—can be successfully treated with a minimum of nonanalytic
intercessions.

Intra-analytic and transference related *acting out* and extra-analytic, defensive *neurotic actions* are two sides of the same coin. Conceptually they are
different, but dynamically there is a continuous back-and-forth between
them. Moreover, both are, like all defenses, of extreme value for analysis if
properly treated. The shift from a drive-focused analysis to one centered on
specific anxieties and defenses cannot afford to make an exception with
action pathology.

When defenses are severe enough, nonanalytic interventions may be
required, whether we deal with a defense by action (and a problem of "impulse control"—whatever that may refer to) or by regression of other types
(severely depressive mood disorder or perceptual disturbance), but such
nonanalytic interventions have to gauge factors like faulty technique on the
analyst's part (overlooking of transference–countertransference issues) and
protection of continued analytic work as far as that is possible.

I have been faced particularly often with this problem of how to handle
actually or potentially calamitous "impulsiveness" or "acting out" in my patients. Part of such frequency may be due to my readiness to take patients
into analysis whom others may consider unanalyzable (e.g., drug abusers and
addicts, patients with strong propensities to regression in perception and

action). Another reason may lie in my style, which is perhaps more active, more outgoing and emotionally responsive (though not conversational or chatty, nor, I believe, intrusively supportive or steering) than that of many present-day analysts. A further reason may go beyond defensible style and pertain to countertransference on my side. No transference occurs in vacuo; all or anyway most transference manifestations are elicited by tendencies visible or invisible, conscious or unconscious, in the analyst. While the distance created by recumbency certainly tips the balance away from such intrusions by the personality of the therapist, I don't think it can eliminate them entirely. Nor should it, I suppose. Ultimately, we cure not by some abstract, cold form of insight and a mechanical form of technique, but by insight as expression of our personality and as part of a very complex interplay of cognitive and emotional factors—"an evocative sort of affection" (p. 26), and "the analyst's deep and lasting attachment to the patient" (p. 31) in Friedman's (1997) poignant challenge.

As so very often in our field we again encounter the principle of complementarity: technique is important, but so is the analyst's personality; transference is crucial, but the "real" relationship cannot and should not be eliminated altogether (see Gedö 1977, Langs 1976, Lipton 1977a,b, Meissner 1996).

Finally, my own extensive participation in teaching activities brings about a relative irregularity in my schedule. While all these absences are known well in advance, they still create discontinuities which realistically interfere with the analytic process and lend themselves to "justify" action on the patient's side.

The material that follows may be somewhat misleading since it shows me as being far more active than I am most of the time. This is due to the fact that I selected "special hours" (kairói)–hours of breakthrough or crisis.

## "A CHILD FORSAKEN, WAKING SUDDENLY"

### The Doubleness

The main reason why Vera, a highly competent and proficient political scientist, but also with broad literary interests and capabilities, entered psychoanalysis at the age of 26 was a desperate dilemma in her love life: she felt deeply attached to a man, Felix, whom she admired, loved, wanted to marry and, most of all, have children with; she felt they belonged ideally together. For several years she even lived with him and was engaged to him, but she could not finally decide on marrying him because sexually she "felt nothing, was dead." His only fault was that he did not offer her "the wall I could bounce off." She found such walls in a series of increasingly coarse, cold, and egotistical men who in every regard stood far below her, sometimes one-night stands, men whom she found uneducated and primitive. They all had the same prominent features: they were very muscular and massive, tall and heavy, even fat, slow in movement and thought—"like walking penises." Several of these Olympians had serious problems with alcohol and mistreated the patient physically and emotionally. Repeatedly she engaged in very passionate liaisons with them; also her sexual excitability was very intense. One of the chosen ones was vulgar, thick, drunk, and stank of garlic, another was uneducated, a third stood her up whenever she was waiting for him. Often, when that man turned away from his girlfriend to her, the patient quickly lost interest in him. In turn, when the man, including eventually Felix, rejected her, she went into a severe depression, a suicidal tantrum, with wild thrashing around and screaming in the session, sleeplessness and anorexia at home, and car accidents or other serious traffic violations jeopardizing her driver's license (and thus risking both her professional future and the continuation of her analysis).

Still, even during such periods of clinical regression, she maintained a high level of professional proficiency. She came regularly to treatment and had to miss only rarely, mostly due to exigencies at work. I saw Vera for six and a half years in analysis (1,050 hours), later on in intermittent psychotherapy on the couch (another seven and a half years, 139 hours, to a total of 1,189 hours).

It was a curious and repetitive split between emotional attachment to one idealized man and, parallel to it, sexual surrender with strongly masochistic features to a series of what she described as brutes. This was in fact similar to the parallelism described by Freud (1910a,b) for men in the two articles on "The Psychology of Love": first, the condition that the beloved woman is already bound, but in a devalued position, and her idealization, the need for jealousy, the repetitiveness, and the rescue fantasy, secondly, the asexual search for the pure woman who can tenderly, but not sensually be loved, and with whom he is impotent. Freud (1910b) traced this compulsive attachment back to the boy's love for his mother and the inability to merge the "streams of tenderness and sensuality" (p. 180). Freud did not remark upon a similar problem in women. In some of the cases to be presented this split is very sharp in women as well, as we see in Vera.

One year after beginning psychoanalysis Vera started another such relationship, one which was to last three years. This time she informed her fiancé about it in order to be able to lead an open and candid life and dissolved the engagement to him. Within weeks it turned out that her new lover, Rudolf, was ill-deserving of her devotion. Whenever she opened herself to him he turned away from her in a cold and unfriendly way. He repeatedly pushed her or threw her through the room and once stomped on her stomach. He had several car accidents while drunk with her, destroyed her car, and repeatedly cheated on her and lied to her. Yet she was unable to leave him. She mothered him, bathed him, dressed and undressed him, pleaded for his love, swore to him that her love would never cease whatever might come. In spite of these vows she decided about every two to four weeks to break off the liaison, but as soon as he wailingly returned the whole thing started all over again. After severe blow-ups they separated for a few days and then rejoined for a few hours of bliss, until he started nagging her about her weight or attacked her for using words he did not know or began arguing about such important things as what the longest day of the year was (he was adamant that it was in August). Concurrently, she treated Felix and her father as her friends and confidants, describing to them her suffering and hoping to receive their criticism, compassion, and forgiveness; she regularly got it. The same kept happening in a more subtle way with me as well.

Neither her friends nor she herself could comprehend why she would forsake her handsome, erudite, extremely bright, and even athletically fit fiancé for such a musclebound, "dumb jock exuding virility, who could answer only with grunts and whose handwriting and spelling were illegible," as one of her friends described the patient's lover, a "bump on a log," as she often called him herself, or "the slug." She could not imagine how she could spend the rest of her life at the side of a man whose highest leisure activity consisted in lounging in front of the TV with a mug of beer and who envied her erudition and tormented her for it.

She used to warn him that with his smoking he would have, at age 50, both of his legs amputated below the knee. And still, in spite of dozens of acts of mistreatment and rejection and in spite of those dangerous car accidents she always returned to him. Only in the later course of her analysis did she finally succeed in breaking with Rudolf.

Vera was an attractive woman. Her movements were rapid and decisive, her laughter and her ire quick and close to the surface, her reactions generally direct, her way of talking clear, often poetic, occasionally vulgar, almost always pointed.

In what follows I shall try to bring extensive, almost verbatim excerpts from this treatment, as from the others, so that the reader may be able, step by step, to consider and investigate for him- or herself its progress, the deepening of insight and success as well as the missing of opportunities. In agreement with what I have discussed, in connection with the questions of epistemology (see the reference to Isaiah Berlin in Chapter 1), I believe that this form of presentation, which strongly deviates from the usual psychoanalytic case descriptions, may better fulfill scientific and didactic demands than brief vignettes.

In regard to these excerpts it is necessary to keep in mind that they usually deal with particularly intense episodes of gaining insight, and that therefore the measure of my activity is considerably greater than it is on the average. All in all, though, I find that with these severe neuroses a pretty active form of analysis is in order. It was also my impression in my talks with Jenny Waelder-Hall, in supervision, that her approach was in general far more active than would correspond to the stereotype of the analyst's "passivity."

Before giving some longer excerpts from our work Vera's background needs to be drawn in a few strokes. Her father, a journalist, was a man of great accomplishments and erudition, soft and sympathetic, somewhat seductive, quite anxious about himself and no match to his wife. She too was successful, as a professor of English literature at one of the universities. The father stood completely under her sway. The relationship between him and Vera, the oldest of three, was highly erotized. This included episodes of spanking that she found very unfair but that held some of the intimacy and physical closeness she otherwise had difficulty finding with him. Later on, there was a lot of shared confidence on his side, of self-punishing rebelliousness on hers. The mother was described as unpredictable in her affects and prone to intense anger, hot and cold, withholding, and throughout as very negative about her daughter's sexuality or wishes for emotional intimacy. Most of all she was always perched to judge with the greatest moralistic sharpness: "You are not allowed to do this! How can you hurt your father in this way!" She is, says Vera, a hard and strict woman who likes to make everyone around her feel guilty.

All three children had emotional problems, feeling blocked or inhibited socially and professionally, and were quite self-deprecating.

Vera herself had been a very active, at times tomboyish child, but had been suffering already since early childhood under states of severe depression and anxiety attacks that were accompanied by a kind of semihallucination—in truth, very lucid fantasies and intrusive egodystonic thoughts. She spoke of a *split*: her parents were seen by her as saintly and good during the day, but robbers and thieves at night, prowling around in the darkness and stealing silverware.

She herself had been an especially rebellious girl. Already at the age of 2 or 3, she pushed and kicked her father away when he tried to hug and kiss her. Fits of jealous anger or envy commenced at age 2, after the birth of the next younger brother. She had many horrible fights with her mother, which always left her completely miserable and contrite. She saw herself as "all alone, ugly, dirty, cast out, unloved, whimpering in the darkness, huddled in the cold, cut off from everybody else and all comforts . . . hated, subhuman, this little sniveling creature" [149]. At age 14, she ran into serious trouble in high school.

Besides the habit and acts of impulsive rebellion and the often high price she had to pay for them, she showed all her life manifold manifestations of phobic and free-floating anxiety. Particularly important phenomena of this kind will come up later on.

When alone, she always had to keep a light on at night to make sure no intruder with a knife was lying in ambush or when she felt the darkness pressing in on her like a heavy moving shadow. Sometimes she hallucinated, as she had in early childhood, that the cracks in the walls would open up and that red bugs or spiders came out—a half-dream she could shake off only with difficulty. These terrors and perceptual disorders mostly disappeared when the manifest masochistic affair started.

While still living with her fiancé, she had attacks of panic after intercourse when she went to the bathroom; she thought he would follow and stab her with a butcher knife. She had to call out to him in order to make sure he had stayed in bed and was not lying in wait to kill her.

In her despair at that moment, she was convinced that only the analysis allowed her to function; otherwise she would certainly kill herself. Yet, one week later when she had gained more distance the intensity of those affect storms was as if blown away, although she might still quietly weep. More important, it seemed to her then as if that feeling were not part of her personality, as if that self were not identical with this self, that is, as if *she were split into two personalities.*

She explained this splitting about eleven months after inception of analysis in the following fascinating way, after we had traced it back to the extent and strength of her anxieties:

"I can't make them into *one* person, I have to divide them in order to protect them against each other. The evil part is so wicked that it could kill the separate good part and I can't understand them together. *They can only be understood if I separate them.* It is so easy to deny that the one exists when it is in descendency [in decline] in regard to the other—just as today, after

I've been in despair, I cannot believe that I ever felt such despair. *When the one rules the other does not exist.* It's the same way with my mother: anger and love are just split, or the good parents against the robber parents. The only time that the robber parents are around is when the good ones are asleep— they are two very different parents, black and white. And the same happens with Felix: the Felix who loves me and cares for me is a good man, against the bad Felix who is mean to me, in a role I have forced upon him."

"And we have observed it even here: that I suddenly would attack you or totally reject you."

"And on the other side it is very hard for me to be angry at you—"

"Precisely because of this."

"You are the good you, above reproach."

"But this is needed because every crack would mean a complete collapse. If you did not idealize me the rage would be overwhelming."

"It is safer to deny it—"

"—and to direct it against work and your father and Felix" [149].

It should be noted how this *"splitting" in absolutely good and absolutely bad parts of her own identity and of that of the others* represents a *complex process,* that it occurs out of anxiety about the intensity of rage and of other aggressive impulses, and is accompanied by denial and idealization. While emotionally fully real, it is intellectually corrected. In the further course it becomes evident that as the main conflicts and the entire defense and affect structure become conscious, this phenomenon gradually recedes.

Thus, in a major theoretical finding of my work, I see in *splitting* itself not an elementary form of defense, but rather the result of multiple defensive processes in severe inner conflicts. Besides that, there are manifold forms of such splits that are not of this type of antithesis of good and evil. For example, she describes two months later how she is dissociating sexual excitement from intercourse in a similar way: "I could dissociate myself from it [sex]; it was separate and secret. It didn't exist outside of that room. . . . When I let my mind drift now, there are surges of sexual arousal, in the memory of last night, as if I sensed the excitement now which I should have felt last night [during a tryst] where it immediately stopped" [174]. This dissociation happened so that she would "remain in control": "I compartmentalize sex in order to control it as something evil" [175]. In this way she breaks sexuality into two parts: "When I make love it is nothing sexual because I don't feel anything. When I have an orgasm it isn't sexual because it doesn't happen during penetration, it occurs outside of intercourse. What appears instead is the monster with a knife: it is anxiety and aggression instead of sexuality" (quasi-quotation).

This kind of splitting is actually above all the form and expression of massive *repression*, partly using violence in order to fend off sexual wishes and feelings [244], that is, by employing one kind of drive as a defense against the other (Brenner 1982). The same refers therefore also to the split between the two men: "The fantasy of taking away and cutting off is possible in a transient liaison but impossible with Felix. The anxiety is too great" [262].

And when Rudolf appeared this split became complete: "Two men and two selves" [273].

"Only the strong man can defend you against your own aggression. He won't be the victim; he will be strong enough to control you, and with that he is safe" [273]—and so would she be.

Together with the radical denial, she needed the outer authority to assist her in the control of overwhelming feelings and impulses that were triggered especially by physical intimacy. She sought *external taming and tying down* as the answer for specific inner conflicts. What those specific conflicts were was only gradually being revealed.

Another version of the split was *depersonalization*, accompanying analysis: "It's a terrible feeling of emptiness: that I cannot feel, that I cannot love, that I feel dead and empty" (149). Already early in the analysis she described how she was stepping outside of herself during her panic and suicidal despair: "My only defense is to step back and to see it as somebody else than me. I began realizing that I would kill myself: this isn't me; this isn't happening to me; I'm not feeling this. I'm like under the influence of a drug that makes me act bizarrely." By the way, although she could have had unlimited access to them, she never resorted to illegal drugs, including marijuana. She was afraid she could lose herself to me and to my hypnotic force and would be unable to regain herself [44]. Frigidity itself was a kind of depersonalization; she was insensible in her loins, like dead, as a defense against the double fantasy of death: "I'm afraid that when I reach orgasm it would be my death, the excitement and the fear [the sense of exploding, of bursting]. And another fantasy: that the man dies in sex, like the female spider that kills the male spider, that he would die between my legs" [54]. In states of anxiety and shame, it kept happening that she split herself into a part observing her from the outside and an experiencing part.

Also, a kind of twilight state occurred sometimes—again accompanied by the inner experience of doubleness. After a fight on the telephone with her father whom she again perceived as self-righteous and smug, whose intellectual arrogance she had subtly attacked, and who, annoyed, had paid back her shaming him with his shaming her, she awakened at 1:00 A.M., convinced her room was veiled by spiderwebs. Reaching for the broom to dust them off she noticed that they were mere phantasmata. Overwhelmed by panic she lay awake for hours.

In these anxiety states she might also see her mother, not only Felix, lie in wait for her with a knife, ready to slaughter her; or she perceived red spiders and ants crawling out of the wall cracks. Unable to turn on the light she often felt the darkness as if it were a monster weighing on her—a frequently recurring nightmare that got intermingled with her sensed reality.

Such panic attacks occurred over long stretches of her analysis, yet they tended to disappear almost entirely during the manifest masochistic relations with Rudolf, but broke in again after the break with him. Only with the solutions to be presented later on did they gradually pale and vanish.

Her chronic attitude showed deep *resentment*: "I have been cheated and deceived." At the same time she was fighting against all injustice, and took the lead in battling for those oppressed and against incompetence. When there was a conflict between her analysis and her professional duties she almost always gave precedence to analysis and insisted that they had to get by without her.

As stated above, this chapter deals with a question of particular relevance for defense analysis: how to approach acting out. In a second part, in Chapter 4, I try to examine the fascinating phenomena of splitting in Vera's identity and in her object relationships. In a final segment in that chapter, I present the core of the neurosis as we understood it at the end of our analytic work.

It will not be surprising that at the start of the analysis and for a long time afterward the *transference* appeared *split* in the same fashion as all the other close relationships. She was idealizing me and by and large dared to admit her aggressive fears and impulses only in the form of dreams where I was sexually importuning her and she would reprove me with scolding and wrath or finish me off altogether. However, she much more clearly attacked her superiors or provoked them into putting her down, and in that way she again shifted her hostility and sadomasochistic relation from me onto those evil forces on the outside, thus very effectively shielding me against them. However, instead of aggressive fantasies on the level of the feelings, she had during the sessions sudden reality-near images of terror, resembling those semi-hallucinations—that I would stick my pencil in her eye or lean over and start sexually molesting her.

This capability for *perceptual regression* remained a part of her makeup even long after termination of the formal analysis, although it had lost most of its punch. Undoubtedly it also formed an integral and eminently valuable part of her creativity.

How these dissociated units of experience referred not only to conflicts, but also to traumata underlying those conflicts or connected with them will become clearer in the course of the presentation. Yet for years, the main problem was the *masochistic acting out*. I turn now to this in more detail and select for it a series of especially revealing hours from the middle phase of the analysis, about two and a half years after its onset.

### "Masochistic Orgy" and "The Wall to Bounce Off From"

The constant ups and downs in her affair with Rudolf increasingly endangered her everyday functioning. She herself had several car crashes and was also risking in other ways her driver's license.

I became therefore more and more alarmed about the extent of her clinical regression as the hours were filled with descriptions of such perilous events and affect storms. Often she felt so overpowered by depression and self-hate that she confessed it was only her intellectual conviction that it would pass that kept her from committing suicide. At times, after a new irruption of frost from Rudolf's direction, she screamed out in her indignation and despair and hammered with feet and hands against couch and wall.

I tried to put her self-destructive acting out in connection with the transference: how she was trying to move me into helping her by strong and effective interventions, for me to become the vaunted "*wall to bounce off from*," so that I would really show my strength in the face of her aggressions; but also how, in contrast, there seemed to be in this constant repetition something like an unconscious intention to show me up as incompetent and the analysis as ineffective and impotent. We were talking about her analytic "*frigidity*," which was analogous to the sexual one.

She herself talked about the masochistic transference—how she was taking on extra projects in order to pay for the analysis, and how she felt I was demanding of her to stop seeing both Rudolf and Felix. "I know it is not so, but I think of you as a cruel taskmaster who wants me to be totally lonely in order to save the analysis."

There was some truth to this, albeit exaggerated, because I had stressed the resistance quality of these masochistic enactments with several men— the self-destructive as well as directly interfering quality of these affairs. While careful about not condemning or criticizing her I had occasionally expressed my concerns and commented upon her attempted provocation—that I would step in and protect her against those evil men—an appeal for, if not the seduction of my love. Both my analyzing and my expression of concern were experienced by her as condemnation and torment—experienced that way, although not intellectually supported.

She agreed: "I turn every facet of my life into a masochistic setup where I torment and destroy myself." In the same way, the payments rendered the analysis itself a part of a masochistic system [441].

This was, incidentally, a good example of the way the transference itself becomes a thematic content and does not need to be pulled in by force. I mean this in reference to Anna Freud's (Sandler and A. Freud 1985) remarks about the defense analytic technique: "It is quite different from the technique of not waiting for transference, but rather of forcing everything into the transference, which is interpreted immediately," and where she warns: "Don't interpret transference before it is transference" (p. 65f.).

In the following session, Vera scolded herself strongly for having spent money on the fabric for a dress that she then disliked. She shifted over to her worry about spending more on her analysis than she could afford. With Rudolf she was frigid—"I just froze." She was berating herself for having spent the money and adduced examples where her mother had furiously attacked her for having wasted a few dollars. I remarked: "Instead of being exposed to your mother's surprising attack you take control by attacking yourself: 'Better I do it first to myself before she does it to me.'"

This *preventive identification with the blaming and condemning mother* is an eminently important special form of identification with the aggressor. It functions as an in-between step in the internalization of the superego-authority.

She went on talking about making love, about her wish to become pregnant, and her very embarrassing urge during fellatio or intercourse to take away, cut or bite off the penis from the partner. This was a topic we had very often touched upon and about which there had been a good number of more or less explicit dreams where she had seen images of a "detached penis" and of "cutting off the penis" although it had not been possible as yet to put it in a more comprehensive context of conflict. I was wondering if it was not rather the pleasure felt by the penis than the penis itself about which she had that overwhelming desire and fantasy during the man's orgasm: "I want to take 'it'! I want to keep 'it'! 'It' is mine." This desire was especially strong when the man was having his orgasm while she herself could not have an orgasm as long the man was within her, only when he would stimulate her clitoris or her nipples, usually before his own entry. Her own orgasm was often experienced like a bursting and a violent death.

She agreed and came back to her inability last night to sense anything, but interrupted herself: "When I was remembering just now how I felt totally dead I had a mutilation fantasy: I was stabbing myself in the abdomen, as if to cut out my womb. The deadness and frustration was so terrible—my inability to open myself, always being dead."

"The forbidden and frightening wish to take from the man, to cut it off—now turned against yourself."

"Instead of castrating him, I'm stabbing myself."

"And the whole *masochistic attitude* seems like a *generalized stabbing fantasy*. The more you despise and hate a man, the more you can allow yourself to feel that wish consciously to cut 'it' off, and then you don't have to be frigid. On the other side, Felix, whom you admired, you had to protect against those wishes."

The sequence was therefore clearly this:

1. "I want to take 'it' away, that means acquiring the pleasure uniquely sensed by the penis, and with that also taking the penis itself."
2. "When I love the man and have real affection and respect for him, this castrating wish is absolutely forbidden. I have to repress it completely. I am frigid, I am dead, I don't feel anything."
3  "The aggression, repressed and turned against the self, reemerges as the stabbing and mutilation fantasy, directed against myself, for example, as an almost irresistible compulsive thought of stabbing myself in the abdomen."
4. "This fantasy becomes generalized into the masochistic attitude and shows itself in a slew of symptomatic actions where I am the suffering victim of maltreatment."

"In contrast, when I feel justified to admit anger, hostility, and contempt toward the man, I may permit myself the fantasy of taking 'it'; and then, those Steps 2, 3, and 4 become unnecessary and I become practically symptom-free—except insofar as I try to provoke enough cruelty in the partner to vindicate my own hatred and contempt. Like, 'If you go on smoking I know that in twenty years you will have both of your legs amputated,' or: 'How can I marry someone who has no interests but drinking beer and staring at the football games on TV—a man with such a high slug potential?!'" With such sadomasochistic interaction in reality, of course, it was unnecessary to protect him against her impulses; he had accomplished this very powerfully for both of them [442].

She behaved analogously in the transference: When she idealized me she had to protect me against all aggressive ("castrating") urges and was, instead, engaged in *her masochistic orgy of acting out.* Thus, more and more she used her love relationship with her tormentor (1) to provoke me into criticizing and reproaching her, so that she could feel freer to confess her resentment toward me and to rebel against me as the now established superego figure; (2) to provoke me into stepping in and protecting her by advice and deed against a more and more dangerous and brutal man, thus into being promoted to be her rescuer, that is, into taking on the protective functions of the superego; and (3), and perhaps most prominently, to show me up as ineffectual, our insights as grand duds, as dazzling but useless, and thus all my skills, knowledge, and powers as ridiculous pretense, in a reversal of the superego relation—now I would be the piteous loser, instead of her. Parallel to her sexual frigidity, there was, therefore, as mentioned, a kind of analytic frigidity, with very similar dynamics (Arlow, personal communication).

Behind her lover and behind me stood her inattentive, absentminded, rejecting, and yet also often seductive father: she must have done some wrong; she could explain only so why he had rejected her and not paid any attention to her. Although his angry spanking of her had humiliated her profoundly, and her impotence and vengefulness had conglomerated into a massive sense of injustice, she also felt it with excitement: "I'm not helpless, I'm not humiliated—I don't feel cheated, I'm not furious—to the contrary, it is pleasurable"—a change by *affect reversal* from pain, shame, and anxiety into lust. "At least he shows me attention, and under the guise of violence I am allowed to feel pleasure" [445].

All these connections were developed conjointly and with her very active and eager collaboration, but they neither seemed to become fully integrated among each other nor did have an effect upon her actions, or at least no ostensibly positive effect.

The next session [446] she did not show up, but about twenty minutes into the hour she called me: she had had an accident on the highway, and her car had been totalled. No, she had not been injured.

Immediately following this newly alarming event the scope of the work broadened. She was not dealing just with castrating urges, but with hatred, contempt, wishes to kill, jealousy, and scorn as well, and more importantly. In turn, all those aggressive impulses, felt and feared and banished, called for that implacable judge within herself who had her destroy much of what she had built up. The incessant voice of that demon within could only be muted if she found an outer comforter—her former fiancé, her current lover, me, her father.

## Search for the Outer Superego Figure and Magical Transformation

Generally speaking, such a need for an outer superego figure is not based on a lack of an internalized superego, but on its too harsh, too radical character; the external approval should function as an antidote to the incessant self-condemnation. This sought-after balance of power forms the basis for many similar "love addictions."

The whole strategy with Rudolf (and with me!) was the one she had tried, though in vain, with her mother: *to make a "bad" mother into a good one, that is, to change an unloving, withholding, uncomforting, cold mother, by her own surrender, by her suffering and giving, into an approving and caring mother.* It was the *magical power* inherent in the *masochistic conflict solution* (see Berliner 1940, Novick and Novick 1996). She had not been able to accomplish anything near this in actuality because of her own rivalry and her "spitefulness." And the size was especially important: that person had to be much bigger, much heavier, even much fatter than she, a portrait of that mother figure she wanted to appease. Rudolf (like her other lovers) was all that—withholding, unloving, unempathic, self-centered, massive, full. Loving him ought to have had the effect of changing him and thus finally also of allowing her to master her painful inability to gain her mother's real, unconditional, empowering love [449].

It was again a piece of convincing insight, but it too remained unintegrated with the previous "complex." It consisted in the dynamics clearly acted out with both men, Felix and Rudolf, the good one who was not bad enough, the bad one who was not good enough, and with me—who was good and kind in her perception, but who would, in her fantasy, implacably judge her for wanting all those horrid things to which she had no right. Again this second major complex showed an inner cleavage between two almost symmetrical relationships of great complexity, like the one we had noted before on the level of the castration conflict.

Yet, just as Vera could not integrate those parallel relationships—the one with the idealized but asexual ("already castrated") man and the other with the sadistic but sexually exciting man, the one with the approving and the other with the withholding and rejecting man—she was unable to integrate these *two levels of castration conflict and split imago* of the other (man, mother, analyst). Nor was I able to at that point. Our understanding always remained fragmentary and lay in big chunks in front of us, the pieces remaining relatively isolated from each other.

At that time she sought refuge with her former fiancé's mother, a woman she probably loved more undividedly than anybody else—a refuge against that pernicious ambivalence she felt with everybody.

## The "Economy of Envy and Jealousy"

However, her self-destructive acts persisted. Rudolf openly resumed his liaison with an earlier girlfriend of his and spent weekends with her while continuing his relationship with Vera, alternatively giving and withdrawing, seeking her out and turning her down, imploring her and shredding her with scorn. She felt as if she were being dragged down with him. "The withholding is what is being repeated. When he is cold and turns his back on me, I flip out. And that *cold withholding* is just what *my mother* used to do; and I have to swear to him that I love him although I'm angry—the same as with Mom: to win her back in spite of my anger. I have to belittle and deny my anger. She could not tolerate it, nor can he now."

"Why do you keep holding on?" Why this obstinate necessity of impulse sequence and denial? That indeed was the question! [453].

She wanted to be determined and kept writing to herself while talking to Rudolf on the phone: "I've already decided it: I shall be firm, I won't give in. I can't go on like that, and I'll be all right." But then the obsessive feeling: "I want to die. I would stab myself in the heart or the abdomen"—clearly a very angry act not only against (herself and) her lover, but also against me (and her family). I mentioned that aspect too: how helpless she was trying to make me feel [455]. From her self-directed aggressions we tried to read off what the original meaning might have been. An image obtruded: a car accident where her pelvis would be crushed and her womb destroyed.

I suggested: "Just like the stabbing yourself stood in for the cutting off of the penis—couldn't we now, in this context, translate this image of your womb being crushed into: 'I wanted to get at my mother's womb, at her ability to have children'? Such a wish, however, would have been far too frightening and had to be turned against yourself."

"And to this comes my conviction that I *had* been cheated. Her love was a limited amount. Whatever she gave to my brother [who was born when Vera was 16 months old] had been taken away from me. And with the third [born at her age 5] it got divided even more."

"So that the envy and the feeling of being cheated would mean: 'I want to destroy the pregnancy and, later on, take away the breast from my brother.' And perhaps: 'How easy would it be to kill that rival brother, as long as he is that small!' And then, as a protection against these horribly frightening wishes, you have to keep stressing: 'I need a strong, big, tall man who can contain me; Felix was just not strong enough and tall enough. With him I had no wall to bounce off.' Meaning: 'He could not offer me enough safety against those frightening urges—against both forms of aggression, castrating the man and killing the rival–brother" (456).

Of course, somebody who had such aggressive feelings and murderous wishes could not enjoy anything but had to suffer with little respite and needed to submit to that harsh inner judge, to those brutal and horrifying storm troopers in her dreams, and those outer tormentors. They had to serve as safeguards and counterforces against all those dangerous aggressions [459]: "I'm my own victim, and I feel a phenomenal self-hatred. As soon as I feel stillness or pleasure the call goes out: Why don't you suffer?" Safeguards? "I need someone who is stronger than I am, to protect me, to keep me from exploding, to make me safe against my rage—somebody who would be the withholding and yet loving mother at the same time" (460).

She spoke with her mother: "I learned one interesting thing which confirmed all we've found. My brother was much more gregarious and got more attention. Once when she was nursing him I hurled a mug full of milk through the room. She saw that something was wrong with me and told her mother that she was deeply worried about me."

She again repeated how often her mother was angry and depressed, and even now when she saw her looking tired she asked herself: "It's my fault. What have I done again?" This perceived inconsistency of her mother's affection must have been the root for Vera's intense *jealousy* and that "*economy of envy*": "'Whatever love he (the brother) gets is taken away from me!'" "Or yesterday: how conditional my mother's love really is. She loves me only when the frying pan is clean."

She again thought about the similarity between her mother and Rudolf: how conditional also his love was and how cutting down, how putting down they both were. I asked whether she doesn't do it too: to him and to me, and I added: "May this not be repeated now—how you competed *with* your brother *for* your mother's love? Isn't it clearly played out with Felix and his mother? You did cut him down and did cut him out and now have his mother for yourself. And with Rudolf it's the loud protestation: 'I love him so much and care for him so unconditionally—because I am afraid I want to do to him what I had in mind against my brother'?" She confirmed how competitive she had been with her brother—how she had to prove her superiority over him, had sought assurances from her mother that her own penis would also grow like his, became a tomboy. "Do I now pick somebody who is dumber than me?" [463].

With all these insights deepening on all fronts, which I also kept trying to link up with the transference whenever feasible without forcing the issue, the "acting out" became ever graver. More and more she saw in her emotionally unavailable and coldly withdrawing partner a new edition of her mother whom she called "emotionally stingy." She talked more about that *"economy of envy"*: mother's love and attention had decreased the more she had to share it with somebody else, particularly her siblings.

Her love-hate toward the unreliable mother, as now recurring with her lover, for a while stepped into the foreground. The acting out continued. It was evident that she hated her mother especially out of *jealousy* and that she had been particularly jealous of the breast that her mother had been giving to her little brother.

With Rudolf she indeed now had reason enough to be jealous, but that had not always been the case; with Felix she had created the reason herself and had suffered a lot when he had taken for himself the same right to infidelity that she had claimed for herself before. Although her jealous fury seemed directed above all at her mother, she likely must have harbored with it the wishes to remove the rival, or at least must have felt anxiety about such wishes. Such castrating and destroying impulses in regard to Rudolf showed themselves not only in locutions and acts, but also in the *defense by reaction-formation* when, in between the quarrels, she mothered and spoiled him in exaggerated ways. Intellectually she recognized how she was humiliating him by this and was robbing him of his manliness, his pride, and his success—de facto, but not as a wish admissible to consciousness.

What happened shortly thereafter in a crescendo of acting out caused ever deeper worry and presented me with difficult technical problems; in a number of subtle ways she fanned her lover's jealousy to such an intensity that he repeatedly abused her physically. I found myself increasingly concerned that her behavior could lead to a catastrophe.

### Role Reversal as Affect Defense

After finally having introduced Rudolf to her parents, who seemed friendly but hardly enthusiastic, something that had escaped me up to now suddenly became clear as daylight: how much she herself contributed to *making her lover jealous*—or perhaps rather, how she had chosen someone who let himself be brought to acts of raging and almost delusional jealousy.

In several steps it became clearer that this was but one of the ways in which she had identified with a specific image of her mother [473]. Now it was not she, Vera, who was jealous anymore, but her lover played the jealous baby. She brought him to wild fury by chiding him: "Stop being a baby; be a man!" Then, she was the one who elicited his jealousy by showing her interest in another man, by playing up her analysis, by disappointing him and showing her cool detachment, but also by having him force her over and over again into admitting her crimes and into apologizing, into saying: "I'm sorry." It was a *role reversal* where now *she was the one who incited jealousy* and the other was the one stewing in helpless jealous rage. He not only tried to forbid her to talk with her earlier friends but also to continue her analysis. When she refused he threw her through the room and threatened to beat her up. From then on she tried to conceal from him when she came to her session. Yet she was ashamed about her double play and decided "to pour him clear wine" (i.e., to give it to him straight) although she was terrified he would injure and perhaps harm her in a lasting way. She was also always very ready to admit how much this "acting out" interfered with her analysis and destroyed it. I repeatedly expressed my deepening concern.

What I, by the way, did not recognize then was that the same might apply exactly to me too: that all along she wanted to *incite my jealousy* by those self-degrading affairs. This may very well also have been the decisive factor in the transference-like relationship with Felix, her former fiancé: the compulsive reenactment of a scenario where *she played the faithless, jealousy-provoking mother.*

Thus, her defense against her own jealousy, in what was condensed into that traumatic scene of seeing her brother at the breast of her ungiving mother, occurred not only by repression and by *identification with the traumatizing mother*, but by action: by *externalization* and *role reversal.* Every piece of memory was linked up with a piece of the sequence of reenactment. Her life followed an invisible script, in endless variations on the same theme. And that theme was most of all: *instead of being jealous she had to make someone else jealous.* That was the defense by *reversal.*

That central meaning of the scenario was of course completely unconscious, as was its link to the original scene; but subsidiary memories—screen memories—had been known all along: her taking on her mother's first name at 5, her breast-feeding her teddy bears, later on her anger at her cat for having babies and nursing them while she at that time did not yet have any breasts, her lifelong career of self-destructive actions and her defiant rebellion against her parents and now increasingly also against me, but also, in some unclearly linked way, her rescue and helping fantasies, the need for a secret relationship, and, finally and most of all, her own recurrent acts of masochistic surrender. But again and again, then as well as now, her defense by action, or more precisely: *her defense by externalization.*[2]

By no means all the pieces of the puzzle had as yet found their place though.

**Robbed and Robbing**

The following material stems from a double session (an expedient we had not rarely to resort to because of the problems presented by both of our schedules) [477/478]. She talked at much length about her seductiveness and provocativeness toward Rudolf and about a new violent outburst between them, which was immediately again followed by her abject and tearful atonement for her sins and sexual submission to him. As if trying to placate me, she quite accurately and convincingly compared this sequence with what used to go on with her mother and more recently with me. I interrupted her: "I'm worried though that you are inviting a catastrophe. We know how violent your friend can be, we know his problem with drinking. I think you are leading him on. Whatever I say and whatever we find out here appears to make it worse, and your own insights serve as rationalizations for the continuation of this very dangerous game."

"The more I know, the more I do it. It's an act of defiance. I project upon you the role of authority—to be out of the affair."

"You provoke a punishment of the first order."

"From him, but also from you—that you'll say: the analysis is over, is destroyed; that I'm kicked out. That is what I'm trying to provoke. It's the same repetition."

I confirmed one part of her fear: "You invite physical injury. We have heard how he has pushed and thrown you, and how he has involved you in accidents before. I'm thinking for example, that you provoke him to punch you in your face, by fanning his insane jealousy and in this way ruin your life. Or worse."

I felt and still feel that such elaborations of her own fears about the consequences of her externalizations were a necessary part of my work because all my interpretations, including and especially the transference interpretations, as far as I was able to give them at that point, had proven insufficient, because I did not yet recognize the *reasons* for her manifest rebellion and provocation of punishment, and its meaning for her *masochistic transference.* The repetition compulsion of these events was evident to her and completely uncanny.

She asked: "Do I provoke physical violence as punishment? Is it a repetition? Where does it come from? It is clearly a pathological compulsion."

"Exactly."

"Did I do that with my parents? To provoke being spanked? Then to get in trouble in school—that was a direct provocation, a rebellion, an indirect act of defiance against the parents."

"And also very destructive."

"It did not just begin when I was 14."

She rambled on in speculations about beating or murdering her brother and then turning this against her self. I felt she was defending herself against the immediate present by an *intellectual "interpretation downward"*—an evasion into the distant past, and again interrupted her: "What's happening now is that you have set up a competition between Rudolf and me. You try to destroy him and are being punished by me. You try to destroy the analysis and are being punished by him. What is repressed is the aggression, the destructiveness in all this. The punishment is conscious."

"His beating me up, that's the atonement."

"You use the analysis to defy him and then get the punishment from him."

"That's something I don't want to look at."

"I have the impression that the present reliving might be covering up what we have found out already."

She agreed: "The sexual and love scene covers my wish to *destroy the rival*—my brother and my father, and in some ways my mother too. I was competing with her, and I was not measuring up. I had neither breasts nor penis. I was not stacking up to her."

"What is being repeated right now is playing out the rivals against each other and trying to destroy them."

"And the punishment for those wishes, by *destroying myself*."

"By inviting some terrible retribution, yes. And thirdly: by *identifying with your mother*—as somebody caring and *motherly*, but also as somebody depriving you and eliciting your bitter jealousy."

"I play it out with Rudolf: that I am a good loving person, so selflessly caring—the good mother."

"Three solutions to the same conflict."

"And all three together or in rapid succession."

"All three act out the primary conflict—the wish, the defense by self-punishment, and the defense by becoming mother."

"The conflict of being jealous at my brother—"

"Specifically at his being at the breast."

"And what was unbearable then was that feeling of deprivation, of being cheated, that something was stolen from me. It is the insecurity: Does my mother love me?"

It is true that she had felt deprived; yet it was even more a matter of her own wishes to take away, to rectify a profound yet always unclear injustice—wishes that had been a threat and were being projected: "You remember your fantasy or belief that at night your parents changed into robbers and went stealing silverware."

"Right! Right! I could not admit that I was robbed, so I changed it into that fantasy."

"You felt cheated and protested against that by acts of defiance, and now I am the robber—"

"—who wants to steal my lover and against whom I rebel. This is the big problem."

"Every interpretation by me is identical with that original robbery."

"Just like that about the swimming pool."

This referred to an incident again around age 2 or not much later. She was with her mother at a swimming pool; while her mother's attention was diverted to something else—again the motive of jealousy—the little child walked into the adult pool, as far as she remembers consciously defying the strict prohibition. Of course, she at once sank to the bottom. She doesn't remember any fear. The lifeguard pulled her out. This scene not only showed already at this very early time the circle of jealousy, defiance, and self-destruction peculiar to her even today, but it may also offer some hint at the attitude of her mother. It is, by the way, also interesting that this recollection, which itself is now rather free of anxiety and pleasurable, has been altered in her memory so that it was not the lifeguard who saved her but her uncle, mother's brother-in-law, a man of whom she had dreamt as a girl that one day he would marry her—probably a disguise for the oedipal fantasy that her father would liberate her from her hatred and vengefulness, and in that sense would save her from drowning in those flooding feelings and thus turn eventually into "a wall to bounce off."

Now she continued: "I feel cheated when I think of breaking with these two men—as if you demanded that I'd be all alone." She praised herself that she had not allowed her lover to pull her all the way out of her analysis—to rob her of that.

I added: "Still, in addition to all the healthy reasons for staying in analysis, is there not also the meaning, that *I am the robber* whom you have to *rob of his success*—by remaining sick, by repeating this scenario, by staying with a man who threatens your safety?"

"Robbing me or you. If I gave up the analysis I'd rob myself of the progress."

"So looking at the three solutions mentioned we can modify the first one. It's more specific than destroying the rival. It's rather *robbing from the rival.* And I'm there too!"

"And it's the same with Felix. I stole from him, I emasculated him, I cheated and deceived him and deprived him." After repeating the connection with that early childhood constellation she added: "And behind all that was a very insecure child, looking for some place to put the blame. Mixed in with all this was wanting to like myself. I don't know all the elements of insecurity, but part of it somewhere was that I felt *robbed of myself*, of self-acceptance, of self-nurture. I don't have yet a good feel for it. But I see a small child standing in a black space, in silence, like on a black stage, standing in an empty theater—that's the part I don't understand. I wasn't a stupid girl, I wasn't slow witted, but it was a terrible sense of not knowing what to do, of having no direction, of standing there without script, without director, without audience, and only to feel very inadequate—to do something and not to know it, unable to do the right thing. It numbs me. I'm hitting an impasse. I feel very cold and I'm full of self-criticism."

**The Core of the Childhood Phobia**

At this point I inquired: "May this not be tied in now with some of your earliest memories?" With this I alluded to the *phobic core of the repetition compulsion.*

"When I was 4 or 5 I lost all imagination. My brother had all those imaginary friends; he invented figures, and I simply wanted to have their big sister, but I couldn't even think of a name. The sewing machine had a big knob, so that became the older sister with a big belly button and without a name. I had murdered my imagination. The door knob had earlier had the name 'Pickles.' Now it was a crippled fantasy."

I became more explicit: "But what were your earliest fears?"

"The cracks in the ceiling, and that a rabbit would come out and run after me, and then the rabbit would be killed by the cat, and I tried to revive it. The rabbit is clearly the little brother being born."

"And then the dead rabbit?"

At first, she took it literally, but then developed the interpretation herself: "I saw its bones under the car. I hadn't always been scared of rabbits. First it had been my friend. But then I asked Daddy to put paper over the cracks so that it would not jump out and get me. It's like Felix's suddenly appearing at the top of the stairs above me and threatening to stab me. The *punishment for my wish to destroy the rabbit.* And the same with Felix."

That was the end of the double session. I should add that in hindsight I see much of the aggressive (sadomasochistic) trend of this dialogue as a powerful defense against, or at least counterpart to, the sexual elements in the transference, that is, the unconscious search for the loving, seductive father. The erotic transference was even more frightening than the aggressive one.

She was sensing the heightening danger. The following hour [479] she reported one of her recurrent anxiety dreams: She was walking around the apartment, trying to turn on the lights, and none went on. She had had a long talk with Rudolf—about the analysis, her fear of his violence and of his drinking. Nothing got resolved. He accused her of betraying him, of not standing by him. He dismissed the analysis as quackery and a waste of money. She defended and described it to him, but he continued seeing me as his rival who tried to steal her away from him, that I was conspiring against him and turning her by this form of mind control against him. She saw clearly the role she played in all this, by provoking and inviting his jealous rage, as a kind of stage manager (this word I add now; it was not used then).

She repeated the "rabbit = brother" equation, with its ambivalence, and I connected the papering over of the cracks with the process of repression already active then (in early childhood)[3] and with the dream last night: "I'm afraid to see; I don't want to see."

"What about that dark space?" I asked.

"I know it's not the womb, but it's being excluded from it." She quoted that beautiful strophe from George Eliot's *Middlemarch* (1871/72): "A child forsaken, waking suddenly,/ Whose gaze afeard on all things round doth rove,/ And seeth only that it cannot see/ The meeting eyes of love" (p. 189).

She continued: "It's the feeling of inadequacy and shame, of being left out and excluded, that I somehow was not worthy. I didn't like to take lunch by myself as a child—that everybody was pointing at me: that it meant I had no friends: 'Nobody wants her. She's an outcast.' Because I was shut out— as we now know from the breast."

"And he was united with the mother, 'eating' from her, while you were alone."

### Death and Resurrection: The Culmination of the Crisis

Yet the crisis came to a head. In the following hour [480], she reported her latest quandary. A colleague had invited her for dinner and for a concert, and she was pondering what to do about this double invitation with Rudolf— whether to lie to him or to abide by his jealous command. She saw herself both as *femme fatale* and as a trapped and *bound victim*. She knew if and when he would find out she could be in terrible danger. "Every time I'm afraid I would suffer irreparable damage." When pressed to specify she explained: "Then he would maim me." She talked about her sexually pleasurable fantasy of being bound and beaten, and how he had at times forced her, against her wish, to have intercourse, and had in a way raped her.

I interjected: "And I think that this need is very active also in relationship to me."

"Right! I made myself feel that way. I always feel bound and beaten, with my affair destroying the analysis. I could act it out. It's so complex." She felt, undefended and unarmed, like having surrendered to the demonic happenings.

The day following her determination to be candid with Rudolf, she did not show up for her session, which barely ever had occurred before. That she also did not call me why she could not make it was unprecedented and very much contradicted her conscientious character. Knowing about her fears and to what extent they were grounded in—albeit self-created—reality, I got increasingly alarmed. So I tried to call her. Her telephone was busy. For about two hours it remained that way. I called at her work place. Although expected there, she had not come to work, even more in contradiction to her great sense of responsibility.

I was at a loss about what to do. I felt there was a real possibility that something serious had happened to her, her telephone being off the hook, either because of a vain attempt by her to call for help or intentionally left so by the attacker. I thought of inquiring with her girlfriend, the only person who besides me was familiar with the entire story, including the potential for violence. At the same time I knew that every such intervention was nonanalytic in nature and posed a most serious problem for any continued analytic work. It would be a kind of counter-acting-out on my side.

When I eventually reached her at home, she said in a desperate voice: "I cannot talk now, but I've made a real mess out of everything."

Because of her and my schedule I was only to see her four days later, but that day she called me to cancel, and the day after I myself was sick.

The next session [482/483], one week after the previous one, she said that Rudolf had indeed flown into a jealous rage. In the face of his wild threats she had seen no other recourse than again to grovel in shame, guilt, and self-accusations.

I let her finish talking, but eventually I said how these dangers she had described to me and the ongoing bondage in which she exposed herself to such risks stood in conflict with the continuation of the analysis itself. I described my own quandary, and how I was forced into a nonanalytic stance, and suggested that we either change to intensive, face-to-face psychotherapy, or that she enter consultation with one of my analytic colleagues and to have that colleague deal with those reality concerns. She preferred this second solution and fully concurred with my concerns and conclusions. At the same time, she acknowledged how she was playing out her relationship with her lover against the analysis and how she was about to destroy one with the help of the other: "I feel poisoned, and it's of my own making. I was not even in love with this guy, but it was like an *addiction*."

"Was?"

"I thought this morning it must be over—to maintain my identity—"

"Haven't we heard that many times before?"

"Oh yes, I know that."

I repeated how I myself became enlisted by her in a kind of rescue mission and added, "one may argue that it was my fantasy" but she interrupted me:

"But it was on the basis of what I had told you. *I turned the analysis into a masochistic bond* . . . My father told me—about what was happening with Rudolf: 'Don't you want a real child, not one that is 28 years old?' not somebody who will compete with my children . . . I wanted so much for it to work, the relationship to Rudolf, that each time I forgot all the bad things. I *ignored the reality* because I wanted so much for *the fantasy to work where I am loved by my angry mother* . . . It's clear, the analysis has become pro forma, my resistance to solving the problem—repeating and repeating."

As she correctly stressed, the *denial*, the ignoring of reality, did play a decisive role in this impulse sequence. I was wondering about that part of the complex "plot" in which I was enlisted as her rescuer: "I'm asking myself whether this was not also part of the overall *reversal*—just as that identification with the jealousy evoking mother. With Rudolf it seems a continuous process of destroying and reviving him, of *death and resurrection*—"

"I think that is very important."

"It might well be the fourth element."

"It makes sense with what I know of myself. Like prodding the little rabbits under the car with a stick, to make them move, so that they wouldn't be dead. And I killed the relationship with Felix and then, as if by magic, salvaged it. This is important."

"And in what is happening right now, it is again the power of reversal. Instead of your own destroying and resurrecting, you depict yourself as the *victim of violent men*, and they are now the ones who do the killing and the ones who resurrect. Just as with the jealousy the whole thing is turned around."

"Oh brother!"

"Literally!"

"I have a much deeper understanding now."

The rabbit meant of course, as she herself recognized, the brother who had emerged from the darkness ("the dark space"!) whom she now wanted to banish back through the crack and behind the wall. The persecutory anxieties in general, today's reprise of the phobia of early childhood, could thus be traced back to her wish to remove this primal rival, and the same might pretty much also hold true for the knife directed against her own womb. The background of phobia and persecutory ideas, her own projected aggression, had to a good part become clear.

I did not notice at that moment, however, how this elicited rescue mission repeated another part of the early jealousy drama—her having walked into the swimming pool and having been saved from drowning.

Still, I resumed: "I also would revise something I said earlier. These *enactments* are perhaps not so much a *resistance* against the analysis, as *a great help for our understanding*."

"My father said that it makes me realize what is at stake for my life and my personality. I did not feel cast out by you, or that I am a bad analysand. I told my father that you were doing your job by pointing out to me the danger and that I do not see it as punitive—"

"—but as protective. Still, it was nonanalytic."

"It's very important for me to speak with Dr. C." (the suggested consultant-analyst).

Subsequently, she remembered a recurrent dream from childhood [487]: "I was leading my siblings down a subway tunnel; suddenly we came to a dead end, a wall. I heard voices from the other side of the bricks, but I could not get through. I had them all by the hand; people were chasing us. I thought we were safe, came to a station. Instead it was bricked off."

"There you were the rescuer."

"But it was 'abortive.' The real wish to—I am blocking—"

"To 'abort' your mother, eliminate her pregnancies?"

"Definitely with the next brother (the third child). We did not want to have another sibling; there should be only two, not three children. So the tunnel would be the vagina."

"The terror about wanting to lead them back?"

"And running away from that, from my wish to destroy them. Isn't that astonishing! And that dream has bothered me for years! And with thirty years I discover what it was. And the word that tripped me up was 'aborted.'"

"And your own compulsive wish to have children?"

"Like atoning for the wish to destroy my siblings."

"Not only atoning. 'I'm safe when I am mother and have children of my own; then I don't need to be jealous.' And I wonder whether the black stage would not be a derivative of the tunnel."

"The womb? It sounds crazy: as if it had already begun in the womb. And my thrashing with Felix—that there was no wall with him, only a gray empty space of nothingness—buffeted by the winds like Paolo and Francesca [in Dante]."

"The triangle again!"

"The wish to bounce off—to stay in the womb—always to remain a child, always taking, and totally occupying my mother, certainly to the exclusion of my father."

"This is not a memory from the fetal stage, but a central and early fantasy about your mother's pregnancy."

"About the exclusion of all the rivals! The feeling: Why am I not good enough? Why doesn't my mother want me alone? Why does she need those other children? And in the dream the construction workers: the womb is where the baby construction goes on. You have seen the maternity T-shirts with the print 'under construction' and an arrow?" [487].

## ACTING OUT AS VICIOUS CIRCLES

This first excerpt is, I believe, particularly instructive because this patient helped to educate me about the great analytic potential of working through even severe and menacing forms of acting out *within* the transference and neurotic actions *outside* of it in form of externalization and their indissoluble correlation. Certainly I have not always been able to refrain from being an authority—"playing superego." Some comments may have sounded critical or were intended to be protective, and it is hard to know afterward whether there could have been better ways of dealing with what was going on. Still, all in all, we were able to maintain the momentum of the analytic process.

Another criticism could be that many of my comments were either quite intellectual or approached the material too much from the drive side—instead of from the defenses. While this is true when some single moments are considered, taken as a whole, I think, the approach was balanced and went back and forth between drive and defense, affect and defense, experiencing and intellectual mastery of very difficult regressive material.

Most of all it became very evident that the main transference—the major transference acting-out—consisted in her attempt *to provoke my jealousy*, and with that indirectly and very unconsciously my sexual attention, just as the neurotic action outside of the analysis had the intent of arousing jealousy in every man. The goal of many of her self-destructive actions was therefore: to *make somebody jealous in order not be jealous anymore herself*, hence the *identification with the jealousy-evoking mother* and, with that, the *reversal* of the entire *traumatic* situation (including *turning from passive to active*). The centrality of this specific, fantasy-fed action schema, which had brought her in seeking analytic treatment, had eluded us before and became comprehensible only in the course of her culminating acting-out. Its components were: (1) an elemental (traumatic) state of feeling deprived, cheated, robbed, and hence jealous and envious; and (2) the need to *make the man of her love just as jealous of her as she had been*, first of mother, later of father; (3) she did this by *uniting* with a rival (the second man) in the same way as her mother had with her brother—at the breast; (4) she was thus forced to *rob from, destroy,* and *resurrect* that rival (the brother, one of the two men with whom she had established a triangular relationship); and (5) she needed to *expiate* for these aggressions by turning the whole range *against herself* in form of all the *masochistic, self-punishing* endeavors; (6) part of what this global turning around involved was that at the end she would be *rescued*, that is, *resurrected*, as in the case of her drowning; but also (7) the renewal of the sense of being cheated. This was one sequence—ultimately a steadily reenacted vicious circle in which internal compromise formations were intertwined with the events in the outside world.

This was the reconstruction of an important part of her neurosis, segments of which kept passing through the transference neurosis in the form of highly disguised acting out—and were only accessible through those actions. I put it here almost entirely (except in the first point) in terms of her triangle with mother and brother; but, as we shall see shortly, this was not the only paradigmatic triangle.

### THE RESENTFUL SELF AND A BASIC EQUATION

Basis for this part of Vera's identity (and the vicious circle just outlined) was the continued existence of that earlier self-representation—the *resentment-laden self*—that wanted to rob from, castrate, and eventually eliminate the rival and to take revenge on her faithless and withholding mother. With her fantasy that her parents and her analyst had robbed her or tried to rob her, there was also ostensible justification for spite, for rebellion, and for revenge. Tied in with that multiply enacted *drama of evoking jealousy*, underlying it in fact, was the conviction that she had been *phallically* and *orally* profoundly cheated: "I have been *robbed of a penis* and of *nurturance*, hence when I am the jealousy-evoking mother I also will possess penis and nurturance" (meaning: the substance of gratification and of love). It implies the basic equation: that *lust = penis = breast = love*, and the sequence of competing for this amalgamated good ® the wish to take it away ® protection against this wish in the strong man = "the wall" (496). Because she had felt robbed of all four and yet helpless about reclaiming them, her *resentment* was overwhelming.

That part of her early self that was rebellious, spiteful, envious, and jealous always invited punishment and humiliation and compelled her to destroy almost all of her often eminent accomplishments, and time and again to break off the development of her great gifts. Just as she had firmly believed as a little child that her parents would wander as robbers through the night and steal the silver, she now saw my remarks as aimed at depriving her of her love toward Rudolf and of any other relation to a man. Was not every aggression, every *defiance* now thus justified—as revenge for the one great damage inflicted upon her, as wiping out her grudge? Her penis envy had basically never become entirely unconscious, and she remembered very well how she had bitterly complained that her brother was owning a penis and that hers was not growing. She indeed needed a strong external figure, "that wall *she could bounce off from*," in order to put a stop to those overpowering wishes of revenge, defiance, and resentment.

With Felix, her former fiancé, whom she had loved and admired, she had to repress completely these taking and robbing wishes, and this was even often the case with Rudolf, namely when the positive feelings toward him prevailed. However, the consequence of such repression was that she felt "like dead." At the same time, the aggressive impulses reappeared, now turned against herself. She was sorely tempted to attack her abdomen and uterus with the knife, or she expected, as mentioned, such stabbings from Felix or from any man. These self-directed attacks were then generalized into her entire readiness to suffer and be the victim—in her masochism, and particularly her moral masochism.

Ultimately, her identification with the jealousy-evoking mother was not only used in order to make up for her deep sense of having been cheated, deprived, and left out, but in order to defend herself against her intense sense of *guilt* about having felt so *murderously vengeful* against her mother— in fact, about having behaved that way. It was, therefore, in the repetition of her original role as the cheated and rebellious child that she had learned to effectively provoke punishment for her "naughtiness," this naughtiness comprising those three steps of *making jealous*, of *uniting with the rival*, and of *stealing from and destroying the rival.*

## IDENTIFICATION WITH THE VICTIMS
## OF HER AGGRESSION AND MASOCHISM

Another very important ego-state, the fifth station in the vicious circle outlined above, reflected the fact that she *identified* with *both victims* of her jealousy, envy, and revenge—with mother and brother. As we saw, she was to such an extent the victim of provoked attacks or of aggressions directed against her self—in fantasy as well as in reality—that we were often able to read off from them almost directly the original impulses themselves. (Read, not interpret! Such direct drive interpretations were at times particularly tempting, and I may have not always resisted that temptation.)

Her masochism was, as Paul Gray explained, not so much engaged in just for the sake of self-punishment as for her intention to *share the position of the victim* and thus to redistribute the terrifying amount of aggression. This *distribution of aggression* must have helped her to get the inner permission to be excited by her father's spanking. Perhaps it may be understood in this way: "Only if I suffer with the targets of my attacks and only if I am equally cruel and vengeful against myself can I afford to be so hostile toward them and to hide my sexual arousal (with father and analyst) behind all the aggressive brouhaha." There would be a kind of safety in spreading the evil. One form this had taken was her identifying with the knifed victim, with the meaning of equating knife and penis and thus reliving and reenacting the sadomasochistically interpreted primal scene [492].

At the same time she could only hope that, by being a victim, she would *obtain absolution and redemption.* By blatant neglect of self-care she called upon "the man" (me, her lovers, her father) to rescue her [495]. The union with her lover meant also, as that with a craved for "addictive" object: "Take away my guilt about my jealous and vengeful feelings and wipe out my shame about being the outcast"—a protective fantasy against the trauma.

In that context her dream about leading her siblings through the tunnel yielded additional significance. More important than having them safely stowed back inside her mother's body was her *masochistic defense* depicted in it: only by sharing her siblings' fate was she enabled to experience those dangerous and frightening impulses of jealousy, and these only in distorted, fended-off form, that is, in this identification with the victim. She could not permit herself to see the light at the end of the tunnel and to abandon them to their sinister fate. She had to entomb herself with them.[4]

At the same time she also felt protected by this masochistic solution against that other drama of jealousy which was alluded to by the scene behind the wall, where she could hear but not see. Her association went to a maternity T-shirt. It probably referred to the intercourse of her parents. Yet, in spite of almost incontrovertible analytic evidence for the *traumatic impact of the primal scene*, she often claimed that she had not been aware of the sexual activities of her parents until late in her youth. As we shall see, there was something very important hidden behind that wall.

In this context, the reiterative metaphor of the *wall* is conspicuous: the wall to bounce off, the wall out of whose cracks the dreaded animals—rabbit, spider, bugs—emerge, the wall closing her off from rescue, the wall behind which those mysterious and ominous events occur. The full meaning of this recurrent symbol was at this point not yet evident; more will have to be said about it later on.

Therefore, this archaic, *contradictory double identification* was crucial. The identification with the jealous-making mother is reflected in the continuous creation of such triangles—a symptomatic pattern of action that both brought her into analysis and almost caused the analysis to founder. The identification with the victim lets her not only suffer, but always wait for a rescuer who, thanks to her many good deeds, would liberate her from the compulsion of deadly jealousy.

## REGRESSION AND RECONSTRUCTION

What all this turbulence, this acted-out, self-destructive and sadomasochistic "tumult" indicated was not a "borderline disorder"—although at this point most readers who take today's literature seriously would hardly doubt this anymore, especially if I add that the acting out as well as the pseudo-hallucinations during the panic attacks, the phobias ("the cracks in the wall"), conjuring formulas ("Mama, Mama") and experiences of intensive depersonalization reach far back into childhood and that her entire life as an adult evinces many chaotic features and much loss of control. Her outstanding social and professional functioning was episodically very seriously compromised and led to several crises in her job, and emotional isolation, even suicidal despair.

In spite of all this and with my far more restricted use of the borderline category, I rather believe that what we were dealing with was a typical, though quite severe *hysterical character neurosis*[5] with strong *masochistic* features,[6] including the sense of a masochistic perversion, and clinically deep *depression* and *depersonalization* states. What manifested itself as splitting and as such was a phenomenon fully admissible to consciousness, turned out to be the result of complex defensive processes, whereby repression and denial, condensation and displacement, externalization and projection, idealization and turning against the self played essential roles that needed to be separately and carefully analyzed. What seems to me by far most important in such a case is the role of *regression* and the function of the *defense by reversal* within that regression. How far regression serves itself as defense will be discussed in Chapter 4. What I mean concretely here is that, instead of being disappointed about me she was overwhelmed by massive rage and vengefulness that she now, deeply frightened, experienced as coming from me and fended off. One drive had to serve as defense against another; above all, violently ravaging cruelty, seemingly storming against her from without, should protect her against her own tenderness, against her own feelings of trust, love, and sexual attraction. Probably because of the seductive behavior of her father and mother's general hostility against sexuality, *sexual wishes appeared to her as far more dangerous* than all the sadomasochistic raging and fighting. They also were far more difficult to deal with in the transference and hid themselves within the idealization.

This is so for several reasons: superego sanction, drive danger because of overstimulation, but most of all because of the perception of reality: "He sleeps with *her*, not with me, and *she* has one child after the other, she, and not I! I want to get rid of all rivals!" Outer reality must have been experienced at the same time as *extremely overstimulating, extremely frustrating,* and *extremely forbidding.*

In her case, the dissociative elements—the sudden moving away into great distance and strangeness, the threatening figures with stabbing knives or blinding pencils—could be traced back to *one* area of meaning, as if she wanted to say by them: "Because of my castrating wishes toward the man I have to feel guilty. All the aggressions motivated by envy and shame are being turned against myself when I rage in a *masochistic orgy* of self-abasement, self-torment, religious contrition, and professional self-sabotage. But I am horribly ashamed about the ensuing degradation. However, this *shame*, this feeling of being pierced by eyes full of contempt, is being repressed and reveals itself on the one side as a general feeling of worthlessness and vulnerability to insult, on the other side as those semihallucinations where I feel pierced." Those piercing, stabbing attacks are therefore an expression of *repressed shame anxiety,* pointing back most of all to the ragefully reproachful eyes of her mother.

Certainly, the manifold regression veils the stormy *oedipal* conflict problematic; what is preoedipal serves the defense against complicated oedipal, broadly triangular[7] conflicts of rivalry, envy and jealousy, craving for power and sensuality, guilt and shame.

The defense by reversal and the processes of regression can also be seen microscopically in the transference; either, as mentioned, by amplification: "Instead of feeling disappointed about you, I talk about murderous attacks"; or by defense against the sexual drive by sadism: "Instead of talking about sensual excitement, I wallow in fantasies of sadistic aggression by you or

Rudolf"; or by ego-alterations: "I detach and depersonalize, I polarize, forget, blur the lines between perceptions and hallucinations, and have transient clouding of consciousness." All this can be treated quite well by careful defense and superego analysis. Instead of my saying: "You are furious at *me* instead of your fiancé or father" or: "You have murderous feelings and intentions against him or me and turn these against your own self," it proved all in all to be better, precisely because of the intensity of regression, to employ a dampening "interpretation upward": "You are disappointed and hurt, and the storm surge of feelings covers what you really feel right now: the sense of humiliation about the fact that these sadomasochistic entanglements are being revealed here." Or: "The rage allows you not to feel so vulnerable anymore—as a defense."

To summarize this section: Vera's defense, in this area of acting out above all, consisted in the attempt to make everybody else jealous. The content fought off by this was: "I competed with my brother for the love of a stingy mother. To see him at the breast was an intolerable insult, full of pain and shame and immense, jealous rage. I wanted to rob him of 'it' (breast, love, etc.) and in turn tear him away from her and eliminate him. As punishment, all this is now being dumped onto me. Ultimately though I will be saved and forgiven once I have a child myself. Then it is my turn to make others jealous and I won't have to be so any longer. Then *I* will be the mother!" The defensive processes aiming toward that result are mostly repression, reversal, identification, denial, and externalization.

Thus Brenner's (1976) advice about early transference interpretations is wonderfully apropos; it surely would have helped me in preventing, with pluck and aplomb, most of the acting out. But that is easier said than done. I simply did not know, nor do I believe I could have known—nor is it even likely that she could have grasped it if I had interpreted it before.

Before? Yes, that is the clincher. It was not understandable to me or to her before it had been repeated many times in action (as externalization): in action outside of the analysis, as "neurotic action," and in action within the analytic situation (or in reference to it) as "acting out" *sensu strictiori*. It was like a secret script that only slowly and reluctantly yielded itself to our understanding, and only after we both had had many chances of watching together a performance that not rarely threatened the safety and the confidence of both of us.

For a long time I viewed these actions as resistances hostile to analysis and also named them that way, since they seemed to conflict ever more strongly with the continuation of therapy. Only when the decisive transference meaning was shining up—in Vera's case, the double play of identify-

ing with the mother who was perceived as jealousy arousing, cruel and judgmental, and with the guilt-ridden victim of the resentment cultivated in the
family—did it become clear that the acting out in the analysis and the neurotic symptomatic actions outside were indispensable for deepened insights.
Their blocking would have made analysis (and probably psychotherapy as
well) impossible, yet the renunciation had to come at her own initiative and
time.

In turn, it had not been possible for me to recognize earlier those specific transference meanings and to prevent those menacing reenactments
by early and appropriate transference interpretations. The only thing that
I was able to contribute was to reestablish the connections that again and
again were being torn asunder, to make her aware in an undoctrinaire way
of what was being "ignored," and to find *with her* less brutal and pernicious
ways by which she might resolve the conflicts as they were becoming clearer.

Our understanding is very limited indeed; in the chaos of the immensely
rich material, it often takes a long time until we may be able to recognize
the main connections and even then we have to ask ourselves how certain
we can be. "We do not know anything with certainty because truth lies hidden at the bottom of an abyss" (Diogenes Laertius).

It was like some secret writing that only hesitatingly and gradually opened
itself to our comprehension and only after we both had repeated opportunities to watch a drama which shook the safety and trust of both of us.

With that, the work was by no means at its end nor did Vera's dangerous
acting-out completely cease. As essential as the insights gained were, they
were but a part of what needed to be known, lived through, and eventually
resolved.

In Eliot's *Daniel Deronda* (1876), the motto over Chapter 35 (p. 455, emphasis added) deals with "uneasiness of conscience" and describes *conscience
as "a fear which is the shadow of justice, a pity which is the shadow of love"*—very
fairly rooting the conscience part of superego in two basic and very
broad affective states: in the *sense of justice* or fairness, and in *love*. Promptly
Gwendolen says about Deronda, as a seemingly outside *personification of
her conscience*: "He cast an evil eye on my play" (her gambling) and enlarges
her seemingly *externalizing* accusation: "I object to any eyes that are critical"
(p. 462, emphasis added). Yet, she internalizes and introjects him more and
more: Deronda "was unique to her among men, because he had impressed
her as being not her admirer but her superior: *in some mysterious way he was
becoming a part of her conscience*, as one woman whose nature is an object of

reverential belief may become a new conscience to a man" (p. 468, emphasis added). "This hidden helplessness gave fresh force to the hold Deronda had from the first taken on her mind, as one who had an unknown standard by which he judged her" (p. 484).

In Vera's inner development, it was thus only the turning away from acting and the turning back onto herself, the insight into the whole depth of her bitterness and of the resentment, which eventually, much later, permitted her to recognize and overcome her attitude of impotence in front of the figure of her conscience. And, as in the relationship between Gwendolen and Deronda, the transference relationship was crucial in it.

Before that we had to ask ourselves, however, What is lying behind that enigmatic, ominous double identification? Does it go along not only with a split in her identity but in her superego? And how is this reconcilable with the very early formation of her phobia? I am going to report about the continuation of this very instructive treatment in the next chapter.

## THE SACREDNESS OF REBELLION

Before I continue with this inquiry into Vera's dynamics and the study of her treatment, I insert a few comments about the value of defiance—a topic certainly central not only to this treatment, but to most of the cases presented here.

It is a sacred rebellion, an inviolable spite, that protects against shame and self-extinction, shielding the identity against unacceptable intrusions—the last line of defense against crushing humiliation. It may be an uprising against unjust blame, whether this comes from without or from within.

I would like to use the powerful words of Eliot to make this point. The first brief excerpt stems from her novel *Romola* (1862/63), which is set in the Florence of the Renaissance. The protagonist Romola, betrayed by her husband, struggles with the conflict between the overwhelming need to leave him and the sacredness of the marital bond, a conflict reinforced by the stance of the prophetic figure Savonarola who himself has revolted against the corrupt papacy, but appeals to her bond of fidelity:

> She felt that the sanctity attached to all close relations, and, therefore, preeminently to the closest, was but the expression in outward law of that result toward which all human goodness and nobleness must spontaneously tend; that the light abandonment of ties, whether inherited or voluntary, because they had ceased to be pleasant, was the uprooting of social and personal virtue. . . . The one effect of her marriage-tie seemed to be the stifling predomi-

nance over her of a nature that she despised. All her efforts at union had only made its impossibility more palpable, and the relation had become for her simply a degrading servitude. *The law was sacred. Yes, but rebellion might be sacred too.* It flashed upon her mind that the problem before her was essentially the same as that which had lain before Savonarola—the problem *where the sacredness of obedience ended and where the sacredness of rebellion began.* To her, as to him, there had come one of those moments in life when the soul must dare to act on its own warrant, not only without external law to appeal to, but in the face of a law which is not unarmed with divine lightnings—lightnings that may yet fall if the warrant has been false. [Chapter 56, p. 441–442, emphasis added]

Eliot was not only presenting and defending the dilemma of Romola, but her own in bucking the social ostracism of her stance as a woman intellectual living in a passionate relationship with George Lewes, whom she could not marry, and more generally as a woman who had stood up for her beliefs against her father, against her family and friends, and against the sacred tenets of her age.

In *Daniel Deronda* (1876), after referring to the "tragic parable" of Berenice and again to Nemesis (Chapter 37, p. 515), she intensifies the stress on tragedy by pronouncing Prometheus' isolation under the power and force of institutions as the real tragic fate:

There be who hold that the deeper tragedy were a Prometheus Bound not *after* but *before* he had well got the celestial fire into the νάρθηξ[8] whereby it might be conveyed to mortals: thrust by the *Kratos*[9] and *Bia*[10] of instituted methods into a solitude of despised ideas, fastened in throbbing helplessness by the fatal pressure of poverty and disease—a solitude where many pass by, but none regard. [Chapter 38, p. 527, emphasis in original]

In culture and psychoanalysis defiance is considered with ambivalence: it has a high valuation when it stands in the service of justice, and is seen as dangerous when it flouts the basic laws of human existence, of community, and of nature.

In Judaism, *chutzpah*, audacity, brazenness, and shamelessness, but very much also defiance, is depicted as one of the great forces of perdition that contributed to the destruction of Jerusalem and is expected to prevail in the times preceding the coming of the Messiah. Still, this *chutzpah klappei shmaya*—the "defiance against Heaven" may be justified, as "an uncrowned royal power and dignity—*chutzpah malchuta bela ta'aga hi*" (*Sanhedrin* 105a). Arguing with God goes through the entire Jewish scriptures, as Laytner (1990) documents; many Hebrew prayers have the character of an appeal before court, specifically of an accusation against God in the court "of a divinely instituted moral order in the world. *Tzedakah* (justice), was the name given to this order and it remains the fundamental concept of the Jewish ethicoreligious world-view" (Laytner 1990, p. xix).

This is a profoundly antiauthoritarian attitude that sharply opposes any abuse of power and all injustice. Here every unquestioning obedience, all carrying out of a command contradicting that moral world order is seen as ethically intolerable. We are reminded of Antigone's appeal to the "unwritten laws of Heaven," and of the encompassing power of Diké (justice) that in Heraklitus determines all of Being.

In our field, we need a respect for the dignity of rebellion, of the inner revolt against irrational exertion of authority from without and from within. Psychoanalysis is unceasingly on the way, dialectically questioning the archaic superego and yet acknowledging the enduring force and fundamental nature of moral and ethical values.


## ENDNOTES

1. I am very grateful to Dr. Ursula Engelhard, Dossingen, for making me aware of this poem.

I shall try to translate it by staying as close as possible to the original:

"Woe to me! My mother tears me down. Here, I have put stone upon stone to myself and I already stood here, like a little house around which the day moves, even alone. And now comes my mother, comes and tears me down.

"She tears me down by coming and looking. She does not see that somebody is building. She walks straight across my wall of stone. Woe to me! My mother tears me down.

"The birds fly around me with greater lightness. The strange dogs know: this is That One. Only my mother does not know it: my face that has slowly grown (has become more).

"From her to me, there never was a warm wind. She does not live there where there is free air. She lies in a high heart-planking and Christ comes and washes her every day" (*Sämtliche Werke*, vol.2. *Poems*, Frankfurt, 1956, p. 101).

2. Externalization = "re-staging his internal (intersystemic) conflicts as external battles," in A. Freud's description (1965, p. 42). An example from another patient: "Their (the parents') disappointment in themselves was externally expressed as disappointment in everybody."

3. Does it not remind us of Strindberg's *Dreamplay*, and of Kristin's refrain: "*Jag klistrar, jag klistrar*"—(I paper over, I paper over)?

4. This is one of the very valuable additions given by Paul Gray to the overall understanding of the case.

5. (Abolished by legislative fiat in the various *DSM* categorizations at the moment en vogue.)

6. (Also currently declared inoperative.)
7. This will be explicated in much more detail in Chapter 4.
8. Narthex, giant fennel (*Ferula communis*).
9. Power.
10. Force.

# 4

## Masochistic Impulsive Action, Resentment, and the Split Superego

*Mais l'envie resta cachée dans le fond du coeur, comme un germe de peste qui peut éclore et ravager une ville, si l'on ouvre le fatal ballot de laine où il est comprimé.* (But the envy remained deeply hidden in her heart, just like a germ of the plague that may break out and ravage a city when the dangerous ball of wool wherein it lies compressed is opened.)

—Balzac, *Cousin Bette*, p. 82

## DEFENSE ANALYSIS OF THE DOUBLE IDENTITY

### Triple No and Triple Yes

In the previous chapter we encountered the intriguing doubleness in the choice of Vera's partners: she entered analysis because of that curious and repetitive split between emotional attachment to one idealized man and, parallel to it, sexual surrender with strongly masochistic features to a series of other usually much coarser men.

There continued to be, parallel to this split in her love life, a split in her self-image; most of the time she felt detached, numb, almost without feelings—a clear state of *depersonalization.* At the same time, she was professionally functioning excellently and effectively. Her powers of judgment and competence, her calmness in crisis caused justified admiration. In contrast, when she was chasing after her lover or was together with him, which still continued to happen although less frequently and far more cautiously, her diminished perception of reality changed to one of painful or ecstatic intensity. It was similarly exaggerated during the panic attacks during which she continued hallucinating that a man was waiting for her with a knife in a closet. Frequently nightmares could be more vivid and real than her waking life. I spoke in the previous chapter of the two part-identities of the jealousy evoking, resentful self and the victim-self. But this dynamic does not fully account for the phenomenology now discussed (Wurmser 1989c).

I believe that there were above all three defense mechanisms appearing in many variants that are particularly helpful for the understanding of these states: identification, projection/externalization, and denial. Gradually, over the course of the analysis, we recognized how depersonalization and mas-

141

ochistic sexual involvement were two opposite but complementary states, the former guarding her against the latter. Already on the surface of it, the state of depersonalization was dominated by *denial and affect-blocking*; virtually all perceptions of self and surroundings were being stripped of their emotional significance, while their factual functioning remained excellent. The second state, that of manifest *masochistic perversion, self-destructive acting-out*, and *depression* (occasionally a kind of rageful suicidal tantrum) was introduced by some act of impulsive rashness and recklessness; in fact, it looked as if it were simply the breakthrough of some masochistic impulse gratification, accompanied by some condign punishment. However, analysis showed that such preconceived notions did not do justice to the great complexity of the dynamics.

She described the motives for her *impulsive acts* of returning to her lover after break-ups: "It always came from inner agitation. I felt extremely uncomfortable, and the impulse was to try to end the uncomfortableness—that things were intolerable and I had to do something to change them, and I had to do it *now*! Twenty-four hours would have seemed an eternity. Something seemed to be hammering at me and nagging at me." What? "The fear of abandonment, of losing his love, his approval, his body . . ."

What seemed essential in this was that the impulsive action, the return to him, had the aim of merging with him, of being totally at one with him who had everything that was forbidden or denied to her. Thus it could be used to circumvent and defy the prohibitions and to deny both her own sense of being excluded and separate and the validity of those profound injunctions. Such overriding of reality and its limitations and prohibitions had immediately to be followed by punishment from without, by doubts and profound contrition, acts of repentance, and perhaps, most of all, shame.

I was, as stated in the previous chapter, again and again shocked by the extent of her clinical regression. For long periods the analytic sessions were filled with descriptions of such regressive occurrences and emotional storms. Yet, despite her often deep depression, self-hatred, and self-disgust, she remained for long periods able to live up to her professional tasks.

As we saw, the *repression* of the aggressive wishes during the act of making love—the wishes to *take away*, to rob the partner of that tetrad of lust, penis, breast, and love—had to be accompanied by the *denial* of a large part of her self-perception: "I am not this being, I am not so envious, angry, cruel, vindictive! Rather, I am like dead, wholly deprived of feelings, of pleasure . . ."

Why? Because all pleasure, all sexuality had become tied to such a gratification of her unconscious envy and vengefulness (the "sadistic" intent) and had to be repudiated with strictest vehemence by her conscience. And this proved necessary because of the original, most intense ambivalence, especially toward her mother (not even primarily toward her father). Sexuality was therefore permitted only under very specific conditions (I shall return to these). It was this sanction by the superego that dictated and kept in place such a broad denial and the underlying repression.

As we have observed before, we have the *No* directed against her *wishes*, mostly those of cruel, vindictive, jealous aggression; this is *repression*. Then there is the *No* directed against *feelings* in general, pleasure, envy, shame, jealousy, and anger in particular; this is the *blocking of affects*. Furthermore, we find the *No* which is turned against *seeing herself* as bad, envious or defiant—the *denial* of the perception of a decisive part of her identity.

In turn, when the man was strong enough to "take" her aggression, respond to her sadistic impulses with a far greater retaliation or at least counterforce, she could afford to counter that triple *No* with a triple *Yes*, in a frenzy of love, surrender, and orgastic pleasure, or in scornful outrage and biting disdain, and finally in desperate contrition and most intense longing. Eventually, this entire intoxicated, Penthesilea-like scenario was followed by a relapse into the inner split with its original triple *No* accompanied by depression, depersonalization, and near-suicidal rage, in what would seem like a verification of some mythical death instinct.

But what did it mean—her feeling of overriding attraction to this man, her addiction-like and often very dangerous dependency on him? It was as if she were to say (explicating even more what we have already found): "I am safe with my wishes to take away from him his penis, his power, to take into myself his defiant forcefulness and strength; and what I thus take into possession I must, of course, according to the 'economy of envy,' deprive him of. I feel secure in doing this because he looks so big and strong and muscular, a wall to bounce off from: I can take away from him, and still he won't be weakened by it. And at the same time, precisely because he has been so withholding and insists on denying me recognition, his love and acceptance would finally confirm that I am not defective, that I am not bad, that I am lacking nothing, but that my secret fantasy, that I do have a penis, is true—that I am not a weak castrated woman nor a wimp like my father, but strong, phallic, aggressive, like my mother. I would finally own what has been withheld from me: lust, power, penis, and breast."

It was clear that the sadistic man was a kind of protector for her. How? "Not I am castrating, but he is. Not I am defiant, but he is. Not I am aggressive, cruel, jealous, but he is. Not I have a penis and orgasm, but he does." Thus he was the carrier of a disowned part of herself—the cheated girl, the "greedy, demanding, spiteful" child in her. Projection and externalization rested on disowning and disclaiming—denial—of important parts of herself.

## "The Miracle of Approval"

What were the genetics behind this sequence?

She said: "The image I had of myself was that of a despicable, wishy-washy, weak, unathletic, depressed little child. Only by rebellion could I counteract this: horrendous restrictions demanded horrendous actions . . . *She* [mother] kept me weak, impotent, castrated. If *he* [Rudolf] accepted me and approved of me it would mean I would not be deficient anymore and stripped and weak. But once I would conquer him and strip him of his penis, he too would be useless."

His attraction for her lay precisely in his containment of her wishes of rebellion and "taking," an attraction relived dozens of times in impulsive acts of greatly self-destructive nature, and sought earlier, throughout her life, with other men.

Still, I believe there is even greater specificity to the links between denial and impulsive action. Her emptiness, her feeling cheated, was undone by his approval, his acceptance, and precisely if it was bought at the price of maltreatment. How?

"By my suffering I have paid for all my evil wishes: to defy, to castrate, and to fill my void. Now I am complete; I have made up my deficiencies. I *do* have power and penis and can permit myself pleasure because now the condemning judge within is appeased, his voice muted. I am not ashamed or guilty anymore."

She was murderously furious at her mother and not only remembers those feelings from the distant past, but even now her anger may approach such intensity. That fury was not solely directed against her mother's withholding of tenderness and her sullen and sulky withdrawal, but also against those "enemies in the womb," the pregnancies (Arlow 1969, 1972). The father had been and still was too weak to protect the children.

Nearly four years after the beginning of analysis, after she had finally been able to detach herself from Rudolf, one Christmas it came to a battle royal with her "pouting, snappy" mother and her "simpering, placating" father—as she perceived them. In the course of this it became clear to her: "You cannot get angry with them. You cannot point out anything to them. It would be taken as a big assault; you'll hurt them. And I played the same with Rudolf: 'You hurt me if you leave.' Now, after the fight, I feel totally unacceptable, barren, and sexless—empty and angry, a fat, ugly, disgusting pig. But one thing has become so clear to me: my mother's withdrawal. Therefore *my anger* was always something so terrible that *it destroyed her. It kills her. She desintegrates.* It is devastating to her. My impulses are therefore so destructive: they could kill her. And I have never seen that so clearly until today—*how horrible and powerful my impulses* are—that they devastate her. My anger, my criticism, my defiance, just *the wishes to be myself.* And certainly they did kill her love for me: she has the mothering instincts of a Samurai. When I wanted to talk with her about [a grave personal loss], the only thing she knew to say was: 'Just don't dwell on it, you'll get over it.' She just turns away. And against that I defended myself as a child. I turned it against myself instead of telling her off. That was safer: to hurt myself with it instead of her" [673].

The whole sequence was repeated over and over again with Rudolf, but in the hope of attaining the opposite outcome—the sequence consisting of (1) seeking love and acceptance, by submission, surrender, and "blindness"; (2) then of hurt, shame, and disappointment, leading to (3) hate, jealous fury, and contempt, then followed by (4) punishment in the form of physical abuse, harm and suffering, even illness, and by (5) overwhelming feelings of guilt and shame and of near-suicidal acts, this contrition and acts of repentance leading to forgiveness and love, thus returning to the starting point of the vicious circle. That is, this entire scenario always culminated in the seeming realization of her fantasy with the longed-for outcome: "Now he does approve of me, of all of me, also of those parts that I had to disown with my parents. Yes, I can be as aggressive, as masculine and strong, as angry and spiteful as my mother, and yet, he is stronger still, and he approves of me the way I am." It is what she calls "*the miracle of approval*" she forever had been searching for: "I am like my mother, and yet I get forgiveness and approval *from* my mother."

It is her identification with a fantasy image of her mother, that she too would become somebody very powerful, defiant, and above all phallic, somebody who is always able to triumph with her angry obstinacy. This is followed by the absolution and approval from the outside, given by the man who is seen as approaching this fantasy image of her powerful phallic mother. It is that acceptance that is being sought by the impulsive sequence.

In other words, the *identification with the aggressor* is followed by *acceptance by the aggressive superego:* "Now all *that* can be affirmed as good because he approves. I do not need to condemn myself anymore for that; now I am good."

In this scenario she can experience all her resentment, her entire cruelty, the whole power of absoluteness and condemnation *vicariously* through him; she can quite consciously identify with him as the attacker. He thus allows her in a very concrete way to unite with her own superego, this brutal executioner in her, and to find reconciliation with that inner figure, which is now embodied in Rudolf. Indirectly, this of course also means the union and appeasement with the original authority figure on the outside, her mother. But *this passage through her own superego* is crucial, as are the intensity of feelings and wishes that contributed by her (to the superego).

## Being Like the Victim Father

Is this the end? No, the reconciliation with the sadistic superego cannot last, reality always breaks in, and the denial is swept away: "No matter what I do, my lover still does not accept me, and he treats me shabbily and with all the withholding of my mother . . ." On this endpoint, the chronic stage, she views herself as hardly better than a powerless wimp, castrated, ineffective, barren, contemptible—as she had partly come to judge her father. It was the image of a father who always had been intimidated by her mother's sullen rage. It is this *depressive identification with the victim* that she ended up with: contrite, suffering, deprecated, and kind—in her words, "without sense of worth, self, competence, assertion—no happiness, no joy, enduring without dignity" [673]. Yet, as a result of the identification with the victim-father, she could also regain a semblance of normality and the actuality of highest accomplishments. It meant not only *his approval* and respect for her intellectual and practical brilliance and ethical superiority, so similar to his own towering achievements in life, but also the approval given by *that* part of her conscience that was fairer and hence far less annihilating and absolute than its first form was.

## Polarized Identifications, Introjections, and Ideals

In this way, Vera's whole life and character had developed into a complicated texture of compromise formations of these stages, over the years actually with a preponderance of the first, the identification with the aggressor.

With that we have access to a deeper understanding of the *identity split* that is such a hallmark of her life.

1. Above all she resembles her resentful, jealous, and jealousy-awakening *mother*; in many respects she has taken over her mother's identity—aggressive, self-righteous, explosive. Yet this figure is also and simultaneously the embodiment of an implacable, vindictive conscience and asserts its presence in Vera's merciless self-castigation. The resentment triumphs in the

internalization of the mother figure. But that entails that she has to see herself as "gross, foul, and disgusting," mother's attributes (in her view).

In technical terms this means:

(a) There exists an *archaic, global identification* with a mother imago that is perceived and feared as *sadistically* refusing and cold: Vera sees herself partly as cold and domineering, and exercises sadistic tendencies in socially acceptable forms, for example, in sarcastic metaphors that she has developed almost to an artform; she knows how to make herself feared by friend and foe. It is interesting and particularly relevant and fateful that this identificatory imago has also become her own *ideal*—which she keeps seeking in a man.

(b) At the same time, she has in an equally *global, absolute* shape, *introjected* the condemning, resentful voice of her mother. This primitive figure within became in addition the carrier of all her own aggressive wishes from early childhood, especially those of an *oral-* and *anal-sadistic* nature that had been *projected* onto mother. Other primitive wishes, based on how she had seen her mother, are now part of the ideal shaped after that mother imago: to be a person of *power: self-sufficient, cold, and untouchable*, an unbending, hateful, and disdainful authority. This *global introjection* lives on now in the figure of the "inner judge," that is, in the judgmental power of her superego, which is exerted with pitiless severity.

(c) Moreover, she views herself as a weak, worthless, dirty infant, and has therefore an extremely degraded image of herself, but also one that relies in turn on an *archaic identification with the despised and hated mother*, that is, with the victim of her own intense aggressions against her mother. This identification with the despised mother figure may be just as primitive and absolute as the identification with the feared mother figure.

This *threefold internalization of the mother figure* had begun very early, presumably during the "separation-individuation phase" (Mahler 1968) (in the late second and early third year of life) but has been since then again and again reconfirmed and even intensified by actual experiences up to the present. It could also be described so that the *self-image* was, because of that *double identification, split* into a *domineering-sadistic and a despised-masochistic part-identity*, and that the *introjection*, in the form of the superego, had internalized and perpetuated the *sadomasochistic object relation* itself with the most primitive drive actions and affect storms. The idealization of power was itself a kind of reversal: "I want now to become as strong as the feared, bad mother. Once I get her power I do not need to be afraid anymore. I admire this greatness and strength and find protection and solace in the thought that I could myself acquire it."

This archaic superego figure is thus the direct heir to the *traumata*, a condensation of many traumatic experiences, whose influence had resulted in this form of self-adaptation and self-splitting and kept reaffirming it. The inwardly and outwardly repeated retraumatization in the form of the rabidness of conscience may best be understood as an attempt at mastery. The inner and re-externalized polarity within her self-experience is that between hangman and victim—between omnipotent, cruel tyrant and despicable weakling, a painting of herself as one filled with *utter shame*. This self-image stands under the dominance of the archaic superego. It is her *masochistic part-identity*.

2. On the other side she can be quite like her intellectual, conscientiously submissive and admiring father; she even deepens and develops his dutifulness and ethical rigor. Yet she perceives herself in her weakness as a castrated "wimp," just as she had castigated him for his obsequiousness toward her mother. She is immeasurably terrified by this image and overcompensates for it with the accentuation of the ideal image patterned after him: his honesty, his sense of justice, and his brilliance, far less than she does with the ideal of unwavering, rigid power and invulnerablity that had been shaped after her mother. The *internalization of her father* is therefore also *threefold* (positive and negative ego-identification and introjection of an ideal), but it owns far less of those archaic-global qualities that mark the identification with and introjection of the image of her mother.

The resulting second inner polarity is the one between *successful competence and competition* and her discontent about her *desire to remove her rival*, a tension which has to result in *deep guilt*. This group of conflicts ultimately shows in her *depersonalized part-identity*. The impulse sequence forms the transition from the second to the first part-identity, from the oedipal triangular problematic to the preoedipal, anal-sadistic, dyadic problematic with mother.

It is also interesting to extend this multilayeredness of identifications to the other defense functions. The turning from passive to active, the denial and predominance of "blaming," some projection of primitive superego, and severe repression appear to be the main defenses of her mother, a predominantly hysterical-depressive woman, and now they also mark Vera's part-identity patterned after her. I presume that it was their shared condemnation and with that their *repression* of large parts of infantile sexuality (especially its oedipal parts) and, closely tied to that, the repression of all competition, that were the main reasons for the formation and the maintenance of Vera's neurosis.

The father appears from her description as a very moral, though thoroughly timid man, with strong obsessive-compulsive and less pronounced hypochondriac and phobic features; his sublimatory capability is particularly strong. Vera's adaptive and effective part-identity, albeit mostly felt as if it were an unreal self, largely reflects this group of identifications with the image of him and introjections of his voice. In the transference she hoped I would personify father's kind of conscience and ideal, but continued to be afraid that I might turn into mother's likeness.

These two forms of identity and superego stand in sharp conflict with each other and each requires for its respective rule the *denial* of the counterpart. If she strives after Rudolf's approval (who corresponds to the superego patterned after her mother), Vera has to pour contempt over her identification with her father. She is ashamed that in spite of all her endeavors she turns out, in front of Rudolf's cold disdain, to always be too weak, too thick, too unathletic, too intellectual.

However, if she craves Felix's friendship (the man who corresponds to the paternal ideal), she can only look with horror at her debasement under Rudolf's despotism and her own addictive surrender to him and can hardly believe it. Then she looks at it as if she were possessed by some demon, quite comparably to the effect of a multiple personality, although without amnesia. But she is scared by Felix's exalted expectations of her; his idealizing of her lets him appear to her as weak, and herself as bad and guilty.

## "EVOCATION OF THE PROXY" AND "FALSE SELF"

*Tout pouvoir sans contrepoids, sans entraves, autocratique, mène à l'abus, à la folie. L'arbitraire, c'est la démence du pouvoir.* (All power that is without counterweight, without fetters, and autocratic leads to its abuse, to folly. Arbitrariness is the insanity of power.)
—Balzac, *Cousin Bette,* p. 233

What is the solution to this inner and outer doubleness, to this split identity?

Although Vera's sexually attractive lover very much resembled her mother in many respects, we assumed that she sought in him rather a kind of superfather, a powerfully redemptive figure who was in all respects stronger and more aggressive than her mother and thus offered her protection against her mother's overpowering presence as well as against her own raging and vengeful desires. In contrast to her father he would have the strength to contain her destructive impulses and to forgive her for them [687].

Yet I believe the key may lie in one very specific part of the transaction, one that many might call "projective identification." What was truly *disowned* in herself and externalized was her *sadism*, in particular her *phallically* intrusive, lustful aggression. In surrendering to the "virile jock" and "gorilla" she "died a violent death"—her self burst and broke into pieces; she became him and enjoyed through him his sadistic thrust, his orgasm, his tormenting her. *Identifying with the sadistic partner* she could *vicariously* enjoy what she had forbidden to herself. In other words, her own sadistic sexuality was, in what Wangh (1962) described as the *evocation of the proxy, projected* onto a man who, already on his own, had strong sadistic inclinations and lived them out without compunction. She could experience them by turning into him, by consciously identifying with him: "I live it out through him. It is his pleasure that I seek and experience. And by becoming like him more and more, cold and defiant, ruthless, not caring what others are thinking, I feel stronger and healthier." At the same time, there is a reversal into passivity during sexual acts: she is now the target of such violence; since *he* does it and she lives it out through him, she feels "good" and free and accepted. She has obtained forgiveness because she has not done it herself and moreover has undergone punishment and received absolution from a man far stronger than her accusatory, "guilt throwing" mother, and far more virile than her "simpering, castrated" father.

In this way she could love, experience, and accept in her lover simultaneously *two parts of herself* that were repressed: the *drive part*, that is, her sadistic sexuality, and the *superego part*, a kind of ideal father who would be far stronger than her mother and would give her the hope of forgiveness and acceptance, thus finally overriding her mother's revenge—fire against fire, force against force.

Thus the identification with the lover happened in two opposite forms—either by the vicarious enjoyment of his (sadistic) power during the act of making love or, after the break with him, by her conscious assimilation of those of his attributes she valued most highly: defiant independence and self-sufficiency, decisiveness, and only in attenuated and disguised form also his sexual sadism.

However, it was necessary to recognize that the core of so much *repressed sadism* lay not only in the described identifications and projections, that is, in defensive processes. Rather it was her intense hate-love especially toward the powerful, sharply punishing, often angrily pouting mother who let everyone around her feel guilty and small—a hatred that had been massively exacerbated by the mother's pregnancies and the advent of the siblings. Already in very early times this exacerbation had found expression in Vera's wishes to murder both the faithless mother and the hated intruders (who moreover were boys!). Since these were fended off and such evil intent only aggravated her sense of being excluded, the next best thing was at least to *identify* with the figures who enjoyed power, special favors, and special equipment, by feeling and making herself the same with them, whether the phallic, ruling, and resentful mother, or a kind of fantasy father and hero, or the more favored brother. In her lover, all three were condensed into one character.

Thus the *doubleness* of her life and the *split of her self-representation* could be understood as follows: on the one side she became somebody who possessed asexual power, was detached, impersonal, efficient, could even be gentle and somewhat feminine, certainly caring and compassionate—her *depersonalized self* or *pseudoidentity* (her "false self" in Winnicott's [1965, p. 358] term, the "pseudo self" in Erich Fromm's [1941, p. 336]). On the other side, living her second identity she had externalized her sexual sadism and could now safely experience it vicariously and without pangs of conscience through her lover under the guise of her sexual masochism—her *masochistic self.* In the first part-identity she *disavowed* any sign of weakness; in the second she denied that it was she who equated violence and sexuality and lived out such an equation. Instead it was: "Not I, but he!"

Since she was in actuality anything but a weak personality this explicit stress on masculine power in the first state and her identification with the spiteful, harsh friend served a much more significant denial, namely of that side of her (that part of her self-representation) she was most ashamed of: the part-identity of the *cheated* girl that would like to *avenge* herself and would be *punished* for it—cheated because it had been excluded from the unity between mother and infant brother, shortchanged because she was not a boy and lacked a penis, slighted as well because she always had felt unloved by mother and betrayed by father, disregarded also because the child had always felt forced to cede her place to mother, and especially also humiliated because her individuality had so often been attacked and squelched (in the form of denial called by Schottländer [c. 1959] "the blinding by images" or what I [Wurmser 1993] have come to see as "soul blindness").

One could also state it this way: in the first, she *accepted* the aspects of phallic power of her sadism, but not its cruelty, yet largely *denied* her own femininity; hers was then a powerful, masculine self, but safe, because her sadism was sufficiently sublimated to be of high professional value. In the second, she denied her own power, but accepted sadism, provided it was not her own; it had to remain disguised (repressed)–projected, reversed in direction, turned against the self, simultaneously pleasurable and painful.

The first self-state showed the *denial of her identification with the victim,* the second the *denial of her identification with the aggressor.*

The conflict was the same in both states but was solved in different ways of defense. It seemed to me that the first was ruled primarily by a defense against *perception* in general, or denial; whereas the second was under the sway primarily of a defense against *drive,* or the repression and projection, specifically of sadism vis-à-vis the pregnant mother (the "heavy man").

## THE SPLIT IN THE SUPEREGO

"Sin"—this is the priestly reinterpretation of the beast's "bad conscience" (of cruelty turned backwards)—has so far been the greatest event in the history of the sick soul: in it we have the most dangerous and most fatal artifice of religious interpretation.

—Nietzsche, *The Genealogy of Morals,* 3.20[1]

Of special interest in Vera's case is the parallelism in the *superego:* from the beginning of analysis on, it had been obvious how much she was suffering under its condemning, prohibiting, and most massively chastizing force. It was a tormentor within with whom she now was perpetuating the old masochistic relationship with her parents. The three main anxieties of early childhood had all become part of her superego and were repeated now as anxiety from within: to be abandoned, to lose love and respect (as rejection, shaming, and exclusion), and to be mutilated (anxieties and threats to be stabbed or to stab herself). The love and tenderness for her father, the wish to eliminate her mother, and later on the desire to get rid of her siblings in mother's womb or in the crib, all led to deep anxiety about these threats, now coming from within. In reexternalized (projected) form, they manifested themselves as nightmares and semihallucinations of retribution.

In the first state, it was crucial that her profound sense of *shame* at being weak and "shortchanged" be wiped out—denied—by her being emotionally unaffected by the world and thus invulnerable, different from that wishy-washy, helpless girl of yore, and now strong and manly, though feelingless and detached.

In contrast, in the second state, it was her guilt for her sadistic murderous wishes toward brother and mother and the castrating wishes toward every man that was being extinguished; since she atoned for them by her suffering as a tortured victim, it should be forgiven—accepted and cancelled. The meaning of her masochistic impulsive action would thus be (in an elaboration of what we heard before): "I am not aggressive, but he is. I am not the one who would like to injure or rob. Quite the contrary: I am the wounded one, and I am even gladly prepared to submit to such injury. He is spiteful and cruel, not I; therefore, I do not need to feel guilty anymore." Here the sequence disavows the *guilt part of the superego*. In that, its endpoint is factual debasement and the feeling of being ashamed.

*Denial is the weapon one part-identity* (more precisely formulated: those ego functions that serve one group of self-representations) *utilizes against the other, and this at the behest of one superego part against the other.* The broader and deeper the denial the stronger the extent of depersonalization in the interval between the impulsive actions, usually in the state of the adapted, externally functioning personality; she was then using her power with the help of her keen intelligence and practical energy, but at the same time she was missing in it that these strengths made her unable to love and to be intimate. Again and again she found herself in the role of a woman who pushed a man away with her prickliness and her mocking, quite similar to the way she had behaved during her third year of life toward her father.

## THE SPLIT IN THE OBJECT REPRESENTATIONS

Felix, her ex-fiancé, with whom she continued her friendship, was ideally suited as a pendant for state one: as an asexual friend, admirer, supporter, and confidant, who made her feel strong, though guilty. But he was unsuited for the aims of her sadistic side, "too weak to contain" her (meaning: unable to live out that part safely for her and with her).

Exactly the reverse held true for her lover: She could, so to speak, entrust him with her sadism for safekeeping by satisfying it through him, but with him she could never feel strong, except through him in the fantasy fusion. Of course, she did not have to feel all that guilty with him, rather to the contrary, because he took care of that; she sooner or later felt humiliated and ashamed instead.

In the first state she could see him as a "slug," a "bump on a log," an alcoholic whose legs would have to come off one day (because of his severe smoking)—a devalued piece of phallic equipment, of curious meaning and low worth, an instrument for her degradation. In the second state, he was the ultimate warrant of reality, worth, and approval—life's main meaning. Only his acceptance meant anything at all, and only in the union with him could she experience herself as a real person, as free of anxiety and aggression. When she knew herself accepted by him she was good.

However, as we discovered only in the course of long and extremely difficult work, his paramount importance consisted in that he had to be the "wall to bounce off from": that is, someone who could "*penetrate*" her without being himself penetrable. And one of the most important and dangerous "penetrations" was the one by feelings—the contagion by feelings. He embodied the *defense against all affects*, especially against anxiety. Therefore the man, whom she wanted to possess but whom she could not allow herself to keep, one with whom she centrally identified, had to be somebody who would stand unaffected and cold in the face of her own anxiety and her other wild affective storms. He should touch her feelings without being touched by them himself. He had to be *emotionally impenetrable*. Only in that way, she hoped, he could contain her so often overwhelming emotions and hold her with his strength as an integrated person, as a whole.

The *impulsive action sequence* meant a switch and transition from the first state to the second. It is difficult to say in general what would trigger it; loneliness, shame and reproof, hormonal fluctuations, exhaustion from her frequent work through the nights and enormous overwork—all played a role in the rising sense of anxious agitation. I presume that anything that would touch upon the deep *equation: "I am cheated, shortchanged = left out = castrated = humiliated"* could act as a precipitant and lead to an increase of the unconscious aggression, hence to more self-condemnation, hence to rising anxiety and depressive affect, and require the second type of compromise formation.

## THE SPLIT IN THE TRANSFERENCE

The *transference* showed both images also: In the state of disavowal (of depersonalization) I allegedly did not mean very much emotionally to her. Everything was disavowed that did not fit into the image of an idealized-ethereal, esthetic and scholarly, benign, though personally somewhat weak-castrated father. What had to do with me seemed impersonal and intellectual, notwithstanding the fact that she saw her analysis as having saved her life and as the highest priority right now. Not only did it exact great sacrifices from her professionally, but also she caused several of her friends to enter analysis. "The analysis" as something that was abstracted from me as a person and as concrete reality was not dangerous. The repression of the sadomasochistic fantasy was the main feature of this transference image, which was all in all prevalent. This was accompanied by a denial of the emotional significance of the insights, her characteristic depersonalization of the therapeutic relationship.

In the second state, however, the one of preponderant projection, I suddenly turned into a sadist who might unexpectedly lean over and stab her in the eye, assault her sexually, or, most frequently, castigate her in the severest terms and cast her out from treatment. As described, her impulsive acting-out also had the purpose of causing me to intercede as authority and to punish her as well as to absolve her, to warn her as well as to give her permission, to condemn her as well as to accept her. Basically she thus ascribed to me the same role as to her lover. The setup of the analysis made me appear untouchable and unaffected, even feelingless, whereas my comments and interpretations could touch and affect her. I was also that wall for bouncing off, even if that meant that at times she had to be the "victim," namely above all of my coldhearted judgment and scorn—something she saw emotionally while discounting it intellectually as blatant distortion. I found myself therefore, just like Rudolf, in the powerful position of her *superego, sadistic* but lending her *structure and stability.*

Thus the transference was entirely shot through by a complex web of negation, disavowal, and repression. For much of our work she could not think that she or I could ever be angry, defiant, *really* aggressive or really condemning of each other, in contrast to her attitude with mother or lover. Nor was it conceivable that I *really* could reject, degrade, expel, or castrate her, no matter how dangerous and provocative her actions, again in contrast to the "bad" part of herself and her conscience, and also in contrast to her mother and her lover. Of course, the structure of the analytic setting also made it unthinkable to her that she could ever see me in sexual terms or in terms of personal intimacy, as seductive or seducible, or as having any sensual wishes. So I ended up and remained approving and ideal, as she *wished* her mother, her lover, and herself to become. It was a sanitized, *depersonalized version*, which left me as a person of benevolent neutrality and idealized rationality, a kind of super-fantasy built upon disavowal, whereas all that was being negated, disavowed, and repressed was safely bestowed upon and acted out with her lover. That relationship therefore turned out be the demonic, but "real" counterpart to the transference relationship—real at least insofar as it entailed a lot of action, not that it was any freer of denial! Thus both relationships showed, side by side, the extremes and the rewards of her bonds to her mother and to her father. Both required not only a large-scale repression of wishes, but the unconscious blocking out of important segments of reality-perception by denial. And both were ways of dealing with profound anxiety and depression. Therefore no reality confrontation could ever counteract effectively such denial or acting out.

Only careful analytic, nonconfrontative, nonjudgmental work allowed the gradual recognition and integration of these two sets of identifications (with the aggressor and with the victim), of these two superego imagos, and of these two groups of wishes and affects—and of all that had been conspicuous by its absence.

How? Through the gradual analysis of the acting out that had seemed like a resistance but was in fact an indispensable part of analytic work.

Seen from the point of view of this split in identity and object representation, the resolution of her neurosis would lie, on the one hand, in the acceptance of her disavowed weakness and shame of the first state, that is, the feeling of being shortchanged and "castrated"; on the other hand, it would become possible if her repressed intense rivalry became conscious and with that if she could accept her repressed cruelty, her envy-filled vindictiveness and the guilt of the second state, the state in which she wanted to take away and reappropriate to herself what she felt entitled to, and where she saw herself as "castrating" or murderous. It had to consist in the integration of these two part-identities.

This defense analysis, which has just been presented in theoretical transformation, took two years and more than 400 hours; these stood between the detailed description of the former chapter and the last part of the analysis. Only now did she feel able to approach the main conflict.

## WORKING THROUGH THE OEDIPAL CONSTELLATION AND RESENTMENT

### "We Can Have It, but You Can't"

One basic trauma, first only inferred (as indicated at the end of the previous chapter), then also relived and remembered with intensive emotional storms, was the *primal scene*; it was mostly experienced as something heard, not seen. In spite of all the later negations and denials, it is possible that she had been frequently exposed to the sounds during the first two years of her life, since it turned out, upon inquiry, that the house had been old and that the sound could have carried.

When she witnessed during a vacation in her parents' home noises and other evidence of their sexual interaction she reacted at first with nearly psychotic panic and consuming fury. "I told my Mom that I had heard that through my childhood, that it was filling me with panic and nausea and I would not be able to stay" [773]. The upshot of the emergence of these very intense memories was this insight: she felt excited about the image of the aggressive, raping, bulky man: "I wanted to take my father away from my mother, but I couldn't. I was inadequate because I had no breasts and couldn't become pregnant." Probably these were later fantasies explaining her being excluded and cast off. His seductive demeanor we had heard about since the beginning of analysis "must have meant to me that I could gain him for myself. I felt led on by him to expect it, and it disappeared all very suddenly again. It must have been a terrible disappointment, and most of all a horrible humiliation, the rebuff after all that anticipation and excitement." This too had often been reenacted with various men [785/786]. Much later she added: "The conflict of the little girl that is wanting to have something and cannot have it. He shows me something that I desperately want, and it is two thousand miles away, with all these obstacles: See, but you can't have it. We can have it but you can't" [950].

An important part of this conflict might have been that in the face of the presumably misleading signals of her father, which she certainly had interpreted as seduction attempts, she needed the shield of repression both for her and for his protection. And the double denial was such a safeguard: "He wouldn't want me anyway; and he isn't manly enough anyway."

**Weaklings and Swells**

Furthermore, her father must originally have been experienced and desired as a sadistic figure. The push and pull of desire and repression showed itself most of all in that she sought her father over and over again (and the men who stood in for him) and then she pushed him away with contempt and dread. When he touched her she fought him off; even today she "freezes" when he gets too close to her and turns away from him when he tries to hug her. She needed to devalue his manliness; she saw him as a "simpering wimp" who deserved all her disdain. Consequently, she divided all of mankind into these two categories of weaklings and swells. The *devaluation* of the man, a sour-grapes defense, was decidedly part of that repression. The more she had idealized him the more strongly she had to protect herself now with this devaluation. How did she bring this about? I believe by *regression as defense*, namely by a form of regression in the image of the ideal: that of having impenetrable armor, of being a figure of power, resembling a wall without any cracks, cold and rejecting, defiant and self-sufficient: *the regression to the ideal of the traumatizing mother*, an *ideal of power and invulnerability*. This ideal guarded her, as we have seen, by reversal against the penetrating feeling of weakness and powerlessness that even now she felt in front of her mother.

She tried, of course, to become a swell herself. The castrating meaning of this *part identity* was emphasized by her luxurious sarcasm.

Naturally, this was only the one part-identity; she was and remained also the rejected girl, a "contemptible weakling," in her role as masochistic victim.

As already mentioned, it was by no means clear that the first, the masculine-sadistic part-identity, would have corresponded to identifications with the father, and the second, the masochistic-devalued one, to those with the mother, nor that it simply would have been the other way around; nor was it merely an identification with the fantasy and projective images of both. It was rather the case that the first identification occurred with the aggressive aspects of *both* parents, and the second with their weak, yielding aspects: "My father was both a powerfully verbal man and a simpering weakling; and my mother was aggressive and strong, but also hysterically out of control and incompetent as a mother" [802].

Moreover, identification and introjection played an especially important role as defense in this conflict. The original traumatic scene (the primal scene, as we recognized it now) and the chronic conflict with her mother were both incessantly repeated in the sadomasochistic identification and the double denial, but this time under her active stage management, instead of her being passively exposed to them. Her superego showed the figure of the (introjected) cruel judge, the heir of both parents whom she hated and desired.

**Three Triangles**

It was the regression by which she defended herself against the *three rivalry conflicts*, that is, against the Oedipus complex in a broader sense: (1) It was the *competition for her father against her mother*—the *early oedipal conflict* that probably can be traced back to the experienced primal scene and its elaboration in fantasy; (2) the *competition for her mother against her brother*—which we encountered in the early phobia, and can comprise as *breast envy* and *sibling jealousy*; and (3) the *competition for power and penis against her father*, and with that the conflict about her *castration wishes and penis envy* that we met with in her frigidity.

She had broken with both of her earlier lovers. Her life consisted by and large of work and analysis. She had largely withdrawn from her social life, completely from all intimate relations. She felt "profoundly suicidal": "The hopelessness—why go on? I had incredible hallucinations [more probably a delirium caused by sleep deprivation]: a shark was gnawing at my side, and

I was all dismembered. I was paralyzed. I woke up in the middle of the room, my body was being dismembered. The room was spinning around. I thought of leaping down from the balcony" [817].

After the severe, at times suicidal depression, again accompanied by a painful superintensity of stimulations and hallucinatory-like anxiety scenes, had lasted several months, she finally started taking an antidepressant.

"I remarked in a conversation with a girlfriend how much I prevent myself from thinking of you as a living, breathing person, how much it is a requirement that you and Felix are stronger than I and have no human frailty."

"Untouchable, impenetrable, to reestablish the lost ideal."

"She said that you must be disappointed. It hadn't even occurred to me." She was referring to a professional change in my life that had then fallen through.

## Idealization and Devaluation

Later in the same double session [836/837], nearly five years after inception of our work, she came back to her need to view me as strong and invulnerable, in contrast to her own deep disillusionment about her father, her anger about it, and the defense by *devaluing* him. All that was now entirely turned against herself, and I needed to remain safeguarded against it: "I need to make you invulnerable and strong."

"To protect me against the devaluation."

"This is absolutely correct, and the problem with Felix was that he could not protect himself. And Rudolf is protected by his withholdingness."

"And what is crucial is the need to devalue the ideal—"

"If I can't have him he isn't worth anything, like my father. He is not as great as he is cracked up to be. However I tried to be like my mother, I could not have him. The embarrassment about it cannot be exaggerated: wanting to be like an adult, without being it, without the equipment, and being exposed as that and mortified. He plain did not want me. I felt neglected in my own right as a child, I was a disappointment for him, he paid no attention to me, he was embarrassed about me. And then my revenge on mother was: 'You have him? He isn't worth anything!'"

I repeated the inner sequence she just had observed and added: "Envy and jealousy led therefore to the need to *devalue* him which you afterwards *direct against yourself.*"

She talked more about these connections in regard to the two parallel lovers: "With Rudolf it was: 'I can't hold onto you, you aren't worth anything anyway,' and with Felix: 'I'm so inadequate, I'm so worthless; I hate myself. If you like this piece of shit you can't be worth anything either.'"

"It was that way with Rudolf as well. He was acceptable only so long as he didn't accept you. The man is only attractive when he rejects you, otherwise you have to devalue and reject him . . . Yet it is decisive in this," I continued a little later, after her metaphorically describing how it was an endless investment in an account with zero returns, "that you incessantly *test* the man if he is strong enough to withstand your efforts to devalue him. Felix has failed the test, and Rudolf leaves you still dangling; he has neither passed nor failed, he is stuck there. And you have protected me against the test. And if you, at least for the moment, succeed in proving the strength of the one you test, you want to acquire it by merging with him."

"That was already my fantasy at 14. I couldn't wait to marry so that the man could take care of all the problems, and I wouldn't have to feel any insecurity anymore."

"Yet the central piece in it is your need to devalue and to *test whether he is stronger than the devaluation.*"

"And the lesson that my father was not that strong, that my father had shortcomings, that he was terribly disappointing, a defeat. That's why I dreamt the parents were thieves. That the things were not the way I had seen them, that I had been deceived by him, used—"

"This is one possible explanation. The alternative might be: he was so attractive, but that he was so unreachable was too painful to bear."

"Both together. It was so embarrassing to want something that I couldn't have. The same humiliation as when the communion plate was handed over my head because otherwise I would reach for something that I couldn't have. I wasn't permitted to eat from it and to drink the wine."

She had often stressed how, in many resounding variants, it had been mother's indignant exclamation, not rare even now: "No, you can't have that! How can you do something like that! A dutiful child wouldn't even consider something like that! How can you do that to us who sacrifice ourselves for you?!" Always, underscoring every word, the refrain: "How can you do this!"

Being a child was itself a source of contempt: "I didn't have a reason for wanting to be a child."

I then summed up the sequence, in an important *reconstruction of ego-states*: "(1) the *conflict* about the man, then and now, the man who is attractive as well as disappointing and prohibited, and the feelings of shame, envy, and jealousy accompanying this conflict; (2) the need to *devalue* him as *defense;* (3) *turning this devaluation against yourself*—how you treat yourself as totally inadequate and worthless and depressed; (4) the constantly reiterated attempt to *put the man to the test* to see if he is truly strong enough to withstand your efforts at debasement; and (5) to *merge* with the strong man and thus, in a kind of *magical identification* through *union*, to partake in his power . . . What we have understood before in terms of phallic power and castration we look at right now in terms of ideal and devaluation."

She found this synopsis a real illumination and added many additions or affirmations, among others also the important broadening that the disappointment had not only been in regard to her father, but also that her mother whom she had set up as her own ideal was a frigid and incompetent woman who in fact had not shown any control over her feelings. This included that "my whole life I have been devaluing her body and mine as far as it was similar to hers: as being not sexy, not attractive, not feminine. She would have been *an ideal to be, instead of an ideal to have.*" Thus she would also have to disparage me as well as guard herself against this tendency for degradation.

She found that the starting point of this sequence was the unsuccessful competition and the compulsively repeated assertion: "I can't and oughtn't compete, neither for nor with the man," and the feelings of humiliation about the defeat involved [845].

**Clytaemnestra and Cassandra**

This led to a reconsideration of an earlier insight that had been overlooked in its significance. Years before she had declared: "I began thinking about my mother. I don't like her, and I don't like the parts of myself that remind me of her. And when I am mad at Rudolf, it is really my anger at her. And it is part of my self-hatred that I feel responsible for my mother's ambivalence: if she doesn't like me it has to be my fault—that there was something I did. And I carry that on with Rudolf, that I'm responsible for the failure of the relationship, because I'm such a demanding bitch, that I close down on him and restrict him" [515].

It was decisive in this that she had to identify with the hated mother, specifically in the figure of the dangerous *Clytaemnestra.* She identified with the hated mother in order not to murder the hateful mother, and even more to the point, *she identified with the resentment-laden mother,* in order to *ward off her overwhelming resentment fueling her often murderous hatred against her.* And, of course: "Electra got Orestes to do her dirty work for her"—again the idea of the *proxy* [515]. It is not surprising then that she compared herself, in a very different context, with *Cassandra:* "a loner, not listened to when she warned, sure in her distress, striding with a core of inner determination to the abyss, unwilling to give up" [946]. I shall return to this fascinating reference.

At this point, late in the analysis, it was less the murderous, and more the blaming, disparaging, always judgmental mother with whom she had at her deepest identified. Thus there occurred behind the mask of the adult and competent woman the constant inner *duel between judge and defendant,* similar to the one between the *accusing mother and the helpless child.* This *double identity of executioner and condemned* was nearly absolute.

### The Shame–Guilt Dilemma

The initial point in this line of inner events was now, even more encompassingly than just in competition, her endeavor *to be herself,* to claim her own *individuality,* but with the certainty that this meant *losing acceptance and love* by her mother, and that this presented such a radical, absolute, final threat (which indeed she can witness even nowadays) that her anxiety (about loss of love) is overwhelming. *Love and acceptance can therefore only be secured if she identifies with the judges-like character of her parents, with their blaming voice and eye.* Otherwise the anxiety would be all-consuming, just as absolute as the alternative of condemnation and utter rejection, forever. In other words, *the absoluteness of the inner demand, this incessant either-or, is the direct consequence of the double anxiety: the anxiety of loss of love, and its counterpart, the anxiety of self-loss* [882/883]. The stronger the anxiety, the shriller the demand. The stronger the demand, the deeper the resentment. *Her own resentment* which pertains to her personal needs is reflected by the *resentment of her conscience,* yet both versions mirror the resentment that plainly cries out from her parents' (especially mother's) whole moralistic attitude. The inner judge has unceasingly to order: "You can't have this; you aren't allowed to see this; you are not strong enough, and you will fail. You are not good enough to have anything good" [890]. The main sin was that she asserted her individuality. But this meant every competition now was just as prohibited as the original rivalry. *Winning was interdicted, yet failing was just as much; the former led to guilt, the latter to shame.* Of course, that was an insoluble dilemma and repeated the puritanical rigidity of her parents, especially her mother: joy and success as well as suffering and defeat caused anxiety and castigation in her family. All three children go deeply bent under this double burden, through life: "All independent thinking and creativity was bred out of us. And with every friendship it was mother's message: 'You can't do this, you will be a whore, you bring shame over the family.' It was a litany of panic and condemnation and judgment" [894/

895]. At this point she interrupted herself: "I should have a tape recorder here and then transcribe it. I could not write this down on my own. It is only possible here because I'm speaking freely, in your nonjudgmental presence. I wish I could do this—simply go home and let it flow—but I don't allow it; it's as if somebody where sitting there blocking my thoughts. Not so here." I replied, almost casually: "Why not?"

## The Capstone

Why would self-assertion, competition, and success be so thoroughly dangerous? "It would mean I would get rid of her." And with this we finally had hit upon the hitherto missing piece of the connection, in the insight we called "the capstone." I said: *"I identify with my mother as accuser in order to defend myself against the wish to get rid of her.'"* It may sound anticlimactic, perhaps trivial, but this insight came with the dramatic feeling that it was very decisive.

She replied: "If you don't beat her, join her."

"Become her."

"And I have become it. The ways how I'm like her I'm so miserable."

"And the prohibition against marrying and having children—"

"—would mean [to be directed against the wish] to supplant her as mother."

"'And I hate myself when I would be like mother: marry and have children.'"

"I cannot be sexual."

"Originally: 'I hate her precisely for this: that she is sexual and married and has children; and that's why I hate myself if I were like her, because I want to eliminate her.' And secondarily, displaced: that you feel frumpy and fat and old and asexual." But this also means: "I'm like my hated, disdained, devalued, and bad mother and have totally *become one with her judgmental and devaluing attitude.* Her approval and acceptance is more worth to me than my life."

This, however, meant that she had dealt with her deep ambivalence toward her mother and with her multiple competition with her and about her *splitting herself into victim and tormentor,* in order to evade the massive anxiety. In lieu of killing mother, her conscience took on all the characteristics of the hated mother. This is the reason for her *split: "I feel like two different people"* [920]. The *archaic, global identification and ideal formation* had therefore above all the purpose of *defending against her murderous aggressions:* "Now she cannot hurt or destroy me anymore; I make myself as strong as she is."

And: "Forgive me now and love me; I don't hate you anymore, but I admire you and surrender to your power in unlimited submission."

This split and, contained within it, the *double form of the narcissism,* as her own omnipotence and as exaggerated idealization, are therefore intimately connected with both major conflicts: the *dyadic conflict about becoming herself, individuation versus dependency,* and the *triangular conflict about the three-layered competition* (oedipal in a broader sense): the fight with the brother for the mother, with the mother for the father, and with the father, or the man in general, for his power and penis. This split is above all also manifest in the peculiar split in conscience and ideal. In each of these conflicts, shame, envy, and jealousy, and with them the feeling of resentment, play a role specific to each particular form of conflict.

Based on this group of multiply *defensive identifications* with, and intro-jections of, the feared and hated mother, her *superego* has become the *merciless prosecutor, judge, and executioner,* all in one; her *ideal* has been shaped as the *invulnerable, impenetrable* muscular mass, and her *self-image* has turned into that of a *miserably incompetent,* shrilly yelling, and sexually vile caricature.

In the outbursts of rage and in her sexual acting-out, her conscience seems to have broken apart. The first part is one that abides by her own resent-ment; in an act of defiant uprising and in the union with a strong hero it seeks (by approval and love) the extinction of all the self-debasement. It tries thus to wipe off all her resentment by attaining that primitive ideal of power and untouchability. The second is its counterpart: implacably and unbendingly it talks to her of absolute duty, vilifies all joy and pleasure, and looks with jeering and bitter derision on her behavior. These two parts are mirror images, insofar as the second speaks with *veiled* resentment and the first shows it *openly.* The flight from conscience has to fail because the resentment, and, dwelling within it, the paralyzing shame, the gnawing envy, and the burn-ing jealousy, follow her like demonic shadows—those demons she had made the leading problem at the begin of analysis, in dream after dream, in im-ages of panic, and in semihallucinations.

**Resentment and Loyalty**

> Power and resentment are seldom strangers.
> —Samuel Johnson

In the course of this case presentation it has become evident how deep Vera's resentment, her feeling of having been cheated, taken advantage of, unfairly treated really was. The attributes of this affect mentioned in Chapter 1 (after Scheler [1915])—envy, jealousy, and helplessness, and the resulting vindictiveness—were certainly present, but I believe we can now go beyond them and have to add something very specific to this analysis.

I asked her about the origin of her resentment [969]: "It's almost as if I were being teased. And there the loyalty issue is so important: I was asked to be loyal, and I was so, a dutiful daughter, but instead of getting the expected reward I was put out and excluded. I wasn't given my due. Somebody had something that should be mine, and it wasn't. And then, secondarily, I saw the reason in that I was so inadequate and therefore didn't deserve it. But that was already afterward."

"And what did you experience as being put out?"

"At first, it must have been when I was in the bedroom of my parents [at least for the first two years of her life, when it was inevitable that she witnessed her parents' intercourse and was the *excluded third*], and then came the birth of my brother, and suddenly I wasn't anymore the apple of my mother's eye anymore, I, that dutiful child, but displaced by that terrible interloper. And my reaction was resentment against his presence and that all of mother's attention was now devoted to him. And my explanation was, as time went on, that I was inadequate, and here this boy was so much better, so much more imaginative, and could entertain her so much better than I could."

"And thus the resentment was the sense of unfairness?"

"My father has commented about that again and again: that as child I had an *overdeveloped sense of justice*, that I always talked of what was right and what was wrong" [969].

Rightly she relates this feeling of resentment to the conscience, to problems that have to do with loyalty and justice. As in the other patients who will be described later on (mostly in *Flight from Conscience*), an important form of Vera's superego conflicts consisted also in *loyalty conflicts*—whether they were now between me and her lover Rudolf, between various men concurrently, in earlier time between the loyalty vis-à-vis her parents and faithfulness to herself (as manifest, for example, in her impulsive acts of rebellion).

It was especially the intense conflict between the loyalty toward the parents and the resistance against her being taken over and steered by the parental emotions that had to lead to her consuming resentment: "I felt the need to be loyal, but my loyalty was being betrayed. I was the dutiful daughter who was not rewarded by acceptance, but shut out and used; 'Fine! You shut me out? So I act the defiant, shut-out outsider!' It was a loyalty conflict: there was an overwhelming command to be loyal, but every sense of self was dissolved; there was no sense of belonging, no identification with the group to be loyal to, and no possibility to developing loyalty to myself . . . Success itself became an act of disloyalty; *to be true to oneself meant to be disloyal to somebody else"* [967].

Moreover, it also is obvious that every oedipal conflict *eo ipso* already includes a loyalty conflict: one is loyal to one parent and betrays the other— or one feels betrayed by both.

Resentment is therefore not merely a synonym for the feeling of disappointment or of being shortchanged, for shame or envy, for jealousy and vengefulness, although all these play into the resentment and underlie it as a broad base, but it is the *sense of injustice*, of unfairness that appears to me indispensable. With that, resentment is really like a counterpart to loyalty, more precisely, to the feeling of *betrayed loyalty*: "I have done my part, and you have withheld yours from me."

It is an affect that, like guilt or shame, could be seen as referring to a particular form of tension between a superego function and an ego function: between the desire for justice based on one's own fulfillment of duty and commitment toward the other, versus the observation and interpretation of an unfairness suffered, that is, a kind of treason by the other.

The stronger the claim for justice, the higher, at least originally, the demands toward oneself, hence also the feeling of entitlement with regard to the other. With that, it is clear that blaming is an integral part of the resentment. The tilt into pathology occurs when thirst for revenge joins up with the demand for justice.

Of course, along with that resentment comes a strong narcissistic component ("Injustice has been inflicted on me!") but it would be too narrow just to designate it as narcissistic injury; the matter is much more complex, and its object-relation character, the wish for love and acceptance in it, is also unmistakeable.

Another narcissistic component is added when resentment, driving from a sense of slight, intensifies to *boundless entitlement*—as observed in Balzac's *Cousin Bette* and in Lagerkvist's *Dvärgen* (*The Dwarf*). "*Men ingen är stor inför sin dvärg,*" says the dwarf in Lagerkvist (Nobody is great in front of his dwarf) (p. 10). "*Alla dvärgars frälsare, må din eld förtära hela världen!*" (Savior of all dwarves, may your fire consume the entire world!) (p. 28).

Chapter 6 of this volume and the book *Broken Reality* (Wurmser 1989a), as well as *Flight from Conscience*, have more to say about these important topics of loyalty conflicts and resentment.

Here I note only that Vera herself reconstructs its origin from the birth of her brother and the primal scene experiences, all prior to the end of her second year of life. Certainly, the sense of justice and injustice is very archaic, and the origins of the superego do not wait for the dissolution of the Oedipus complex.[2] I rather tend to see its development over longer periods, in fact throughout her growing up, the temporal fixation functions perhaps somewhat like a condensing, telescoping screen memory, here as a summarizing reconstruction that now has a decisively important *organizing function.*

In all this, the *resentment invested in the superego* appears to be crucial, more important than her own resentment about feeling cheated—a mighty figure of defense which haunts the entire family, not only some individuals. "That demon is the archaic identification with the mother," with her outrage: "How could you do that to me! No dutiful child would even consider that!"—crushingly experienced. It is more: a family demon [915]. *The resentment is like a ghost binding the generations together in shame and hatred,* "binding with briars my joys and desires," in Vera's Blake quote (Chapter 1). It is the *spirit of the avenging inner judge demanding the absolute, "la recherche de l'absolu"* (Balzac): "How could you be, have, and do this?! How do you dare?! No, you can't have this, you can't be so, and can't do that! If you stand by yourself you will be absolutely rejected and excluded! By being an individual you flout your duty toward the family" [926].

### Affect Modulation

Yet even this complex piece of inheritance is only part of the truth. Besides this, Vera is also the curious researcher and the effective and highly conscientious professional, the therapeutic collaborator in the analysis and the trusted friend, the highly gifted, very articulate teacher, rich in metaphors, a woman capable of great sensitivity and with patience to *feel herself into others* (in fact, we may confer this last, *consciously employed gift* with her great propensity to *use, unconsciously, identification* as a major defensive device). "Felix still only sees the old me, and he behaves so as to bring it out, the unself-confident, cheated, tortured me. I can't make him see the new me" [924].

The transformation now finds expression also in the fact that, in the hour which followed the "capstone" insights, she indeed brought a tape recorder to the session, and from now on recorded most sessions. She not only listens to them again at home, but she transcribes them into her word processor—a new *identification with me as "regulator and moderator"* (her own words) for the feelings which otherwise so easily slip out of her control. At the same time, this inventive form of self-observation and working-through represents a potentiated acquisition and deepening of her insight which, as she herself states, has become of dramatically transforming strength. This was the deepest significance of that "wall to bounce off from" she had been seeking in every man: the *regulation* of her overwhelming feelings *without condemnation*, the *taming* of her ferociously aggressive and sexual wishes without scorn and humiliation, the *binding of overstimulation*. She was looking for a conscience that would be strong, but without resentment, sympathetic and understanding, but firm and decisive.

**Untying the Mind-Forged Manacles**

Technically speaking, it is of the very highest importance for the analyst not only to avoid being condemning, but not even to *seem* so, when silence and every technical rigidity, every emotional coldness may be perceived as judgment. The theoretical conclusions of these insights in regard to the primacy of affect disturbances and the new view about the nature of splitting will be taken up more thoroughly in the coming chapters.

Vera asks me now to review with her the most important hours of the entire analysis, its high points, step by step—which, with the help of my stenographic notes, is not very hard. "This is the first time that I can look down from the top of the hill and see the end of the way. For a long time it seemed to me that, like Lot's wife, I shouldn't look back. Now it makes sense as long as I don't allow it to paralyze me but see it as a help to free me from the past. It is itself a wonderful metaphor for the analysis" [907]. She sees the taping as a sign that "I'm independent of you. I can also gain power over the material and handle it. I'm identifying with you. It's a helpful acting out of that pattern."

She now feels "intact, full of courage and self-confidence, willing to take control over my life." She is satisfied with herself and feels attractive; she has started dating men without falling back into her masochistic entanglements and is also trying to rebuild her relationship with Felix on a more mature basis. "My life is so different now that I'm not so absorbed anymore in the details of my conflicts; many are resolved and more comfortable. Life is a progression on a different level now. I'm able to experiment. This is a wonderful period of discovery for me" [970]. "I stand on the threshold to a new phase of my life . . . It's the first time that I know my own mind and know what I want, and that I'm not trapped in the pattern of repetition anymore. My intellectual curiosity has awakened again, and I think much more and enjoy my life." In spite of the severity and long duration of her illness, there grew from "the intact core of honesty, the wish to be myself and autonomous, and the curiosity" a healthier and more integrated personality: "These had to become unfettered by prohibitions and preoccupations, 'the mind-forged manacles of fear,'" she added, again quoting Blake (975).

Epicritically, it should be mentioned that she developed a full and largely fulfilling love relationship. She did marry, had several children, and built up a successful career.

From the identification with the hated rival and judge there has very slowly grown a much freer self. Apace with this, that archaic set of identifications has been replaced by the identification with the analyst as a nonjudgmental, rigorously nonauthoritarian observer and as a warrantor who gave support and helped to resolve the affective storms. And being such a warrant, such deepest vouchsafing of inner growth is the profound meaning of the word *auctoritas* (authority), withal one of the main tasks set not only for the analyst, but for our conscience as well.

## THE NATURE OF REGRESSION

Now some more general thoughts concerning the basic theme of this book.

"Their every desire turned into rage, and their rage ranged boundlessly," says Iphigenia about the race of the Atreids (in Goethe's *Iphigenia on Tauris*).[3]

At issue are those demonically overpowering, uncontrollable, endlessly repetitive breakthroughs of impulses and drives: What about them?

What Vera, like all the other patients described here, showed in a particularly strong way is the prominent tendency to *clinical regression*. It affected the functions of the ego as well as those of the id and the superego and evinced itself perhaps most impressively in regard to the affects. The question posed itself then how far this regression was itself a defense, or whether it may not rather have been one of the results of those massive conflicts and defenses, engendered by recurrent traumatization, and particularly whether it may not be the massive dissociation of states of consciousness and their contents, caused by repression.

As mentioned, partly it was indeed an issue of a genuine *defense by regression*, namely, I think, above all of the avoidance of rivalry (of the "triple competition" presented) by regression to the level of an anal-sadistic ideal of untouchability and impenetrability, embodied in the "ruthless muscle mass." Thus all of life's relations changed altogether into concepts of power and impotence, that is, those mostly of *anal narcissism*.

In contrast, examining the *impulse sequences* and the accompanying *clinical* regressions, we might come to a different conclusion. This *global regression* was rather the *result of other defensive processes* than a form of defense itself; rather a resuscitation of earlier forms of functioning the way Anna Freud (Sandler and A. Freud 1985) meant it when she spoke of "more a revival than a regression":

> I would call it an overwhelming of the ego's controls by the strength of the emotion. . . . But at some point passion may overwhelm the individual, and the ego's control is lost. I think that it is essentially a quantitative matter, and what we see is that for the moment the affect and the impulse are stronger than any of the restraints which usually keep them in check . . . [the crime of passion] is a release, not a regression. [pp. 118–119, 123]

This jibes with what Gedö (1986) describes as Freud's "lifelong conviction that at the core of every insoluble intrapsychic conflict there lies an archaic propensity for psychoeconomic imbalance—in Freud's terms, an 'actual neurosis'" (p. 162)—or what he considered "trauma." It is identical with a disturbance of affect regulation or modulation.

We will be able to observe this in all the cases presented here: *severe neurosis means overwhelming affects, either manifest or rigidly held back, and that means underlying, deep, and chronic traumatization.* Certainly biological factors play an important role in this. Chronic, severe, early traumatization has biological consequences. There is no question that this had been the case for Vera. She herself observed that any form of sleep deprivation would precipitate affective decompensation, with all the emotional storms and rabidly exacerbated conflicts entailed, a decompensation that very quickly would turn into a massive vicious circle, because the affective storms strongly reinforce the insomnia. In turn, selective medication has been, in addition to the analytic work (and later recurrent episodes of nonintensive, supportive/exploratory psychotherapy), capable of breaking open that circle. In addition to that, there was possibly a constitutional (inherited) disposition, since the wider family shows many persons with affective disturbances, mostly in form of anxiety, although it could be argued that family dynamics rather than genetics could be involved.

But there is more to this. With Vera and in the other cases of severe neurosis presented here, and in *Flight from Conscience,* it was not a question of crimes of passion but of frequent alterations of consciousness and addiction-like, often perverse acts that asserted themselves over and over again in spite of all intentions. What was it, therefore, that regularly had the effect of "unleashing"? The direct answer can be found in the *severity of the superego pressure,* as evident in the intensity of feelings of self-condemnation and self-overtaxing (*Selbstüberforderung*). Under certain conditions, namely those which brought about an additional exacerbation of self-criticism (hence superego demands), this inner pressure became intolerable; I have mentioned the particularly important function of loyalty conflicts in this.

With this it is thus exactly and again a matter of *quantity*, requiring the application of certain economic assumptions, as negatively charged and unacceptable as the economic model as a supraordinate explanatory principle has become today. However, as long as it remains close to description, it is indispensable. An overwhelming feeling that is stronger than any conscious intent and volition is a phenomenological fact. Yet, why this happens, that is, what the explanation is for the question why these patients suffer under such affective storms, goes far beyond what is descriptive in economic terms and changes to the question: Why do these patients show the repetition of such demonic possession by the intensest emotions and other states of consciousness? More exactly: Why this quantitative excess? And in turn (from the opposite vantage point): Why does the ego control collapse under the assault of these affects? In other words, the question only begins with the description of the central quantitative aspect; it is, by no means, yet an answer. But the careful description of the changes that often occur dramatically during treatment may bring us closer to such an answer.

Usually it would be premature and inadmissible immediately to conclude that there must be an ego defect (a circular reasoning anyway: the description itself is being used to explain). It is rather of the essence that we can observe here not so much a basic "weakness of the ego," but a particular *intensity of the conflicts*. As soon as these can be reduced, the controls automatically strengthen.

Furthermore, it should be doubted that what is involved in these breakthroughs of impulses is "the dissolution of the superego,"[4] as Anna Freud suggested in this context, and not rather a matter of *superego regression* as Sandler brought up in the discussion. Connected with this is certainly also the question: From what point on in the development should we even start talking about the superego—if only in the late time, after the "dissolution of the Oedipus complex," or already in the early stages of internalization of outer authority? As stated, I myself hold the latter view.

However, it is certainly the diminishing of the superego pressure in therapy that is experienced by patients as *unspecific* help, somewhat in the sense: "Finally, not only am I not condemned but some of the most tabooed and awful secrets about me and my family can be told and thought through without my losing affirmation and approval by the authority. This gives me, maybe, also the permission to treat myself more tolerantly and forbearingly, precisely there, where in the past I had to be especially implacable, and thus it enables me to renounce those wild breakthroughs that seemingly gave free passage to my desires." Vera expressed herself in this regard in this way: "I spoke at length with my father when I visited him in the vacation. He wanted to know loads about the analysis. I told him that his entire life was marked by paralyzing anxiety and that his own mother had not helped him when all his life she dumped her own burden on him and treated him as her parent. That's why he felt so comfortless. I told him, and he could see it, that he and my mother fed each other's anxiety but totally missed that the same had happened between them and me: how strongly we children have partaken of *their* anxiety."

"Now you yourself become his parent," I remarked.

"That is all right. I have had the analysis and have found my safe parents in you and in Mrs. N. [the mother of Felix]. I'm ready to move on. I have gotten the security and protection I had missed in my own parents so that I feel myself stronger than him. I don't need him anymore as a source of protection against anxiety . . . He is a wonderful man, and he can't help it either that he is in certain regards inadequate. It is a function of his neurosis. He's thinking of going into analysis himself, in spite of his age" [949].

Still, this is the unspecific impact, the general, psychotherapeutic efficacy, not the claimed specific effect of psychoanalysis. The former resides in some suggestive influence where an enormously harsh regressive superego is replaced by a milder one, that is, as Vera alludes to by rights, in a kind of "after-education" by parent figures who are more indulgent and promote independence.

In contrast, what is claimed to be *specific* lies in the exact observation of the defensive processes, of the fought-off wishes, and of all the emotions arising in this conflict in such overwhelming form. These aspects can best be observed in the study of single, repetitive, often circular sequences.

Surprisingly, it is noted then that these severe neuroses more or less clearly have a *phobic core*. Each of the cases I present here, or can remember beyond them, had early phobic symptoms or attitudes of avoidance. It reminds one of the postulate ascribed to Wilhelm Reich, that "behind every character trait lies a phobia" (Sandler and A. Freud 1985, p. 215), a compulsion to avoid something, thus alleging that such phobias are also part of "normal" psychology. Here again it becomes a matter of quantity as to whether we would see it manifestly as pathology but it also raises the deeper issue of what constitutes psychopathology, which I shall take up in Chapter 6 (see also Wurmser [1978]). In most of the cases presented there, and in *Flight from Conscience* and

*The Riddle of Masochism* (1993), the intensity of these phobias of early child-hood was striking in hindsight, and alarming at the time of occurrence.

Later on, this avoidance becomes part of the observable sequences. The doubleness of object and situation of *anxiety*, and object and situation of *protection*, the categorical, absolute nature of both, that is, their mythical quality and intensity, largely determine the inner life of these patients and stamp their fate. The *repetition compulsion* consists in the avoidance of anxi-ety and in the quest for protection, namely in a series of compulsively suc-ceeding feelings, actions, and interactions—a vicious circle of succeeding compromise formations as I analyze it further in *Flight from Conscience.*

Thus these individuals flee from the mythical realm of the terrible into the sheltering reservation of what is impetuously longed for. This frantic flight, experienced as demonic drivenness is only a first approximation to what this case can teach us also in regard to more general interests.

## A NEW DYNAMIC CONFIGURATION

The more we immerse ourselves in the complex and difficult dynamics of cases like Vera's, the more we discern a pattern emerging out of the bewil-dering multiplicity of phenomena and underlying dynamics, which then may be rediscovered in others—as a constellation of archaic elements:

1. It is built upon those just-mentioned observations of the *phobic core.* In Vera's case these were, in early childhood, the rabbit which had turned into an animal of terror (a "killer"-rabbit), and with it also the cracks in the wall which made her scared. Later, the phobic anxiety shifted to the wall itself: every instance of being closed in, whether in physical form or much more importantly, as closeness, as intimate relationships and feelings, or whether as professional obligations, evoked in her a restless tension that she tried to master by acts of breaking out and rebelling, often causing much harm to herself. This *claustrophobia* often found sudden concrete expression in the delusional figure of the persecutor sallying forth from closet or wall. This shading over into what was paranoid cannot deceive us, however, about the enduring basically phobic character of the disturbance. In the phobic core, drive-, reality-, and superego-dangers are *condensed* into an outer object. Her own drive wishes and affects are experienced as if they came from without, and in reversed direction (her death wishes against the brother, now turned against herself); they are being *projected.* The anxiety caused by the traumatic events in the surroundings (as noted—overstimulation, frustration, and pro-hibition), and hence the *reality anxiety* (*Realangst*), *shifted* from the trauma-

tizing objects and situations (the intercourse of the parents, experienced against the foil of her deep ambivalence, especially toward her mother, the advent of her siblings, her mother's outbursts of cold rage, and her father's seductive, yet soul-blind attitude, at least as she had experienced it) to adjacent or otherwise mythically linked things which more easily could be evaded or altered: the darkness and the cracks in the wall, the rabbit; they were being *displaced*. At the same time, the phobic objects and situations may have powerfully served the symbolic representation of the *superego anxiety*.

2. Standing opposite to these objects and situations of dread, there are always those that seem to promise *protection and redemption*. The lovers as well as the analysis were being sought as protective figures, compulsively, or in her words, addictively, but they constantly threatened to flip over into their opposite. These protective figures have just as much of a *total and mythical* quality as is the case basically for the anxiety objects. They own the power of safeguarding only by dint of their (hidden) capacity for violence and cruelty. Like the numinous powers of religion, they still show clear traces of hatred and fear. Freud (1913) spoke of their *"dangerous sanctity"* (*gefährliche Heiligkeit*, Germ. ed., GW 9, p. 53).

3. Both aspects live on with particular force in *archaic superego constellations* that persist side by side with more adapted, milder configurations. This must perforce lead to massive *superego splits and superego conflicts*, that is, to conflicts about values and ideals of often tragic dimension, precisely due to the overwhelming intensity of the feelings involved. Under the impact of these massive contradictions in the superego, there arise those typical *identity splits*, that doubleness in the experience of self and world. Particularly characteristic are the juxtaposition and the opposition of guilt- and shame-conflicts. In Vera's case it was the paternal ideals of competence, of ethical sensitivity, culture, and erudition that stood in sharp contradiction to the archaic ideal of untouchability and impenetrability, of emotional coldness and invulnerability, the values and the ideal of maternal power: "There they stand, the heavy cats of granite, the values of antiquity: Woe, how do you want to overthrow *these?* . . . Scratch-cats with bound paws, here they sit and look venom" (Nietzsche, "Fragments" in *Twilight of the Gods*).[5]

These fundamental superego conflicts inevitably lead to severe forms of the affect of resentment, be it as the expression of one's own conviction or as an attribute of the superego itself, as what Nietzsche (1887) called "the resentment in the structure of moralities" (*das Ressentiment im Aufbau der Moralen*).

4. The repetition compulsion shows up in demonic irruptions of certain sequences of behavior. The avoidance of anxiety objects and the driven

search for saviors determine action sequences, usually of an impulsive nature; to the outsider they give the impression of a sudden massive personality change, in fact that of a *demonic possession*. These *impulsive actions*—the hunt for the lover, in other cases for drugs, for revenge, for power—carry in themselves the germ of thwarting exactly that which is striven for most: the deliverance from the pressure of anxiety. It is an integral part of the impulsive action sequence that it must lead to defeat. Just as the expression *repetition compulsion* indicates, these impulsive actions have a peculiarly compulsive character; the attributes of stereotypy, inappropriateness, and irresistibility, which mark the neurotic process generally (Kubie 1954), are especially prominent in them. It is also inherent in them that they are circular. What this means dynamically will be taken up later on, in Chapter 6.

5. An essential external sign of the split of self and world consists in the conspicuousness of the defense functions ("mechanisms") of externalization and projection, of turning passive into active, and particularly of *denial*, the blindness in the face of the emotional significance of broad parts of reality. Denial and turning passive into active have also been called precursors of defense, or defense forms directed against the outside world, not against the drives or the superego (Sandler and A. Freud 1985).

Vera often described the blatant disavowal of reality by both of her parents, especially by her father: "It is the denial of reality: He makes stupid little jokes that one day I'll come down from the mountain married. He can't face it that I'm alone and 33 and unmarried; it is simply not true for him that I suffer under it and am depressed and suicidal. He can't see it, he denies it—a total lack of vision. Instead of listening he is lecturing me and gives me useless advice. I'm the result of their denial . . . There is no recourse, no acceptable way to express grievances. The result was always to be cut off, to be condemned; the feeling of impotence and humiliation was overwhelming . . . I was left with my impotent fury and full of shame" [952–954]. Her own pounding on the sinister reality could not be heard: "It was most important that she [mother] and my father never listened to me" [955]; that they *could not hear.*

The emphasis on the just-mentioned defensive processes should in no way detract from the central significance and power of *repression* shaping the entire process.

6. The repressed conflicts are both of oedipal and of preoedipal origin. They always have to do, though by no means exclusively, with *competition*, not only in the triangular relationship with her parents, but very much also with siblings (and substitutes for them), and are thus reminiscent not merely of the tragedy of Oedipus, but very much also of Cain. Yet, as commented

upon at least briefly in the case discussion, the conflict between the wish for self-assertion and *individuation* versus the wish for love and *dependency* turns out to be just as relevant. This conflict is often presented in connection with the separation and individuation phase and encompasses of course also the anal conflicts about power and submission, defiance and cleanliness. This conflict about individuation and dependency, about separateness and belonging, about autonomy and self-object relation gives, with its sharpness, their full brisance to the rivalries. In some of these cases, the disturbance could anamnestically be traced further back into preverbal layers. The characteristic *affective storms* appear to be the heirs of this earliest (oral) time and speak for the faulty affect regulation between child and environment (Lichtenberg 1986, D. Stern 1985), although this can of course not be compellingly proven.

Certainly, however, oedipal and preoedipal conflicts are intertwined with each other and cannot be cleanly teased out. Pathogenesis appears to be rather *panphasic* than only attributable to regression from oedipal conflicts, as attested by the presence of oral, anal, and phallic conflicts in the structure of the neurosis and the early history of symptoms.

7. An otherwise *rigid character structure* serves as a safeguard against these six factors, especially against the demonic irruptions, and allows patients to function quite well in circumscribed areas of their lives, at times even excellently. This character structure may be obsessive-compulsive, hysterical, depressive, or phobic, and correlates with the above six factors in specific ways. There is no gap between them. Rather, the character structure is a further development of the same protective structures, the same defense forms, the same anxieties, and the same conflicts, a development that, at any given time, takes into account the changed developmental phase and surrounding. Yet, these character structures break down in the situations described before as clinical regression. The *double life* between the episodes of demonic drivenness and an existence of orderliness and adaptedness that is a hallmark of all these patients is what I have above all tried to anticipate with the original title of this book, *Flight from Conscience*, although in addition I wanted to hint with it at other versions of doubleness and complementarity to be brought up later.

If we look once more over these six main factors, which are set against the "normal life" as the seventh, their repetitive occurrence from patient to patient is striking:

1. Phobic core with affective storms and taboo objects;
2. Mythical protective system and mythical belief;
3. Radical and irreconcilable value conflicts and split identity;

4. Impulsive actions of a nearly ritualistic kind;
5. Denial (blinding) and reversal (especially from passive to active);
6. Multilayeredness of core conflicts.

These six recurrent factors appear to make up a largely unconsciously motivated and motivating "complex" that is not completely identical with the Oedipus complex, but also cannot be clearly severed from it; the "complexes" overlap. In contrast to the Oedipus complex, we deal here rather with a formal ordering principle that recurs in the severe neuroses and, at least in the form presented, does not have to be universal. Each part is in itself already a compromise formation, and the entire constellation a series of solutions to a coherent group of conflicts.

I was wondering whether this important and often reencountered "complex" could be earmarked with a poignant term. To begin with, even the concept of the "complex" is unclear, historically weighed down and too narrow, not to speak of possible rivalry with the "Oedipus complex" and the "inferiority complex." "Syndrome" is too much slanted toward diagnostics and phenomenology and not sufficiently dynamic. Therefore it would be better to speak of a *configuration* or *constellation*. To specify these further, the concepts used up to now, like "phobic core," "demonic possession," or impulsive action sequence, do not suffice because they always only select part of the whole and describe it without explaining it. I was also thinking of some encompassing mythical symbols; although they are not explanatory either, they are rich in meaning and thus may, as concentrated ideas, point to these recurrent connections. I was thinking of Cain, of the character of Philoctetes, of the figure of the demonic double, of the Biblical system of *Havdala* (the division between pure and impure, sacred and profane, good and evil, protection and danger)—or, like Freud (1913), totem and taboo. It was, however, finally the patient's own suggestion which seemed to me most evocative—the image of *Cassandra*, in its powerful shaping by Aeschylus and Schiller, united most of the mentioned elements.

Cassandra, the daughter of the Trojan king Priam, refused to conceive from Apollo, and as a punishment her gift of prophecy, earlier presented to her by the god, was changed so that while she anticipated all the calamities, but that no one would believe her—"the horrible pain of the correct prediction—δεινὸς ὀρθομαντείας πόνος" [deinós orthomanteías pónos] (Aeschylus, *Agamemnon*, v. 1215).

And they scold my plaints, and they jeer my pain; I have to carry lonely my tormented heart to the desert, avoided by those who are happy and an object of scorn to those who are glad! You, Pythian, have assigned to me a hard lot, you malicious god! Why did you throw me, with the unlocked mind, to pronounce your oracle, into the city of the eternally blind? Why did you give me the ability to see what I cannot avert anyway? What has been imposed must happen, what is dreaded must approach.[6]

She flees from the joyful marriage celebration of her sister Polyxene (the "hospitable one"), who weds Achilles. How can happiness be possible? "Who could enjoy life who has looked into its abyss!" "Wherever I wander, wherever I walk, I see the ghosts surrounding me."[7] "And, lost in her pain, was only *one* soul. Joyless in the plenty of joy, unsociable and alone . . . Everything opens itself to joy, all the hearts are happy . . .".[8] It will be her brother Paris who will insidiously bring disaster over her family and her world and ruin her, her sister, and her brother-in-law. "And I see the murderous steel glisten and the murderous eye glow, I cannot flee to the right or to the left from the horror; I am unable to avert my sight, I have to complete my fate, knowing, seeing, steadfast, falling in the foreign land."[9]

Troy falls, and Cassandra is abducted to Mycene. In Aeschylus she appears as a foreign slave and "chosen blossom" (ll.954/955). In wordless terror, in inarticulate stammer and outcry of lament, "ὀτοτοτοτοῖ πόποι δᾶ— *otototototoi pópoi da*," she sees the imminent horror, perceives the spirits of revenge dancing on the roof of the palace of Atreus. She struggles against being dragged into the house of the "fatal coils" and laments the little children who had been slaughtered and roasted, served up to their own father Thyestes. She knows she herself will now be captured in the deadly net of the murderess, slaughtered together with her master. "Pain floods my song of suffering" (l.1137).

> What use is it to lift the veil where horror nearby threatens? Error only is life, and knowledge is death. Take away from my eyes the sad clarity, the bloody vision [or: the sheen of blood]! It is terrible to be the mortal vessel of your truth. Give back to me my blindness and the gladly dark mind! I never sang joyous songs since I have become *your* voice. You have given me future, but you have robbed me of the instant, robbed me of the hour's glad life—take away your perfidious present.[10]

Here we find all the elements gathered together: the core of anxiety and the flooding quality of pain and horror, the yearning for the protector, idealization and devaluation of what is prohibited and sacred, nearness to the godhead changing into curse and doom, the doubleness of knowing and refusal to believe what is being announced and thus the doubleness of reality, that is, the denial of the dark prophecy by the others, but also her own inability to see and experience what is good in the present, the kind of denial typical for the depressed; the rising up in revolt in an act of defiantly throwing off the power of knowledge and conscience ("and angrily she threw the priestess' band down to the earth") (*und sie warf die Priesterbinde zu der Erde zürnend hin*) and the multilayered nature of the underlying conflicts: spouse and lover, motherhood and prophecy, perdition of the family and joining as victim of slaughter the slaughterer of her own family.

In this, a very particular motive appears to me to shine forth thoughout: that of the *slaughter of the children*. It is the killing of the siblings that again and again resonates as a main motive both in the Trojan and in the Mycenean scene—Polyxene, Paris, Thyestes and Atreus, Iphigeneia. And, looming over it, stands Nemesis, the cry for justice, the profound sense of injustice, and punishment at its absolute and extreme.

Strikingly, the same motive of the slaughter of the children occurs also in Vera's core phobia: in the shape of the rabbit pursuing her. The *killing of the children* by siblings or parents is a motive that we shall encounter also in several of the later cases. Although this motive is closely linked with the Oedipus complex (in fact, it is part of the Oedipus motif, since Oedipus himself had been mutilated and exposed in the wilderness, after the father's wish to have him die), it does not appear to be reducible to it and possesses its own dignity and importance. I mean with that above all the wish to kill one of the siblings, especially one that is younger, in order thus to (re)gain love, power, and special position as child, and the fear to be slain in turn by the parents or at least sent away by them, expelled. The affect of resentment and the archaic intensity of the superego is strongly bound up with this motive.

In contrast to the Oedipus conflict, the configuration probably has less to do with impulses of infantile sexuality than with the wishes for self-affirmation, the other strong drive that in the later theory of Freud has been, in my view wrongly, "devoured" by the "instinctual drive" of aggression and the concept of narcissism and only now, with the investigation of early infancy, may regain more of its dues.

If we put this postulated *Cassandra configuration* in relation to the Oedipus complex, I believe that the either-or, as in so many other regards, is mistaken. The one does not replace the other. This configuration, which is built upon the phobic core and often contains that motif of infanticide, is a valuable model in its own right. With that, though, I do not want to claim that its phobic core always has to refer to the murder of siblings and children. Frequently it is the oedipal conflict that makes up the content of the phobic fear and with it also determines the protective measures and the other factors of the configuration. We have only to remind ourselves of Little Hans (Freud 1909). It is rather the case that the *phobic core gathers in itself the anxieties resulting from all the conflicts of early childhood.* It is probably typical that all three rivalry conflicts outlined in Vera's case have gained entrance into the phobic core and that, as with her, earlier and earliest conflicts are drawn into it.

The intrapsychic perspective does not suffice; that of the family dynamic needs to be added: the image of the cold and condemning mother as murderous avenger, Clytaemnestra, accompanies that of Cassandra, as it does in Vera's imaginative account. So does the figure of the hero of rape and pillage who sacrifices his daughter for the purposes of his leadership, Agamemnon, and the cruelly seductive, yet disdainfully rejecting, indignant God, Apollo. Then there is the spirit of grave injustice done and suffered, and the craving for revenge and punishment haunting the preceding generations down to the present—the Furies dancing on the roof of the Atreids.

Our observations led to a second central conflict that also was involved in this patient. Frequently, it goes under the heading of the separation-individuation phase: "When I assert myself and turn away from my mother I lose her love and my belonging that I need so much. But when I retreat into the shelteredness with her I run the risk of dissolving myself in her, and losing myself again." *Merger* and *defiant independence* are the two poles of this conflict—and it is a very basic and cardinal conflict—and many trials at safeguard and solution are employed in order to satisfy both of these so essential needs.

As the modern research of early childhood shows, there are good reasons to view this doubleness of individuation and object relation as something given from the very beginning, although, of course, not necessarily as inner conflict nor in form of mental representations of self and object (Lichtenberg 1983), and not merely as something arising at the end of the second year of life (D. Stern 1985), although there is a culmination of it at that time.

Moreover, there are at least some hints that pronouncedly neurotic phobias can be observed already in babies under 12 months of age (Cramer, in D. Stern [1985], p. 224ff).

Other conflicts derive from the overwhelming affects inherent in overstimulation and still others from early perceptual-expressive interactions.

To be sure, the earlier conflicts are recognizable in analysis only in their derivative versions as remembered from later times, not in their primary shapes; in Vera's case, for example, in the form of conflicts between wishes of primitive identification and union versus those of defiant self-delimitation, or the conflicts between global affects, commands of unconditionality, and judgments of absolute correctness versus those of reasonable limitation and human restrictedness—that is, conflicts commonly called "narcissistic."

To what extent this Cassandra configuration can be detected in other cases and whether we might not uncover other repetitive configurations the next case examples (see Chapter 5 and *Flight from Conscience*) will show.

Would it not be conceivable that some of the other life-determining conflicts we just spoke of (basic needs for separateness and individuation versus those for love, dependency, and belonging) would lead to characteristic configurations ("complexes") which would be frequently and powerfully combined with the "Cassandra configuration"? The experience with Vera lets us assume this as likely when we think of the contradictory identifications, the massive and primitive introjections, the role reversals, the radical antithesis of archaic feelings of shame and guilt, and the anal-sadistic (not only phallic-sadistic) ideal formation. The next case will give us more information about this.

Before we turn to this, I would like to give some deepened thought to the more general questions of trauma, defect, and conflict, and with them the entire structure of psychoanalytically relevant causality. Not only does the just-presented case circle around these issues, but so do all the studies to follow. Logically, these considerations would fit best in the concluding chapter. Yet they are so fundamental and form so much of the background to everything that follows that I have decided to let them follow here.

## THE COMPLEMENTARITY OF DEFICIT AND CONFLICT

In the discussion about the nature and origin of the character and personality problems of severe neuroses, the question often arises: Are they caused by conflict or are they the result of developmental deficits? As basic explanatory paradigms for severe neurotic as well as for psychotic illnesses, both concepts are significant and useful. They fail, however, if they are forced to serve as shibboleths between different diagnoses and approaches. As so commonly in our field, it is a matter of complementarity, of as-well-as, not of an either–or choice. All neuroses show superficial or deeper defects. They are derived from conflicts, or they lead to new conflicts. More important, however, than ascertaining such defects are the manifold *fantasies of defectivness* that themselves lead to deep shame. Shame fantasies are in fact such inner convictions that we have a flaw reaching to the very core of our being, a fault that cannot be repaired, a stain that can never be removed. In the case I am shortly going to present in detail this will be presented in sharp profile.

The question of deficit versus conflict also led me to consider its technical implications. The sharpness of this debate goes back to the split between Kohut's (1971, 1977) self psychology and the mainstream of psychoanalysis. I always decidedly took my stand on the side of the latter, specifically putting conflict entirely in the center of the psychoanalytic model of causality, and hence also the primacy of defense analysis, in the tradition of Anna Freud. Above all, it was the judgmental quality in the concept of deficit and defect that impelled me to employ it only with great restraint. The risk with it is always that we fall into blaming and accusing. Moreover, the leap from description to explanation seemed to me far too quick; the entire neurosis standing in-between is jumped over. Visible "defects" in the control of affects and impulses are results of highly complicated processes, and we can state only at the end of a well conducted therapy, above all an analysis, if and why these "defects" were lifted or have remained. Hilgers (1996) notes by right that "impairments of reality testing, of affect and impulse control, of perception, of memory, of motor functions, etc. [all of which he counts as 'ego structural deficits'] lead perforce to secondary shame conflicts, regardless whether there was a primary causative shame dynamics as well" (p. 30).

Conflict was central in my explanatory schema but trauma gained more and more importance in it. But the recognition of the ubiquitous causal significance of chronic traumatization not only had theoretical relevance, but also consequences for the technique. A technique revolving entirely around conflict gives pride of place to insight and the solution of conflict ultimately by cognitive means, and views in these the Alpha and Omega of therapeutic change. Yet in my work with severely ill patients, it was always clear to me that change occurred not only due to insight, with all its huge complexity, but also, parallel to it, thanks to factors of the interpersonal relation in the treatment. Always and inevitably, psychagogical, that is, suggestive interventions played a role, and very much so with decisive, long-lasting effectiveness, not merely as momentary adjuvants. Here too a one-sided either-or turned out to be wrong. Such one-sided emphasis is anyway not what most serious thinkers present; almost always it is a matter of "weighting."

Still, the rethinking of this question led me to see many phenomena and problems of technique in a new light—not in the sense of some great confession, but in that of a gradual shift in thinking.

To begin with, the concepts of "deficit" and of "defect" are used in practice as if they were synonymous. They are not, although they overlap. Both stem from the Latin *deficere*: "to detach oneself, to be diminished, to vanish, to start lacking"; *defectus* means "weakened, having lost power." "Deficit" (the active, present form) means according to *Webster's Unabridged Dictionary* "the amount by which a sum of money is less than what is expected, due, needed, etc.; shortage." On the other hand, "defect" is not only a "lack or absence of something necessary for completeness; shortcoming," but very importantly also "an imperfection; fault; flaw; blemish; deformity." In our context, "deficit" refers to the fact that too little comes in from without, whereas "defect" means the fault or flaw in product or development. Thus, deficit may very well lead to defect, but they are not identical. This same doubleness of meaning we will encounter shortly with the trauma concept.

Recently Merton Gill (1994b) wrote a review-essay with the title "Conflict and Deficit," in which the main thoughts are worked out in a particularly clear way, although he appears to use "deficit" and "defect" synonymously. I give here some thoughts from this paper that have struck me as particularly pertinent. He suggests that the use of the idea of development is a disguised reference to deficit, inasmuch as deficit is, in the view of those who give it explanatory preference over conflict, the intrapsychic consequence of trauma. He proposes that the real theme in the dispute between concepts of conflict and deficit is that of the relative roles of drive and experience, and cites Anna Freud (1974, p. 70):

> We can . . . differentiate between two types of infantile psychopathology. The one based on conflict is responsible for anxiety states and the . . . infantile neuroses; the one based on developmental defects [deficit?], for the psychosomatic symptomatology, the backwardness, the atypical and borderline states. [p. 758 f., added by Gill]

Classical psychoanalysis has (in Gill's view) minimized the role of experience, whereas self psychology has been accused by many of assigning too much importance to experience and empathy. The preponderance of the therapeutic relationship over insight corresponds (in Ornstein's essay) to this stress on experience, hence on outer reality, on potential trauma and deficit (Gill 1994b, p. 762): ". . . the word trauma emphasizes the external event, whereas the word deficit emphasizes the intrapsychic effect of the event" (p. 765). In Gill's view the struggle is really about the relative importance of event or drive:

> Mainstream analysts . . . use different words than deficit to convey the same idea. They are willing to speak of ego weakness, even of Freud's concept of congenital ego vulnerabilities, but then do not recognize the equivalence of such concepts to the concept of deficit. [p. 765]

He answers his own question as to the reason for this by opining that, in addition to their negation of the existence of drives,

> an important one is that the idea of deficit connotes to many . . . an absence of something, a hole in the psyche. The notion of a hole in the psyche, of course, makes no sense. Psychic structure may be other than desirable, but it cannot be absent. . . . The idea of a hole in the psyche can exert a pernicious effect on both theory and practice, because a manifest subjective sense of deficit or absence on the part of the analysand may be accepted by the analyst without further investigation [pp. 765–766],

a criticism leveled by rights against some of Kohut's assumptions, for example in regard to fragmentation. A second reason for this rejection of the deficit concept by mainstream analysts is the implication that a deficit calls for remedial activity, on the analyst's part, to make up for what is missing—namely as "corrective emotional experience"—something forbidden in recent classical psychoanalysis as contravening "neutrality." Gill suggests that this attitude against the concept of deficit begins to waver. In the words of Boesky, in the volume discussed: "My prediction is that as we refine our criteria of evidence and learn more about the interrelation between insight and relational factors we will discover that the sharp distinction between these two categories masks the complexity of the manner in which they are related" (p. 766). And, "In my opinion the profound importance of the interaction between the patient and analyst is indisputable" (p. 766; quote from p. 187 of the book reviewed). Again, in Gill's view, this dispute is not a matter of either-or but of the *relative weighting* of drive versus experience, hence of interpretation and insight versus therapeutic relationship, of neutrality and anonymity as the attitude in a one-person model versus interaction and a two-person model of the psychoanalytic situation; and, last but not least, of the theoretical valence of inner conflict versus trauma. As Gill (1996) explains in another essay, "the dispute is about whether instinctual drive, an innate factor, or interpersonal interaction, an experiential factor, is the primary organizing principle" (p. 129). The answer is to be found in their *complementarity*. He refers to the decisive statement by Freud in "The Dynamics of Transference" (1912, p. 99):

> . . . in connection with the idea of a series in which constitution[al] and "accidental" (experiential) factors are complemental, Freud writes of "the restricted

nature of what men look for in the field of causation: in contrast to what ordinarily holds good in the real world, people prefer to be satisfied with a single causative factor." [Gill 1996, p. 127][11]

Gill (1996) talks therefore about "complemental interaction" (p. 133).

## TRAUMA

As already mentioned, the understanding of deficit and defect and of trauma is very tightly correlated. In the book reviewed by Gill, Arlow defines "trauma" as "a special vicissitude of development, seen in the context of continuing intrapsychic conflict" (Gill 1994b, p. 757), whereas we just came across Gill's calling it simply an external event.

I would like to briefly review now the development of the trauma concept.

The Greek word signifies "wound, injury" and also "defeat," from the words *troein*, "to wound, to pierce, to charm," and *terein*, "to rub, to torment, to torture."

In the Preliminary Communication Freud (1893) notes that the causation of hysteria usually lies in "psychical trauma," and he defines this so: "Any experience which calls up distressing[12] affects—such as those of fright, anxiety, shame or emotional pain—may operate as a trauma of this kind" (p. 6). He adds that often "instead of a single, major trauma, we find a number of partial traumas forming a group of provoking causes. These have only been able to exercise a traumatic effect by summation . . ." (p. 6). It is then of greatest importance

> *whether there has been an energetic reaction to the event that provokes an affect.* . . . If the reaction is suppressed, the affect remains attached to the memory. . . . the injured person's reaction to the trauma only exercises a completely "*cathartic*" effect if it is an adequate reaction—as, for instance, revenge. But language serves as a substitute for action; by its help, an affect can be "abreacted" almost as effectively. [p. 8]

In the Discussion (*Epikrise*) of the case of Frau Emmy von N., he and Breuer state: ". . . we regard hysterical symptoms as the effects and residues of excitations which have acted upon the nervous system as traumas. Residues of this kind are not left behind if the original excitation has been discharged by abreaction or thought-activity" (p. 86). Conversion is being defined as "the transformation of psychical excitation into chronic somatic symptoms" (p. 86). Usually such transformation occurs incompletely; in its place we encounter "alterations of mood (anxiety, melancholic depression), phobias and abulias (inhibitions of will)" (p. 86). These symptoms are seen by Freud as due to trauma, not, as claimed at the time by French psychiatry, "as stigmata of neurotic degeneracy" (p. 87).[13]

In the case description of Miss Lucy R., Freud takes a decisive step ahead when he refers to experiences "in which opposing affects had been in conflict with each other" (p. 115), and he states poignantly: "The conflict between her affects had elevated the moment into a trauma, and the sensation of smell that was associated with this trauma persisted as its symbol" (pp. 115–116).

> The actual traumatic moment, then, is the one at which the incompatibility forces itself upon the ego and at which the latter decides on the repudiation of the incompatible idea. That idea is not annihilated by a repudiation of this kind, but merely repressed into the unconscious. [p. 123]

The result is "a splitting of consciousness" which is "a deliberate and intentional one. At least it is often introduced by an act of volition" (p. 123). He notes later that "it was a peculiar state of knowing and at the same time not knowing—a state, that is, in which a psychical group was cut off" (p. 165). It is theoretically crucial that the traumatic moment is one in which the conflict is conscious (pp. 167 f.).

Thirty years before this description of trauma by Freud, the great English novelist Eliot wrote in *Romola* (1862/63, p. 425) how her protagonist, informed about the infamous treachery and adultery of her husband, "sat paralysed by the shock of conflicting feelings."

Thirty years after the "Studies on Hysteria," Freud (1926) calls more generally "a situation of helplessness that has been actually experienced a traumatic situation," distinguishes between "physical helplessness if the danger is real and psychical helplessness if it is instinctual" (the former being traumatic), and adds that "anxiety is . . . on the one hand an expectation of a trauma, and on the other a repetition of it in a mitigated form. . . . The ego, which experienced the trauma passively, now repeats it actively in a weakened version, in the hope of being able itself to direct its course" (pp. 166 f.). The repetition refers here not only to the anxiety signal ("reproduced . . . as a signal of help"), but to the much more general "changing from passivity to activity," which is now equated with the earlier understanding of "abreacting a trauma" (p. 167).

Krystal (1988) asserts incisively: ". . . trauma refers to an overwhelming, paralyzing psychic state, which implies a loss of ego functions, regression, and obligatory psychopathology" (p. 145). I have already quoted in Chapter 1 the definition of trauma from Moore and Fine (1990).

Similar is the formulation of Inderbitzin and Levy (1998): "Trauma is regularly defined as the ego being overwhelmed by internal or external forces that render it helpless in its immediate adaptive efforts" (p. 38).

If we look outside of the confines of psychoanalysis we see that at present this question of psychic trauma has assumed new actuality in the modern psychiatric literature. Herman, Perry, and van der Kolk (1989) describe the very close relationship between borderline pathology and severe traumatization whereby they restrict this term to physical abuse, sexual abuse, and witnessing domestic violence. What is omitted are other important traumata, like early abandonment, severe physical diseases, and operative interventions, and above all emotional abuse that has, as we know from our work with patients, a particularly persistent effect. I remind you of the words of Goethe: "Doch ein gekränktes Herz erholt sich schwer" (*Torquato Tasso* IV, 4) ("But an offended heart recovers only slowly"). Freud (1896) also says that small slights at present trigger the symptoms, but behind them lies a long series of earlier perceived slights, "behind all of which there lies in addition the memory of a serious slight in childhood which has never been overcome" (p. 217).

Moreover, those investigators take only severe forms of such traumatization into account. Even so, they find such severe traumata, especially in the first six years of life, in 81 percent of borderline patients (those that I usually would rather call "severe neuroses"), whereas they find this in patients with other diagnoses only in 35 percent. They conclude therefore that "the hypothesis that childhood abuse has a major formative role in the development of the [borderline] disorder is strongly supported by our findings" (Herman et al. 1989, p. 493). In another study, van der Kolk and coworkers (1996) bring the symptoms of *dissociation, somatization, and affect dysregulation* in close connection with long-lasting and severe traumatization, particularly in early childhood; they view the damage done mostly in terms of defect.

Disturbances of affect regulation consist of "unmodulated anger and sexual involvement, self-destructive behaviors, and chronic suicidality" (p. 85). They note (again as defects):

> An impaired capacity to process information and to differentiate relevant from irrelevant information may be at the root of the disturbed memory and concentration in PTSD . . . as Nemiah proposes, dissociation (i.e., "a disruption in the usually integrated functions of consciousness, memory, identity, or perception of the environment" . . .) represents the core issue in PTSD. [pp. 90, 91]

In my own view, we could define trauma as an overwhelming, unsolvable external conflict between self and environment whereas Freud, as we found, saw it as moment of a conscious inner conflict. I do not believe that these two are contradictory, but that they are two sides of the same coin: *In the trauma the conflict between self and outside changes to a conscious but unsolvable inner conflict.* The affects battling each other overwhelm the capacity of the ego to master them, a failure that leads to the split between the groups of ideas and to the act of making the connections unconscious, about which Freud originally was speaking. Dissociation and even hypnoid states, for us, are also important concepts for the understanding of the traumatic genesis of the severe neuroses. However, these phenomena themselves should be comprehended much more importantly as expressions of the attempt to deal with inner conflict rather than simply as defects.

Accordingly, Richard Gottlieb (1997) views dissociation or the "multiplicity of selves" due to traumatization not as the result of a mechanical process of disintegration, but as the expression of a powerful and organizing defensive, protective and wishful fantasy of being owned and controlled by other persons.

Inderbitzin and Levy (1998) criticize the literature on psychic trauma for its onesidedness, especially for its disregard of the severity of *conflicts about aggression*:

> In our view, what is regularly absent from such formulations is a consideration of the intense frustration and ensuing aggression such trauma generates and the opportunities for aggression provided by "re-experiencing trauma." The trauma appears to take on an instinct-like role that really belongs to the aggression created by the trauma. [p. 41]

Therefore, the manifest disturbances are then ascribed to defect and damage, instead of conflict and compromise:

> We wish to underline the vast, complicated array of defenses against aggression that are poorly regulated and integrated when trauma has significantly interfered with ego development and object relations. In such instances, fantasy cannot be utilized to transform the traumatic disturbances. In the stereotyped victim and victimizer repetitions that ensue, turning of aggression on the self and identification with the aggressor are central. [p. 45]

Part of the appropriate technique consists therefore in the "systematic interpretation of the massive defenses against aggression" (p. 49). Repetition compulsion, postulated as an elementary force and a basic cause, is a pseudoexplanation.

Marion Oliner (in a yet unpublished study, "Analysts Confront the Holocaust: the Unsolved Puzzle of Trauma" [1998]) examines closely the one aspect of posttraumatic disorders that is most frequently attributed to a defect: dissociation. She stresses the defensive quality of the shift in experience from *representation* to *presentation*:

> . . . one of the most important residues of trauma resides in the creation of duality caused by the persistence of unchanging and unassimilated *presentations* alongside the normal memories that change and fade with time. The apparently factual nature of the memory of these events, their denuded reality, wards off their integration into psychic reality and lends itself to be used for purposes of defense . . . , especially against guilt. These clearly remembered events can serve as a screen against the awareness of the manner in which they are *represented symbolically*.

Depersonalization as defense appears in the form of hypnoid states or autohypnosis. The duality consists in the parallel existence of presentation and representation; the former wards off the latter. For Oliner, it is also the role of conflict, specifically about omnipotent aggression and the corresponding feelings of omnipotence of guilt, which causes the duality.

## EXTREMISM

At present this question of psychic trauma has assumed new actuality with the controversies swirling around the alleged frequency of repressed sexual abuse.

On the one side there are those who believe in the almost ubiquitous occurrence of severe sexual traumatization which, although repressed, is said to exert an uncanny power. On the other side there are the critics who want to destroy the concept of repression altogether and, with it, deny psychoanalysis its right to exist. In the first group are zealots of repressed memory, who are convinced that they can infer from superficial symptoms and single dreams the suffered sexual seduction and violation of their patients. They then impose those interpretations with great suggestive powers upon their patients and induce them to accuse their fathers and mothers of heinous crimes.

> While Andrea Dworkin and Susan Brownmiller were hypothesizing that American fathers regularly rape their daughters in order to teach them what it means to be inferior, Bass and Davis set about to succor the tens of millions of victims who must have repressed that ordeal. [Crews 1994b, p. 49]

Families are torn apart, marriages destroyed, men and occasionally women sent for decades to prison, without recourse to further evidence. Wright (n.d.) says therefore: ". . . whatever the value of repression as a scientific concept or a therapeutic tool, unquestioning belief in it has become as dangerous as the belief in witches" (Crews 1994a, p. 59).

In the second camp we find nonclinicians, like Crews (1994a,b) and Grünbaum (1984), who assert that the concept of repression is without empirical support, and that the power of suggestion is such that all the claims of psychoanalysis for scientific truth are without basis and its character not much better than demonology.

Obviously and unfortunately, the criticism of the practices of the first camp are only too justified; they can very well be accounted for by the realm of mass hysteria. The polemics by the second group induce us again and again to reflect on the epistemological foundations of our own work and understanding, although their anankastic quibbling and *pars pro toto* reasoning leave them strangely uncomprehending as to what really goes on in psychoanalytic work and hence make them remarkably irrelevant, in spite of their clamor for attention.

## TRAUMA IN THE SEVERE NEUROSES
## AND AFFECT DYSREGULATION

How does the question of repressed trauma relate to my own experience with the severe neuroses, with an approach where I am particularly careful with interpretations, particularly cautious with the factor of suggestiveness? Most importantly, how can we understand the consequences of severe traumatization and their treatment?

Almost all my patients with severe neuroses (and even those with less severe manifest pathology) have been massively traumatized, often chronically so throughout childhood, and even later on. But it has *not been my experience that even with these patients those traumata have become unconscious,* and that their lifting out of such amnesia would have been the decisive mutative factor. I don't claim that this does not exist, but it has not been my observation. It was rather the case that the main affects and the attempts to gain control over them, the main anxieties and wishes engendered by those traumata, and with that the conflicts derived from them, have become or remained largely unconscious and are at the center of our therapeutic work. Their transformation into words (and other symbols) and the partial resolution of those conflicts have clearly had the mutative effect and justify the psychoanalytic endeavor.

As already noted, in our experience as psychoanalysts, in contrast to the methodological presupposition of the research mentioned before, verbal-emotional traumata are in their pathogenicity at least as important as the concretely perceptual variants, like physical or sexual mistreatment. Therefore, those sensory processes, the repetitive intrusion of specific perceptions, recede in importance in this type of cases. The amnesia affects the emotions rather than aspects of the physical facts.

There are, of course, many forms of traumatization, but of special importance is what we can call *soul blindness* and *soul murder*. *Soul blindness* is a systematic, chronic disregard for the emotional needs and expressions of the child, a peculiar blindness to its individuality and hostility to its autonomy. It shows itself as the peculiar dehumanization of the other person, as that which Francis Brouček (1991) has called "objectification" and postulated as the core of the shame experience. As to *soul murder*, Shengold (1989) defines it as "the deliberate attempt to eradicate or compromise the separate identity of another person . . . depriving the victim of the ability to feel joy and love as a separate person" (p. 2). It stands "for a certain category of traumatic experience: instances of repetitive and chronic overstimulation, alternating with emotional deprivation, that are deliberately brought about by another individual" (p. 16). The first term refers to something that is too little, the second to something that is too much; yet they cannot be clearly separated and belong clinically closely together. Also, trauma and inner conflict are complementary concepts.

I return now to the concept put forth by van der Kolk as central for traumatization: affect dysregulation. I believe that by definition it is entailed in the word trauma, specifically in the sense of *affect regression.*

Henry Krystal (1997) distinguishes sharply between the effects of infantile psychic traumatization and the one occurring in adulthood. With the former, it comes to "maximum excitement": "Because of the *nature of* the affect *pre-cursors* (*Uraffects*) and the immaturity of a child's general development, if the mother is unable to relieve the baby in a fairly short time, the affects tend to snowball so that virtually every part of the mind, indeed the whole organism, is in a state of maximum excitement. Eventually the baby becomes virtually *inconsolable.* This represents the onset of infantile psychic trauma state" (p. 131, emphasis original). Severe, repeated traumatization means that every emotional experience resonates as if it were the recurrence of the trauma. It leads to the standstill, usually partial,

of affective development: the differentiation, verbalization, and desomatization of the emotions are blocked.

Thus, in traumatization, by definition, the feelings, once roused, very
rapidly become overwhelming, get out of control, are *global* (*"dedifferenti-
ated"*), *beyond symbolization* (*"deverbalized"*), and are being experienced, as if
they were physical (*"resomatized"*). These three concepts of dedifferentiation,
deverbalization, or hyposymbolization, and of resomatization represent,
according to Krystal (1988), *affect regression.*

He contrasts this with the trauma in adulthood:

> In contrast to infantile psychic trauma, adult trauma *is not brought on by intense
> stimuli or intense emotions.* . . . that is subjective helplessness in the face of what is
> experienced as unavoidable, inescapable danger, and the *surrender to it.* Once
> the *surrender* takes place, the affective state changes to a catatonoid reaction that
> has certain commonalities with cataleptic responses, which in turn have the
> following attributes in common with trances: the more one submits, the more
> one obeys orders and *feels* unable to resist or escape and the more one goes into
> profound surrender. This vicious circle is the initiation of the traumatic pro-
> cess [1997, p. 133]

There is a numbing of physical and emotional pain, an automatonlike
obedience (*Kadavergehorsam*) and increasingly dissociative phenomena. All
mental functions become severely and progressively narrowed down and
switched off, leading to psychic death. Part of this turning-off is alexithymia,
the suppression of all feelings—similar to the one observed in infantile traumatization: "Many alexithymic patients act like those untouchable mothers.
They avoid emotional and physical intimacy." After traumatization and in
the transference, powerful figures are adored like idols who possess everything good and have the power of healing: "idolatrous transference." If they
fail the victim has to suppress his rage, to transform it into guilt and shame,
and to sacrifice his rage in order to appease the increasingly cruel idol. The
function of self-caring is particularly compromised.

I find much in this very valuable. I still believe though that all that he
ascribes to infantile trauma, specifically the enduring affect regression, forms
part of the reaction in adulthood as well. Only in extreme circumstances
(Krystal refers to catastrophic trauma), that "Musselman syndrome" he describes is added to it and eventually may supersede it.

But there is something else of great importance, especially in the recurrent traumatization in childhood: These affects tend to appear in sexualized form. *Sexualization is an archaic defense set up to regulate affect.* The *affect
flooding,* combined with this very primordial *defense by sexualization,* leads,
however, to an overwhelming sense of humiliation and embarrassment. Not

to have any control over one's own emotional life is just as shaming as the loss of sphincter control, if not more so. *Aggressive* wishes are then being used to reestablish control, a form of further archaic defense to deal preventively with a further spiraling out of control, an important way of *turning passive into active*. In this connection it is also very important to see not only the passivity toward the outside, but, even more important, the *ego's passivity* vis-à-vis the affects, the drives, and the lashings by the superego (cf. David Rapaport 1953, see below).

The result of such severe *disturbance of affect regulation* is the archaic equation of (1) *overstimulation* by something on the outside which is being experienced as traumatic, as intolerable, and to which one feels helplessly, passively exposed; (2) *overwhelming, but usually contradictory feelings, the sense of bursting, "I cannot stand it anymore," the traumatic state (that inner state of passivity)*; (3) something *devouring, consuming,* i.e., the imagery of *orality,* like rapacious animals or elements (fire, floods); (4) *sexual excitement; and* (5) *aggressive fantasies and violence, even cruelty.* This archaic equation of traumatogenic affective storms, sexualization, and aggression, which is in turn again deeply frightening and humiliating, calls for equally global defenses, and eventually to massive counteractions by the superego, in form of pervasive and global forms of guilt and shame: ". . . and conscience, turned tyrant, held passion by the throat" (Brontë, p. 238).

Losing control over the affects, the *collapse of affect regulation* and the *conflict between global but opposing affects,* is indeed a *primary danger,* evoking a most profound sense of helplessness, of "fragmentation" and "splitting," and thus deepening in circular form the basic anxiety and shame; it is not even necessary theoretically to resort to fears of abandonment, rejection, castration, or self-condemnation to explain this anxiety. All these latter dreads give, however, very often concrete and specific form, rooted in personal history, to those overwhelming, repetitive traumatic experiences.

## TRAUMATOGENIC SHAME

We have found before as prominent among the frightening affects induced by trauma the feeling of shame in its multilayeredness and depth. Much of psychoanalytic work may consist in listening to the sense of current slights that seem to confirm the feeling of one's own unworth. In fact, the analysis itself can be traumatizing as a repetition of this original link between trauma and shame within the transference, or rather within the real relationship with the therapist. What is this link, however?

One indeed may be massive shaming as part of the trauma, and that seems to be a self-evident connection. But there is far more that we uncover in our analytic work.

Very commonly it is, as noticed above, *the shame about the intensity of feelings* in general, the great anxiety to express them, and the anxiety of inner and outer loss of control. It is so often the premise in the family, supported by cultural prejudice, that it is a sign of disgraceful weakness and thus of vulnerability to show, or even just to have, strong feelings. This causes a great tendency to be deeply ashamed. The body, especially sexuality, may be far less strongly shame inducing than this alleged weakness of having strong feelings: feelings of neediness, of longing, of tenderness, of being moved, of being hurt. Many look then for a partner who is an *anti-shame hero*—someone emotionally untouchable, impenetrable, invulnerable, a disdainful ruler, as we saw in Vera. Looking for acceptance by such a figure and merger with him or her would remove the shame of feeling and wishing too strongly, but it means an almost incorrigible masochistic bondage.

Shame is also caused by the experience that one has not been perceived as a person with the right of his own feelings and will. The *soul blindness* of the other evokes the conviction of great worthlessness; the contempt by the other expressed in disregard for one's own inner life is matched by self-contempt. I mentioned how analysis itself may be shaming and thus inadvertently repeat the traumatogenic shame. There are many ways of doing this: Sometimes it may be the silence to a question, sometimes a sarcastic comment, often direct drive interpretations, and—what I see particularly in my supervisions in Europe—the unempathic, forced relating of every aspect to transference. All this can be felt to be soul blind. Incomprehension and tactlessness are experienced as a renewed deep insult and shaming.

Then there is a fourth important reason: Every kind of excitement turns, as affect regression, into overexcitement and overstimulation, and this has to lead inevitably to a crash, to a very painful disappointment. This traumatic, passively experienced process is again and again turned around into something actively reenacted. How so? It happens in the way that every joy, every gratification, every expectation, everything good has to be broken off and changed into something negative and bad. It seems as if an unconscious guilt makes it appear that one does not deserve to be successful. This may certainly contribute. But that dangerous and mortifying excitement appears to be more important. Thus the inner judge, the archaic superego, has to prevent all pleasure. This too can be observed both macroscopically and in "close process monitoring," and can be explored together.

Closely connected with this is a fifth reason: that of the *intrapsychic passivity*. David Rapaport (1953), as briefly mentioned before, wrote about the passivity of the ego, of that part of our personality that is weighing, considering, deciding, and hence "willing." Often, what appears as ordained from the outside is in truth an *inner passivity in regard to affects and drives*, but also and no less so a *passivity vis-à-vis the threatening and hammering superego*. There is not only profound anxiety about being helplessly delivered to these inner powers, but also shame for such *inner ego-passivity*. Outer victimhood is very often its externalization: a repetition on the outside in the vain attempt to resolve it within.

The result of these developments is a *double reality* within and without: on the one side a world of omnipotence and impotence, full of magical expectations and experiences, a basic masochistic attitude and world orientation (Novick and Novick 1996a,b), which is being determined by the omnipotence of suffering and the omnipotence of responsibility; on the other side a world of competence, of real power through mastery of problems and resolution of conflicts.

In the extreme case we see, as with Vera and Thomas, the alternating invalidation of the feeling of reality. At one time, that whole first world of omnipotence and helplessness is experienced as unreal, like a shell. Only the second world, that of competence, of work, of creativity, retains its character of reality. Only this adaptation is felt to be good; it permits them joy and protection. It is like a railing holding them back from falling into the abyss. Then a massive disappointment occurs, a "narcissistic crisis," and now it is the reverse: only the world of global affects and of the radical either-or dilemmas is experienced as real, and with that the centrality of global guilt and global shame.

Such a split in the experience of reality presupposes the force of denial, and with that the search for magical transformation (Wurmser 1999b).

## CONFLICT CAUSALITY

Obviously, there are several important elements that greatly help us to obtain effective (mutative) insight: conscious and preconscious conflicts, intense affects, the great variety of transference manifestations and reenactments and transference-like repetitions in current outer reality. Yet in our effort to reach the deeper, causative layers they point back to some central, largely unconscious *fantasies*. In the search for psychic causality these form *indispensable bridges* between the phenomena and their sources in unconscious, life-determining conflicts.

However, a few words are in order here on my understanding of psychoanalytically relevant causality, so that the position of the fantasies in this structure becomes more understandable. The more detailed study of the core conflicts will follow later on.

The causality relevant to the psychoanalytic approach to problems of psychopathology is that of the centrality of unconscious inner conflict. The entire structure of such causality could be formulated in the following way: The more severe the traumata, the more overwhelming the affects. The more radical and overwhelming the affects, the more intense the conflicts. The more intense and extreme the conflicts, the more encompassing the defenses and the more totalitarian the contradictory demands of "the inner judge," that sadistic version of conscience. Thus the trauma lives on in the severity and pitiless character of the conscience as well as in the split character of the superego (conscience, ideals, values, loyalties). The more extreme the aggression of the superego, the more life-determining are the narcissistic and masochistic fantasies and the more prominent the core phenomena of the neurotic process (compulsiveness, globality, and polarization), meaning, in turn, the broader are the problems of "narcissism," of "splitting of identity," and of compulsiveness. Traumatization and severe inner conflict belong together as two sides of one coin.

In reverse order, the psychoanalytic path from description to explanation proceeds from the *core phenomena* of the neurotic process—compulsiveness, polarization, and absoluteness—as they typically are reflected in preconscious conflicts, affects, and self-protective behaviors. It uses with particular benefit the bridges of the *core fantasies* in order to reach the *unconscious core conflicts.* The recognition of them and the new attempt to resolve them brings about the effective change; their place in the inner chain of causal connection is at the very center. Beyond the conflicts we deal with *core affects* of a traumatic or physiologic origin that often determinine the severity of the conflicts we deal with. The core fantasies and core conflicts are specifically set up to deal with, to defend against, *central affects of a primary and global nature.* Behind those four layers of psychopathology—*core phenomena, core fantasies, central conflicts, and main affects*—there looms like a monster, in every case of severe neurosis, the fatal power of *trauma.*

What impresses in this layering of causality particularly as "defect/deficit" is the deficient defense against overwhelming traumatogenic affects and their appearance in the form of unsolvable inner conflicts. The absoluteness of inner experience is then described as "ego weakness." We could call it also the *narcissistic dimension of the neurosis*; Freud (1914b) called overvalu-ation (*Überschätzung*) the "narcissistic stigma," the criterion for narcissism. In our understanding, narcissism refers to a "too much," a transgression of limits in value, truth, and deed (for a detailed study, see below and *Flight from Conscience*).

It is important not to succumb to premature schematizations that block our view of what is novel. Every single patient may, if studied in sufficient depth and detail, help us unveil new connections.[14] It is above all the respect for the individual, the interest in his present as well as his past and the resulting understanding of the anxieties and pains accompanying him like a second shadow, that reopens for him the obstructed path to the future.

"Life teaches us to be less strict with ourselves and with others. . . . Also we are not charged to doom [judge] ourselves" (Goethe).[15]

## ENDNOTES

1. (*Die "Sünde"—denn so lautet die priesterliche Umdeutung des tierischen "schlechten Gewissens"* [*der rückwärts gewendeten Grausamkeit*] *ist bisher das größte Ereignis in der Geschichte der kranken Seele gewesen: in ihr haben wir das gefährlichste und verhängnisvollste Kunststück der religiösen Interpretation.*) Nietzsche, *Zur Genealogie der Moral*, 3.20, 387.

2. Gedö (1986) endorses Parens's (1979) finding of "the acquisition of some superego functions *before* the onset of the oedipal conflict" (p. 158).

3. (*Zur Wut ward ihnen jegliche Begier,/ Und grenzenlos drang ihre Wut umher*), *Iphigenie auf Tauris*, Act I, Scene 3; Goethe dtv vol. 10, p. 89.

4. The precise wording is: "a dissolving of the superego" (Sandler and A. Freud 1985, p. 120).

5. (*Da stehn sie da, die schweren granitnen Katzen, die Werte der Urzeiten: wehe, wie willst du die umwerfen? . . . Kratzkatzen mit gebundenen Pfoten, da sitzen sie und blicken Gift.*) (Nietzsche, *Bruchstücke zu den Dionysos-Dithyramben*, p. 558 [1888].)

6. (*Und sie schelten meine Klagen, und sie höhnen meinen Schmerz, einsam in die Wüste tragen muss ich mein gequältes Herz, von den Glücklichen gemieden und den Fröhlichen ein Spott! Schweres hast du mir beschieden, Pythischer, du arger Gott! Dein Orakel zu verkünden, warum warfest du mich hin in die Stadt der ewig Blinden, mit dem aufgeschlossnen Sinn? Warum gabst du mir zu sehen, was ich doch nicht wenden kann? Das Verhängte muss geschehen, das Gefürchtete muss nahn.*) (Friedrich von Schiller's *Kassandra*.)

7. (*Wer erfreute sich des Lebens, der in seine Tiefen blickt! . . . Wo ich wandre, wo ich walle, stehen mir die Geister da.*)

8. (*Und in ihrem Schmerz verlassen war nur eine traur'ge Brust. Freudlos in der Freude Fülle, ungesellig und allein . . . Alles ist der Freude offen, alle Herzen sind beglückt . . .*)

9. (*Und den Mordstahl seh ich blinken und das Mörderauge glühn, nicht zur Rechten, nicht zur Linken kann ich vor dem Schrecknis fliehn; nicht die Blicke darf ich wenden, wissend, schauend, unverwandt muss ich mein Geschick vollenden, fallend in dem fremden Land.*)

198 THE POWER OF THE INNER JUDGE

10. (*Frommt's, den Schleier aufzuheben, wo das nahe Schrecknis droht? Nur der Irrtum ist das Leben, und das Wissen ist der Tod. Nimm, o nimm die traur'ge Klarheit, mir vom Aug' den blut'gen Schein! Schrecklich ist es, deiner Wahrheit sterbliches Gefäss zu sein. Meine Blindheit gib mir wieder und den fröhlich dunkeln Sinn! Nimmer sang ich freud'ge Lieder, seit ich* deine Stimme bin. *Zukunft hast du mir gegeben, doch du nahmst den Augenblick, nahmst der Stunde fröhlich Leben—nimm dein falsch Geschenk zurück.*)

11. (*Ein solcher Vorwurf stammt aus der Enge des Kausalbedürfnisses der Menschen, welches sich im Gegensatz zur gewöhnlichen Gestaltung der Realität mit einem einzigen verursachenden Moment zufrieden geben will. Die Psychoanalyse hat über die akzidentellen Faktoren der Ätiologie viel, über die konstitutionellen wenig geäußert. . . . Wir lehnen es ab, einen prinzipiellen Gegensatz zwischen beiden Reihen von ätiologischen Momenten zu statuieren; wir nehmen vielmehr ein regelmäßiges Zusammenwirken beider zur Hervorbringung des beobachteten Effekts an.* Δαίμων καὶ Τύχη *bestimmen das Schicksal eines Menschen; selten, vielleicht niemals, eine dieser Mächte allein.*) (Freud, *Gesammelte Werke* 8, p. 364 f.)

12. In German: *peinlich*; its translation would be more like "embarrassing, damaging to self-esteem, shameful."

13. By the way, this was the general, so-called scientific view in the Victorian age. Frederick R. Karl (1995) describes this view, in his biography of George Eliot, that: "because of the female sexual and reproductive systems, women's cerebral evolution had been arrested at a certain undeveloped point . . . she lacked the element that was thought to contain the 'will'." Therefore, it was held that "women were more subject to diseases of excitement, that is, hysteria and related nervous ailments. This, too, was held as 'scientific,' despite evidence that men outnumbered women in such nervous diseases" (p. 324).

14. As Gedö (1986) very rightly states: ". . . almost the only efforts at validation to take place within psychoanalysis are the individual activities of clinicians who apply specific theories—more or less faithfully—in the therapeutic arena" (p. 142).

15. *Das Leben lehrt uns, weniger mit uns und andern strenge sein . . . Auch sind wir nicht bestellt, uns selbst zu richten.*(Goethe, *Iphigenie auf Tauris*, IV, iv, vol. 10, p. 123.)

# 5

# The Need to
# Destroy Success

Our doubts are traitors,
And make us lose the good we oft might win,
by fearing to attempt.
　　—Shakespeare, *Measure for Measure*, I, iv


This chapter describes some of the highlights from a particularly difficult analysis which reached its successful conclusion only after six years and 1,092 hours.[1] It illustrates many of the issues I have put forth in the introductory chapters as being of special interest in regard to therapeutically mutative insight and the obstacles standing in its way in this group of patients, the severe neuroses: the layering of affects, particularly of shame and guilt, and more generally, the layering of conflicts and of defenses, the central importance of a careful superego analysis—precisely in patients often looked at as "narcissistic" or as "borderline"—and the value of great flexibility in management and of combining several treatment modalities. Moreover, it gives us an opportunity to study a character type that is rather neglected in the literature though frequent among the severe neuroses, namely the diagnostic category of "phobic character," now often subsumed under the "avoidant" or "schizoid" personality disorders (Axis II). It provides us with deeper insights into the nature of "the negative therapeutic reaction." It will end with the analysis of a literary text representative for some of the dynamics developed.

The patient, Jacob, whose analysis furnished several excerpts for *The Mask of Shame* (Wurmser 1981a), was a businessman in his late twenties when he entered analysis, the younger of two sons by three years. He was a tall and very slim man, most of the time somewhat anxiously bent over, his eyes behind eyeglasses and averted, his mouth hidden by a beard.

He had repeatedly sought treatment before because of generalized and severe anxiety and depression, psychosomatic gastrointestinal spasms with vomiting and diarrhea, an almost complete blocking of his love life, and grave concerns about homosexual propensities. Several treatment modalities had failed. Although highly gifted in a number of areas, he had broken off all higher education.

He lived isolated; except for his close but deeply ambivalent relations to his family he had hardly any social contacts. Because of overwhelming anxiety states, he had had to break off several attempts at university studies out of town. He was suffering under a severe travel phobia that made it impossible for him to go away even on vacations. Apart from several homosexual experiments at the age of 15 and a little later a few dates with girls with whom the excitement had been so great that he had ejaculated into his pants, his sexual life had remained entirely restricted to fantasies and almost completely homosexual. This predilection caused him, however, deepest unease.

His anxiety when engaged in something new seemed worse to him than the depressive realization when he saw himself shut in within a life of little joy and no hope, within an empty, gloomy existence.

I begin with the depiction of the role played by shame in his tremendous phobic inhibitedness, before I address in detail the process of resolution of his neurosis.

## THE LAYERING OF THE SHAME CONFLICTS

I shall try to summarize these layers in a sequence from surface to depth as they emerged in the first four years of his analysis. Some of the material had been easily accessible to consciousness all along, some of it had only gradually and grudgingly been delivered. I put these in quotes, in quasiquotes, or in editorial comments.

1. "I am ashamed to express my feelings and possible wishes. I might lose control over them, and I would be ridiculed for them. Expressing feelings and desires leaves me exposed and vulnerable to contempt, instead of joyous and excited—having an erection." *All excitement was dangerous*; it would rapidly get out of control, and it had to be prevented.

    Almost from the beginning of the analysis his *castration anxiety* had been prominent and accessible to some conscious and explicit scrutiny. It was an attitude: "Please, don't cut me down. I don't want to cut you down. And anyway, I have already cut myself down." This *pre-emptive stance* had become a general character attitude, that is, the pervasive *avoidance* inherent in the phobic character: "If I am withdrawn and unloved I can safely remain at a distance from all those dangerous stimulations. True, I always expect shock and disappointment, instead of excitement and erection. But by such anticipated disillusionment I prevent dangerous arousal and hence overexcitement." Thus the fear of being intruded upon and penetrated by man or woman, of being invaded emotionally, stimulated intellectually, or aroused sexually, had frozen him into a state of *general inhibition* and nonperformance. His tremendous musical and intellectual gifts had become almost completely blocked. Although having reached a concert level of performance, he was now functioning at a level of mediocrity in the family's business. He had turned to generalized passivity as a protection against his dangerous active impulses.

2. "I show my weakness and failure inherently in my overall passivity and whining dependence, in submission and subservience. I have retreated from all competition with other men. Not competing means not being competent. I have lost out a priori. I am a born loser." All his relationships had the tinge of his victimhood. In bitterness he blamed others and himself as a failure. No one had helped him, everything was worthless. There was a sexualized quality to this position of victim and blame. Such a *masochistic* attitude was a very potent motive for shame in him, as it is more generally one of the most frequent ones. It meant: "I express my spite by proving that my parents and you are all failures. I fail in order to prove *you* to be impotent. What do you have to show for after more than 700 hours of effort? I'm worse off, the chasm separating me from success is even wider than before I started. You are a pathetic fool. I prove you to be such a fool by being a fool myself. It all ends in shame." This was his *masochistic triumph*—both an attack and a victory attained by suffering and failure. It was endlessly repeated in life and reiterated in the analysis as "negative therapeutic reaction." Every success *must* be followed by dismal failure.

3. All expression was equated with excretion. "What I show of myself may overwhelm and flood me. I'm not sure whether I can hold it back once I start." It was the *anal* or urinary view of emotional expression and of releasing some of the inhibitions about his drives: "It's dirty to express myself, to show my affects, to communicate my desires"—shifting from phallic to anal conflicts—defense by regression.

4. "My own defiance and rebellion against my parents is reciprocated by everybody else. Therefore I can remain safe only if I am largely inhibited. But because of this overall inhibition of feelings and actions, my overall *inauthenticity, estrangement,* and self-consciousness, I'm not a real human being, but rather like a loathsome insect, caged in by the armor of numbness and unreality." He had frequent anxiety dreams and

a phobia about insects and compared himself with Gregor Samsa in Kafka's story "The Metamorphosis."

5. "I'm ashamed of my parents—my mother's social ineptitude and superstitiousness [she hid her own phobic nature behind much compulsive avoiding], my father's dismissal of anything serious. I'm ashamed for their sexual activities or emotional display. I'm afraid of my curiosity in general, ashamed of it in regard to what I might find out about what they are doing at night"—ashamed and inhibited, that is, rather than watching, being excited, or being aggressive.

## THE SPLIT IDENTITY

The basic damage to his development appeared to have been done by his mother's and grandmother's frightened overintrusiveness and bossy, angry dominance, especially in regard to his bowel movements. Time and again, his self-esteem, his identity, his autonomy had been injured. That imposition of *fearful authority* was now perpetuated in the voice he called the "*drill-sergeant within.*" Accordingly, withdrawal and defiant rejection had extremely early been chosen as self-protection. They were being endlessly repeated in the transference as silence and in the negative therapeutic reaction.

Thus the internalization of the mother figure played a crucial role in his character development, and this in a double form: both as a *devalued identity* and as the imperative voice of his conscience, that is, the internalization represented by an aspect of the superego, as *introjection* (Meissner 1970, 1971, 1972, Sandler 1960). On the one side: "I'm as bad, as worthless, and terror-ridden as she is. And I am just as incompetent, just as contemptible, and castrated as I see her." In other words, he *identified with her as a victim of his own hostile wishes.* On the other side he had *introjected* her as an authority commanding taboos into his superego, the "inner sergeant."

Against this paralyzing identification with the anxious, superstitious mother stood one fantasy, one large and grandiose protection: "Against all this I have the *homosexual fantasy*: there my partner and I both have such a grand and nourishing penis, a monumental penis, great like the Washington Monument [in a dream]. We can assure each other: we do have a penis, penis, penis. It is phallus, phallus *über alles!*"

One consequence of this solution was the *deep split in his self(-experience)* and the marked disturbance of his identity, as was evident in his swings between considerable achievement and very severe clinical regression, especially during the panic attacks, a split quite similar to the one we encountered in the case of Vera. On the one side, he saw himself as being just like his despised mother, as pathetic and phobic. On the other side he looked to his father, an older brother, and to me for an answer: the wished-for, idealized identity. When he felt unreal, *depersonalized*, it meant: "I don't want to be the one, and I cannot be the other." Since "being with" and "looking at" were equated with "becoming like" he had to shun being with a woman in order to avoid becoming emasculated altogether—a fantasy that was not at all deeply repressed but quite close to consciousness and articulated early in our treatment. This equation represented a kind of primitive identification, a hallmark of *mythical* thinking, namely of *being together = being one*, based on the *merger through the eyes: looking and being looked at = becoming the same*. "This explains," he said, "the unreality of my own being. I'm defined by the identity of the other" [732]. Instead of this frightful togetherness, he attempted to become strong, successful, and proudly defiant by approaching the stronger man, especially his older brother, then also other men who resembled the latter in their fanatical interest in sports. Thus he could not get enough of sports events, of course almost exclusively as a passive spectator. The only exception consisted in his playing golf, but this game had also to fall prey to his compulsion to annihilate every success, to his "*phobia of success*," just like the piano playing and his analysis.

His *depersonalization* was an expression of that inner split, specifically of *denying that shame-filled part of his identity*: "I am not this, I don't want to be this. But who am I? I cannot be whom I want and aspire to be. Why? Because excitement and spiteful self-assertion—hence success as a man—stand under absolute interdiction and would bring about intolerable guilt."

Thus he was caught between the *Scylla of shame* (in submission) and the *Charybdis of guilt* (of standing up like a man and confronting reality).

The split in his identity and the clinical phenomena due to it (depersonalization and derealization, impulsive actions, especially of avoidance, "nervous breakdowns," including near-suicidal episodes of despair, actions of self-sabotage, sudden and "inexplicable" setbacks in all the forms of treatment undertaken) could be seen above all as the outcome of a conflict between opposite parts of the superego, the one represented by guilt versus another one represented by shame.

Genetically seen, his sense of self, his identity, was all along violated by intrusion and disregard of autonomy. In turn, withdrawal and defiance, now endlessly repeated in the transference, as both silence and negative therapeutic reaction, became, probably extremely early, his brief of protection. Under a veneer of subservience he showed that "obduracy of the spirit" described by Dickens (1846/48) in *Dombey and Son*.[2]

## EXCERPTS FROM THE TREATMENT

You are thinking how to *act*—*talking*, you consider, is of no use.
—Charlotte Brontë, *Jane Eyre* (1847)

At the time of these excerpts Jacob was in his mid-thirties and still worked with his brother and his (mostly retired) father in their small factory. The almost complete blocking of his sexual life was still coupled with a profound uncertainty whether to follow his homosexual or his heterosexual penchants (with a marked preference for the former). The treatment remained burdened by an almost unremitting "negative therapeutic reaction": every success in the treatment, every new insight, every advance in his outer life was followed by a setback, a crushing and at times nearly suicidal depression, and the violent protest that analysis had not only been unavailing, but also actually harmful.

The insights into deeper connections were often dramatic, but remained for the longest time without similarly dramatic improvements in affect or behavior, although there was, as he occasionally allowed, a very gradual lessening of anxiety, an opening up of certain paths of activity, an increased willingness to meet others and even to go on some smaller trips—as adamant as he was in disclaiming that there had been any *real* improvement. Usually, every such sallying forth as well as all major new insights were followed by intense outbursts of despair and rage against me—that nothing made any difference and that he was at least no better off than all along.

This isolation, this mutual partitioning off of insight and factual, visible change, was less attributable to an obsessive-compulsive defense against touching (also present to some extent) than to the phobic avoidance of success and the "masochistic triumph." In spite of the anankastic features, the severe and tenacious depressivity, and his masochistic sexual, social, and transference orientation, the patient can best be described as a phobic character: *avoidance* was what altogether determined his character and his fate.

I now give several quotes from the later treatment, which should show the major reconstructions, first of the main anxieties in their hierarchy, then of the major underlying conflicts. Again, as the other quotes reconstructed from my shorthand notes taken during the sessions, they are in a condensed form, and it has to be kept in mind that what appears as one statement may have been given in a somewhat more disjointed form, often with repetitions, false starts, interruptions by hesitation and long silences, or as grammatical fragments.

### Excerpt 1: "Nothing Makes Any Difference"

In the weeks preceding the sessions to be depicted, about four and a half years after onset of the analysis, he described his frequent, though never carried out threat to break off the analysis, and that he was feeling as if he were closed in and wanted to flee. It was the same as with the breaking off of his studies and friendships with girls.

In hour 821, the one preceding the first session I would like to present in more detail, he talked about how he was afraid of any kind of decision, as if such a decision would exclude all others and hence would present a loss of freedom. And the deeper he committed himself, the less freedom he would have. I used another metaphor at that point, one of innumerable little interpretive comments: "Like a closing door, a *claustrophobic situation*, like with breaking the silence here."

He equated his fear of decision and hence commitment with being *locked out* from everything else. I went two steps further and equated those two members of his equation with a concrete image—*closing the door*—giving it a clinical, though popular name and tying it in with a frequent difficulty in the analysis: his long silences that he could not break because talking would mean to choose one content over all the others—another decision, another closure.

He responded: "That's a good word. That's a pattern. The urge to flee. It was so with . . . [he mentioned two former girlfriends], it was so with my need to break off my studies, and the wish to break off the analysis. I feel closed in . . . Also my interest in prisons and prisoners. . . ." These connections were looked at in several contexts, and I expressed my own surprise that we had not seen this so clearly before. He mentioned how every attachment or commitment immediately became so frightening that he had to withdraw, and how this freedom limited all his other freedom. I said that the "freedom from" became so important that there is virtually nothing left over for the "freedom to."[3]

I would like to give in much more detail the following session, 822. He began: "I think more about the connection that has become clearer since yesterday, how the threat of leaving here is similar to what happens in my relationship with women—feeling *trapped*, as if a wall was closing in, the claustrophobia. Why would a relationship evoke that? Every other week I'm threatening here to leave. We have talked about my losing the sense of self, of merging, that I'm afraid of that. But it's more than that. The more revelations take place, the more *ashamed and embarrassed* I become. The more you know about me the less I want to be in your presence, out of shame. And the same in other relationships, when there is shared intimacy. Instead of that I would feel closer, it acts as a wedge between me and the other person. The more intimate I become, the less I want to remain intimate. And that element of fear—that seems to suggest that I have a reason to be afraid of revealing myself, to be close and intimate."

"And the anxiety would then not be so much of merger than of shame?" I simply repeated here the interpretation *he* had just made and the refutation of a connection made sometime in the past.

"That seems more powerful, more likely to drive me away. The fear of merger is too abstract. The *fear of exposure* is concrete."

"Yet still not concrete enough: the exposure right here—or with that woman next Saturday?" I was referring to a possible date. This was an explicit defense interpretation, as if to say: "By not being specific and concrete enough you avoid the fears right now."

He took it up: "You are well aware of my difficulty in communicating feelings. And when I do it my speech is broken. Once I reveal something personal it's followed by silence. Or I change the subject. I feel so uneasy—as if there were some dark secrets, and if those were revealed it would change the relationship; that I'm embarrassed that I've told you this or that, that I'm sorry I let you in: 'Why did I have to tell you that?' I don't like people knowing things about me, getting close to me. [silence] Perhaps this is revealing. I've often thought for myself: if I had a wife or a girlfriend I would have to worry that something would happen to her—if she got sick—morbid thoughts like that. The fewer attachments, the fewer chances to be hurt. There would be an extension; it multiplies the chances for tragedy. Being free from such attachments minimizes that, but also the chances for shared happiness. It's as if I had made a conscious decision: not to have such shared tragedy, but also no happiness. It seems a strange decision." Here his insight had suddenly deepened very much, as if to state: "I avoid, by all these measures of evasion, thoughts of tragedy, of death, of loss." It is as if he had reached such a decision consciously and that *the fear of loss* was much greater than the *fear of loneliness*, that it always was the expectation of disappointment. "Why do I always assume the worst? Perhaps I had built up my hopes. It sounds as if I had gotten attached to somebody who then died or left . . ."

"And the fear that you have caused it, that you have killed or driven away the person."

The patient engaged here in a kind of thought experiment: he extrapolated from his current fear of losing somebody a historical event, a guessed trauma, that had not occurred, as far as was known, and I expanded the thought experiment by adding a mythical contribution by him, the fear of his *magical wish.* He was silent for a while, then resumed: "I've occasionally mentioned the thought that something would happen to you before the analysis would be over. I've got mixed feelings—that it would be terrible, in the middle, to begin again with somebody else. On the other side, that it would be a way to get out of the analysis without breaking it off myself."

"Except probably again for the fantasy, 'I've magically brought it about myself.'" My comment connected his feared killing magic of the past with the present fantasy.

"Right. That secretly I had wished it."

"And perhaps revelation is so dangerous—because of those secret wishes?"

He deepened it: "And these repeated statements to get out of the analysis—the panic there is the fear of my own wishes."

I reiterated this and asked: "What wish with me—or with the woman next Saturday?"

"When I'm close to a woman I'm worried that she'd get in an accident. The fear is that I wish that . . . that the closeness arouses the fear of such harm—" He halted.

"—that the closeness would *reveal* the wish and lead to retaliation." I finished the thought. The withdrawal manifested itself also in the way of his speaking.

He asked himself repeatedly about the origin of this wish and after a while answered his own question, in his stilted and forced way, his hesitating, chopped-up style: "I cannot ignore the body of information about the feelings I have toward my mother . . . given the perception I have . . . with somebody with whom there was much intimacy . . . physical closeness, in early childhood . . . who sends out contradictory messages: that of a loving mother, who on the other side can be a tyrannical, violent, hysterical, physically abusive hag, who would provoke wishes that she would go away, or even more violent ones: that *I would kill her.*"

"And then the *fear about them.*"

"And with women in general. *The* woman."

"And so with everybody whom you get *close* to, like me." Quite peremptorily and suggestively I gave premature closure to what had just been uncovered in regard to the very pervasive claustrophobic nature of much of his character: "This is the whole conflict, and the symptom is set up to deal with that conflict, the claustrophobia, and then the running away to deal with that symptom. This sequence is repeated in every close relationship."

"The claustrophobia is the signal: I have to run away. I feel boxed in. In slang 'box' means vagina. Even the sexual act, the anatomical area has these claustrophobic overtones."

"And there is another meaning for the box—the ultimate of being boxed in."

He: "The womb."

"That's true too."

"And being in the coffin," he added. "Beginning in a confined space and ending up in a confined space. The impulse is: to get out. The fear of death is that claustrophobia. Both *sex and death are seen as claustrophobic experiences.*"

"And you often equate both."

"And the woman's womb. I associate that too with death. That she is a confining being. And she acts as the cause of the claustrophobia."

At that point I repeated the conflict once more that *he* had elaborated so clearly a little while before. I added how the conflict solution itself, the symptom, led to new defenses against that: new fears about that fear, in derivative forms, without myself giving examples. He was silent for about three minutes, then he resumed: "Perhaps it's not only the fear of those wishes, but also the *fear of being humiliated,* for example in the intimacy of the analysis, that I would say something that would provoke condemnation from you, anger and censure. I always expect rebuke" (an expectation, a form of superego transference, known to us since the very beginning of the analysis). "That is something that is characteristic for my relationship with my mother: that I expect to be rebuked for everything, that there was this overall tone of disapproval."

"And what would be the response in you?"

"Either to remove myself—flight. Or to remove the other person—my mother or you."

"You have dealt on your own with the question I had just wanted to raise: how to tie in the new insight with your statement at the beginning of the session."

He responded, "You could almost say that the object of my feelings of love and attachment is more like a *two-headed monster*—that the same person provokes the love, but also the hate, and is loving and hating towards me also." This would recur in all intimate relations and with me as well: "That I expect that both sides have to be present, and that I'm provoked to hate as well as to love . . ."

"I would say that of all we talked about—most difficult to deal with and most pathogenic—is the *fear of your own violent reaction*" [822].

A few sessions later [825] he said how angry he was that I was withholding help and was cold, and spoke of his frustration, but countered by the feelings of hope and trust that I did care—again the deep *ambivalence conflict,* this time as part of the transference. I asked directly: "When you think of the conflict, what is the resistance [against talking]?"

"Whether it's not the fear of expressing my outrage? The wish to strike out in frustration at you, and the anxiety to allow those feelings—not only to be expressed, but even just to be felt."

"Exactly. Because if you felt them and expressed them to the fullest, what would happen?"

"That I would be punished. The retaliating response."

"And what would be the worst retaliation?"

"Being sent away, disowned." He was reminded of his grandmother's saying: "If you say a lie you'll be sent to heaven in a handbasket." "I imagined flying without control away and could not come back, being sent off, like by a Banshee, or in the carriage with the headless horseman. Nightmares—to be taken off to unknown places, unable ever to come back."

"And would it be fair to assume that this was not only for lying?"

"Definitely. It was not connected with a specific offense like lying, but reflected a more general fear. That it was not safe—that at any time that carriage would come and I would be sent off—"

"For doing what?"

"The image is: like that my mother could suddenly turn on me, so hostile. It was an insecure environment, I never felt protected."

"What would cause her hostility?"

"My disobeying her, my resisting, my defiance—and I feel, like yesterday, the resistance right now. Instead of expressing the anger at you, I get depressed, I'm angry at myself. I put myself down; God forbid that I would put *you* down."

I repeated his words about the fear of the carriage coming for him. He replied that the symptom of claustrophobia expressed wanting to run away from the anger at the person whom he felt close to. I added: "And the resistance is the same: showing the anger and withdrawing from it at the same time."

While in the previous sessions there had been a prevalence of slowly emerging insights without very much affect, the next hour [827], which followed a trip with a friend to an ocean resort where his parents were staying, showed an outpouring of feelings (his date had been put off). He reported that those three days away had been an emotional roller-coaster—apprehension, depression, feeling comfortable, finding with his elderly parents a refuge from the world, an escape to a fantasy world without any demands on him. He called himself regressed, as wanting to be a child again, and berated himself as not having grown emotionally; "I feel very unhappy. Feeling safe and protected, and enjoying a leisurely way of life, that's denied to me." He went on castigating himself until I interrupted him: "So you notice again a force within yourself denying you pleasure."

"Self-punishment."

"As soon as something goes well, this voice rises, this force, telling you: You should not have this or enjoy that."

He was silent for a while, then said: "It's again the feeling that I'm such a child." At that he choked up and began crying; for the rest of the session he cried intermittently and heavily: "If something happened to my parents I would be totally cut off—unable to stand on my own. —I don't understand why I feel like that just now . . . Yesterday, leaving them, there were such fears."

"The fear of loss we talked about?"

He replied that he had seen a movie with his visiting friend where two college students murdered one of their friends, as a mark of their own superiority. "One of the two immediately felt guilty—the sense of *permanency of guilt*, that there was no way to undo it. That for the rest of his life he would have to pay for it. And I *identified* so strongly *with the guilt*. I wish I had not done it, and there is *no way to undo it*. That it is permanent and cannot be erased, regardless of what. Which leads me to think that the guilt that so pervades my life has the meaning: *nothing can be done about it*. Whatever it is, it is so horrendous that it cannot be undone. That I have to live with it for the rest of my life."

"And what is this guilt?"

"It obviously has some connection with *murder*, something irrevocable that cannot be undone. But if I only wish it?"

"Why would it be so strongly experienced as a deed?"

"That is what I cannot understand," said this usually extremely self-controlled man, with heavy crying, "and why I'm so choked up as if somebody *had* died." The impression was so real that he was wondering about the *confusion of fantasy and reality*; it was the *consciousness of a real guilt*. I surmised that "that confusion itself speaks for something from a very early time."

He mentioned the incident where his mother, wanting to beat his brother, dislocated her shoulder and cried out aloud. "I keep going back to that episode, that I perhaps had wished it, and when it happened, that I wielded the magical power."

"That is certainly a powerful event, but we know a much more powerful one." He remained silent for several minutes; so I resumed: "Your father's illness."

"That did cross my mind." It referred to the father's very serious cardiac insufficiency when Jacob was 5 years old.

"Which was about the same time [as mother's injury]. And you said the Kaddish." He had gotten up in the synagogue and, to the horror of the family, started saying the Kaddish.

He added: "And the fuzziness of details; that I remember very little about it is an important factor."

"And the only other time that I remember your crying here was when your father was told that he needed a bypass operation."

He corrected me: "The other time was at the beginning of the analysis when my friend [upon whom he had a homosexual crush] began his relationship with his later wife. The sense of loss, the separation. It has the connotation of death, my having the fantasy of killing, and then seeing it realized as the end of the relationship."

"In the context of your *rage* at him. So that we have three memories. The crux is: it's not only the loss, but the *real sense of guilt*." He repeated the last words and went on: "That I am punished for something that I might not have done. I punish myself as if I had done them [the deeds], while I never did more than think them or seem to cause them, and only by wishing.'"

I reiterated this and added: "That is it exactly where it is *at*. And your entire phobic life can be explained on that basis—namely how?"

"That I'm *afraid to act because I'm afraid that the angry wishes would be translated into something like*—as if I were afraid *I would kill* somebody. The passivity is defending against performing 'another' murder, against having another brush with causing somebody harm. And it is the continued punishment. But also the continued *preventive measure* against acting upon aggressive wishes."

"And you remember last week when we talked about it: that you had the fantasy that *I would suddenly die*."

He replied: "And the *passivity* here is a similar defense against taking responsibility if something happened to you: 'I don't have to take any blame because I'm so passive; I've never expressed any anger or rage'" [827].

We both left out the major defense here: the "not touching"—touching either by any form of intimacy and closeness, or by having thoughts and feelings touch each other: *the defense by severance of thoughts and affects.* We did address it in the following hour [828] when *he himself* talked about avoiding the conflict by shying away from intimacy, and I connected it with the formal aspect of that defense. Then I asked him to observe the *tone* he was using throughout that hour. He noticed the desperation, the crying in it. Only when I imitated it as well as I could he noted the same as what I had perceived: "It's more *protesting* that the analysis has done nothing."

I agreed: "It's an angry protest, besides the dread and despair, the accusation: 'You haven't done a damned thing for me!'" And I added that this seemed to me like another part of that forgotten memory, severed from the content of the last several sessions, as if those two should not touch each other at all.

He replied that he tried now to have the love and affection and care he had missed.

"And the angry protest," I said. "'I don't want it from you, I want it from my mother and my father, not from you'—me, girl friends, other friends . . ."

"Desperately wanting it from them because it never was there when I grew up."

"Or it was so intermingled with rage and guilt, that double-headed monster, and on both sides."

The following hour [829] finally allowed me to make a second important and comprehensive interpretation (after the one regarding claustrophobia), and one that much revised my last conjecture. Pondering the material I had strongly come to the feeling that something important still had been left out; I had a hunch what it might be. After his normal long silence at the beginning, he slowly and interruptedly repeated some content of the previous session, adding that he felt deep resignation. Referring to his need for self-isolation due to his anxieties, he said, overwhelmed by despair: "This is something that runs so deep that it cannot be overcome, that I have to be so for the rest of my life. Almost five years of analysis have only chipped away at the surface. In terms of change it has hardly done anything. It would need another five years to do more, and it doesn't seem worth it."

"I wonder if the *reality* of what has happened that you mentioned is not so much with the parents, but with *me*—and the crying expresses your sadness: 'You've disappointed me. You haven't helped me at all.' And that it was shifted away, onto your parents?"

He confirmed it and elaborated: "And the absence of spontaneity here is an effort to fight against any growing feeling of intimacy. It is representative of the shell. In the last few days, I should mention, I've had passing thoughts of *suicide*—to shorten the misery, turning all the hostility against myself; *instead of killing you I kill myself*; that is what I deserve. It would also relieve the anxious feelings and the despair and the hopelessness." Again there was a long silence.

I interrupted it: "And what is the anger at me all about?"

"The main thing is that I'm now as much or even more paralyzed in my actions than before. I feel less free to act—with women or traveling—even more frightened. I'm disappointed that things have not changed more. I feel worn out by anxiety and not willing anymore to fight it. I'm sick and tired of being depressed about things and dreading those that should be exciting." Again a long silence.

I: "To prove what to me?" [silence]

He: "That the analysis has been a failure."

"Perhaps more specific?"

"That *you* have been a failure."

"In regard to—?"

"Alleviating these profound anxieties."

"About?"

"Intimate relations and traveling."

"No. These are the symptoms—as if firemen rushed to combat the heat, not the fire."

"Probably the anxiety about the deeply felt anger, the inability to express this and to deal with it—and the wishes that go with it."

"Concretely?"

"The violent wishes we have spoken about:—*wanting to get rid* of—people who are close to me, and the *guilt* about it."

I reinforced it: "It's even more concrete: '*You don't help me, and I wish you dead, go to hell!*'—with all the feelings that entails." I spoke out what he meant and still was afraid to say. "And I cannot even say that, not even express it in words."

"Exactly. And what is in the way there?"

He explicated the conflict: "The fear of driving you away. You are right. There is the lingering *wish for love* and *closeness*, and to say: 'Go to hell!' eliminates any hope for intimacy, for receiving love, as remote as that already is—the desire not to drive away the person whose love I want."

I repeated the first part of the interpretation, the wish to send me off to hell, perhaps in a handbasket, and asked him how he would put its antithesis now. His response was: "'I don't mean that. I want your love and affection and evidence that you care about me and that you don't hate me—and that you do something to help me.'"

I reiterated his words verbatim and continued: "And what you say is: 'You don't show me enough that you do love me and admire me, and I'm very hurt, and I'm very sad and desperate about it. And I'm paralyzed by this double feeling [more accurately: the wish for love versus the feelings of pain, sadness, and rage]—certainly with all the persons I'm close to, but with particular intensity right here.' A word more about how you deal with this conflict. You were very right about the passivity and turning against yourself in despair, but the *main defense is by severing the connections*—especially not to feel *here*, with me."

"The success or failure in the analysis is equated with the degree with which you show love or withhold it, seem to care or don't care," he replied. "Success means that you do care and love me and failure that you don't care."

I enlarged the field of meanings, addressing a broader conflict: "I wonder whether this does not also entail another link: that the *love* you crave for from me enters dangerous territory—the *homosexual* implications."

"Engendering a whole new amount of guilt and anxiety."

"When I care and love you it means homosexual submission. So you cannot win. Wherever you turn there is a no-no." There was a long silence which I interrupted: "But to repeat: the main defense is *not to feel here, now*. The feeling is *displaced*."

His whole mood had radically and visibly changed; he spoke quite freely now and even said the following sentences with some chuckling: "Just before, you said that I thought how much I feel like an *unfeeling robot*, or rather, like somebody who had the capacity for feeling removed, like a being that is unable to feel anything, although I certainly feel all the negative things—the despair, the anxiety, the sadness, but I am unable to feel pleasure or joy and warmth. *It is the inability to love*. . . . It's ironic, I don't even feel comfortable using the word *love*: it seems so alien to me."

"Again: what feels so alien to use it here, with me, about me?"

"*Embarrassment*. I don't know how else to explain it. As if I got somewhere the idea that there is something inappropriate or dangerous pertaining to the feeling of love. That somehow love is tied up with the feeling of danger."

"And what is the danger with me?"

"I guess the danger is always of rejection and disappointment, being spurned or turned away: that you would be indifferent. That is what the accusations are all about: that you don't care. I come to you, pleading for care and love, and that it's dismissed as meaningless, met with indifference, or even outright rejection. And that brings us to the area of *homosexuality*: that it is *wrong*."

"So that, very specifically, what do you ask from me?"

"I have the image: wanting you somehow *magically* to affect a *transformation* in my life—that you wave your arm and, like with a magic wand, eliminate all the anxious feelings."

". . . I think what you're saying is: 'I want very direct proof of your love, be it in form of praise and admiration, or in other forms of direct love and care, and the magic wand is one of those proofs.' And the desperate protest and plea is: 'Give me the proof!'" It was, implicitly, again the fantasy of the mighty penis, of the Washington Monument.

Still, we had left out two very important aspects to tie in the interpretation and make it more truly effective, but I did not realize this. The feeling was very upbeat and hopeful. The deeper was my own disappointment in the following session [830] when he again repeated, with long silences, with protesting whining and blaming: "All the effort here is for nothing. Five years wasted. Everything is fought and resisted. The rage that analysis is a dismal failure—that's my constant feeling, underneath everything, always. Regardless of what we do here, even when we progress and have new insights. I always feel: '*But what difference does that make?*'"

Here I could not suppress my own feeling of hurt and exasperation: "You notice how terribly aggressive, even sadistic that is, and how you try to wound me to the core."

He allowed: "It is very cynical, but I often have a hard time not to see it so. I don't know what difference it makes. It does not appear to make any difference."

"You do now to me what you feel had been done to you: to make *me* feel utterly impotent, utterly helpless, and cruelly dealt with, as you felt cruelly dealt with and made helpless." This had clearly been a drive interpretation, meant by me as criticism and experienced by him as that, an expression of my countertransference; but now it was being turned into a defense interpretation.

He talked more about his cynicism out of despair and self-pity, and I replied: "But what you conveniently leave out: that you *do* it, that now it is not you who is the victim, but I am the victim."

He rightly and ambiguously countered: "I do what I am capable of doing."

Again, I chose one meaning, the interpretation of the all-encompassing defense of *turning passive into active* with *role reversal:* "Exactly. You do what you are very capable of doing: to make me the victim as you yourself had been. And you are splendidly succeeding."

He responded: "*The neurosis is more powerful than the analysis.*"

I felt we had once again come up against the wall, and I saw no key to the door leading through it. At that point I consulted with Dr. Paul Gray, with whom I had repeatedly discussed the analysis of this case, and he had what I believe to be the key. It was a double interpretation:

1. The need to fail, the aggression itself, the guilt were, as the patient himself had stated, *preventive.* They were a *restraint* needed against his ag-

gressive wishes in the future. What was the meaning of such restraint? "*As if I could do that again!*" There must be a source to that conviction explaining the intensity of that need for restraint. That is, there must have been an event confirming to him in the remote past that his *murderous impulses would be so dangerous*—either in the form of severe injury to someone else when he wished this, or that he was almost able to implement such a design himself at one point. While we had dealt with this just a few sessions before, it had not been tied together with the more comprehensive interpretation in the previous session [829], nor given in that precise form.

2. The anxiety mentioned at the end of that session had not been explicated: "What would he be afraid of were he to love me, passively as it were?" That had to be fought off by reversing the danger, as if he were to say: "I am the attacker, I make *you* helpless and castrated, I make you into the victim." Based on the child's misperception and misjudgment that the woman is, as he often had come right out in declaring, castrated and having but a bloody hole, he feared I would inflict such injury on him. Hence his protest: "Nothing is different. It is not true that I am passive and castrated. Nothing has changed. We are not moving in *that* direction. I have not gained such dangerous freedom, such a danger of loving—here. There is no difference!"

To the following session [831] he came prepared and determined to break off the analysis. But in one dream he was left alone, abandoned in a house, and in another driving in a canoe down a river, all alone, running without control and at dangerous speed. It was very conducive to give the first interpretation: "That's why the restraint seems so necessary," and strongly postulating the *reality of the danger* motivating that need. And then, mentioning the danger inherent in loving, I added the second interpretation. He focused almost entirely on the first, but the mood had again completely changed: from despair, anger, and wish to break off to that of active collaboration and curiosity.

In the following hours we entirely focused on this one fear: "*As if I could do it again—or as if it could happen again,*" whatever "it" might be, and the desperate protestation: "No, *nothing has changed, nothing is different.* There is no difference!"

The necessity to hide, something having to remain covered over, hidden, not exposed, as if there were a *deep, dark secret*, a source of *shame* and *guilt* that poisoned all success, that was the refrain. Why would every wish for power, for self-assertion, for triumph turn into a fear worse than of death, and each evidence for such success have to be undone? Why was the intimacy with women so particularly to be shunned?

An important new part of the solution came unexpectedly in session 834—unexpectedly as to actual content, not as to time (we felt very close to it).

His parents came to town, and his father inquired how he was doing in his analysis: "I took the opportunity to pose the question whether there had been anything special, traumatic, influential, serious, which I may not remember. They brought up several things, and one that I had not remembered before: When I was 4 or 5 I went to day camp and had no problems. Suddenly, from one day to the other, I refused to change into swimming trunks and absolutely refused to go swimming. The counselors offered me a separate room, but I balked at the very idea. It gives the impression that something must have happened."

"Internally," I chimed in, barking up the wrong tree, and he complied by adding that he had inquired about earlier events, fights, and so on, without a yield, although the negative response did of course not preclude it. I stressed *their* [the parents'] likely defensiveness.

He came back to that incident, though: "What I remembered was the sudden awareness of shame. Like Adam and Eve—about more than just the idea of success."

Perhaps prematurely, even suggestively I threw in: "Standing out as a potent male?"

"No, what I've thought: that there was some external event—perhaps that a camp counselor did something to me? Physical abuse or a careless comment? —that made it so frightening."

"This is a very good conjecture."

"There are two elements," he said, "one, the fear, if abuse was involved and I was naked, and on the other side, that I felt a certain *responsibility* for what had happened, and then the shame, most of all. It brings to mind the later fears in high school when we had nude swimming, the fear of erection."

"So that *success would recall successful arousal where you felt derided?*"

"Rather: when somebody older, a counselor, did something—that it was wrong, shameful, but that I felt excitement about it. And I would tend to believe that it was an *external* event, not only something internal—"

"—that there was no prior inner conflict?"

"And from that I would extrapolate all the withdrawal, my lack of initiative, my inhibitions, and the fear to be assertive, beating myself down."

"Let's see more how you see the story—"

"The sexual excitement with F. [a boy, at age 15]—that was only a repetition. The same when wrestling with my brother. There must have been a counselor at camp. I remember little, but I do remember—suddenly not

wanting to go through with it, the sudden turnabout, mostly about the un-
dressing, the sudden shame. That I do remember. The shame about the penis—that it was not to be seen by others, or exposed. That there was suddenly
so great embarrassment, so strongly, and that I was crying about that too."

I asked him for the exact details of the scene.

"A room, with little cubby holes. It was not segregated by sex either, probably, boys and girls in the same room."

"Entailing what?"

"Certainly the awareness of the *difference.*"

"Which would entail—?"

"That they had no penis."

"This suddenly casts a new light on your protestation here: '*There is no
difference! Nothing has changed! Nothing is different!*'"

"The *denial* of the difference."

"Entailing—?"

"It entails the fear that that would happen to me, that I would lose mine.
And if this hypothesized incident of abuse happened, that because of my
participation and excitement I would be *punished by losing* it. And to undress
and change suddenly became impermissible. The punishment—to be vulnerable to its falling off or being cut off. I would not undress so that nothing like that would happen."

"And why would it happen when you undress?"

"Because of the exposure of the penis."

"Perhaps of the erect penis?" He nodded. After a longer silence I inquired
again about the details of the camp and the counselors and encouraged him
just to let his imagination, his fantasy play, but we did not get any farther. I
interrupted one of his silences with the inquiry: "A thought that keeps coming to *my* mind—and perhaps it is farfetched—that threat of your grandmother about lying and the handbasket, whether to heaven or someplace
else—if that is not connected here?"

"That I was told: '*Don't tell anybody!*'—to be threatened—?"

"And as antithesis: '*Don't lie!*'—the danger of lying. And it did not have to
be a counselor; it could have been a kid, a girl or a boy, and then you had
this *deep, dark secret* that put you in direct *conflict* with your grandmother's
saying of the handbasket." [silence]

"There is so much evidence," he eventually said, "to me it is obvious that
there was some single incident that had that element to keep quiet about.
And this whole mentality of keeping something secret has come to take over
so many aspects of my life, it must stem from an incident of this nature."

"I can't agree more."

He enlarged the interpretation: "And the *danger of success* is: that it brings attention, which is equated with *exposure*, and that is dangerous because the *secret would be exposed*."

"Exactly. That is a very good point. And add to this the verification of the anxiety of castration as punishment, by seeing the girls naked, that would fit too . . ."

Obviously, I didn't know whether this hypothesis reflected historical truth, nor did he. It should also be noted how he kept correcting me and kept steering our dialogue in that particular direction where someone else did something to him, in other words, where there was an external event (as befits his phobic nature) and one more or less inflicted upon him (as befits his passive, masochistic orientation). So he could rush into finding that one event, both to please me and to relieve himself. To please me? Or rather: to tease me on, and then to disappoint me and show me up the more radically as a quack?

Still, these hidden motives did not invalidate the intense conviction in him, as if to say: "Finally, this hypothesis starts making some sense out of the most troubling parts of my personality which have destroyed nearly everything I have tried to accomplish. Moreover, it fits together innumerable fragments of history, memory, and of incessant repetitions in one way that makes *emotional* sense, not just as a cognitive construct. True, this hypothesis will have to be refined, recast, perhaps even repositioned again, but it has a *convincing truth value* because it seems to unite all the major conflicts of my life as if in the focus of *converging* beams of light."

The next session [835]: "I ruined the whole day's effort in golf—a totally *mangled hole*. . . . It's indicative for what the problem is: You can't do that, you can't succeed, you're not so good, you'll mess this up anyway, and all the effort seems to go down the drain. . . . Success must be punished. I almost forgot the dream: I was very young—with my parents—a car accident— I or someone else had a broken arm or leg—and *a broken penis*. My parents discussed whether it could be fixed or had to be amputated. I was afraid they were talking about me. . . . Protesting my innocence: it's not my fault, I didn't do anything!"

Again, this partial uncovering—or rather surmising—of all these important connections was to be followed by the recurrence of depression and "resignation" [837]: "No change, I give up."

"So I gather *your brother* is back." During the latter's brief absence due to illness, the patient had appeared much more relaxed and far less subdued, a connection that had occasionally emerged earlier also.

The patient remained silent for six minutes, then replied: "You're sarcastic and try to embarrass and humiliate me."

I remarked on the role reversal and his turning passive into active by putting down the analysis and me: "Making *me* feel helpless, ridiculous, and a fool: 'Not I, but you!'"

In the following session [838] he added that these spells of "resignation" and protest really contained a "*plea* for help, a wish for some help": "Do something, once and for all! Hear me, listen to me!"

In the context of our hearing about the "*deep, dark secret*" and the "*threat of punishment for lying*," in the form of some nefast trip, I wondered whether this plea did not mean: "*Forgive me!*"—interpretively connecting the new element with the main conflict guessed at.

He shot back at once: "That's it! To *unburden myself of some sense of guilt or shame*, and yet so that it would be too dangerous to reveal the secret itself, but equally dangerous to lie about it. And in the scene at the camp: not to swim was a similar signal of a plea, drawing the attention to the fact that something was wrong, and I couldn't say what it was and demonstrated it by this behavior."

"And one may argue that the closer you come to that deep dark secret, to these hidden impulses, the stronger would have to be the plea for forgiveness and the protest: 'I'm not any better.'" The whole inquiry was gradually shifting the focus from outer to inner reality.

He replied: "Your comment yesterday about my *brother* suddenly brought out the feeling that my self-deprecation and attacks upon the analysis may be due to something *I had suffered literally from his hand*, like the assaults by tickling or some similar sexual attack or exploitation upon me."

"Which you suffered *passively*, and yet for which you felt guilty."

"Because of the *associated excitement*."

"And what may have been *traumatic* in the camp was your seeing the girls: 'Yes, the *penis can be taken off*, as punishment.' And it is perhaps also significant that there seems to be a particular taboo against talking here much about your brother, including even calling him by his name, or inquiring with him about your childhood."

"It must be kept unspoken, covered over, ignored, that whole topic . . . And perhaps what is the secret is not only what he did to me but *my wishes for revenge against him* that my mother implemented for me, by *beating him*."

The brother was repeatedly severely beaten by the parents. The patient himself is convinced that he himself had once also received such a belting although this is vehemently denied by parents and brother. He had kept contending that he always had been the good child who had never deserved or received a thrashing.

I responded: "And all this—all four aspects—is lived out here with me, symbolized by the silence: the secret and the *need for hiding*, the *fear of lying*, the submerged wish of *revenge*, and the *plea for forgiveness* in your helplessness."

The following session [839] brought a further piece of denouement. This one was contributed by me, by picking up on what he had mentioned, the element of *excitement*: "I wondered after what we heard about the excitement, and yet the feeling of helplessness with the tickling, whether there may not have been an *erection or some peeing* with it, as is almost inevitable with tickling—and that your brother ridiculed you deeply for it. Not only is it likely that such a thing would happen with such merciless tickling but both the water in the dream of the canoe [being out of control on a river, 831] and the refusal to swim [in the camp memory] refer to water."

No, he could not recall any such actual event, but he added: "What would fit though: I had such an *irrational fear that I might wet the bed* that I always refused to spend a night in any friend's house. What tremendous humiliation that would have been! Although it never happened."

"All the fear of excitement and exposure—"

"and with that of ejaculation—" He gave a number of examples where he actually had in a panicked way equated ejaculation with urination during his teens, and several examples where, to his infinite shame, he had, while on dates, ejaculated in his pants. "—and the danger in every successful encounter with a woman."

I pulled it together: "So what is equated is this: *Excitement and success = erection and ejaculation = peeing and exposure = humiliation, ridicule, and shame.* We find this equation of excitement with humiliation in regard to physical play and the wrestling with your brother, we heard about it with your playing golf or playing the piano, it happens with the insight here or with a woman, in your studies in college and at the university. Every *success* is seen as an *exposure* that has to be undone, changed into something shameful."

"And because of this fear I had to deprive myself of everything, of every success and any enhancing experience; all because of this overriding sense of shame—the need to keep myself inferior."

"As *preventive restraint—not so much as punishment.*"

Here he recalled a complicated dream of the night before where a customer refused to pay his bill, adding: "Where is the payoff? Where is the result? It's again about the analysis: after all I've put in, all the effort I've expended!"

"That is true, but may it not also, or even rather directly, refer to what we are working on?"

"I have difficulties to relate it to it. Except for all the delays, putting off opportunities—?"

"The wish to be *finally relieved* of that restraint, of those delays, and of all the guilt and shame, which would make it possible for you to be *liquid.*"

He laughed out, having caught the pun at once, the equation in the word "liquid" for "ready money" with "being free about urination and ejaculation." I added that the man in the dream actually might be not only me, but even more the brother as the force of humiliation, and that he finally would free him, pay his due to *him,* Jacob.

He went back to the "wet dreams" in his early teens and the curious mixture of pleasure and terror with them: "Something is not right; it's out of control!" and he spoke more about that tickling, at age 3 or 4: "I almost fainted, I couldn't breathe. I felt completely powerless and helpless. It was mixed fun and pain, playful and scary. It was a very suffocating feeling. I was begging for mercy."

"Like with me, when you feel I've not helped you. And what is perhaps omitted is not an *event* of peeing, but the *fear* that it might happen: 'It *almost* has happened.' And then the *restraint*: 'Don't let it get close to that danger again!'"

"It also reminds me of how each time I had had intercourse I had to flee right after the ejaculation. That was the feared thing." During the analysis, he had several times started an intimate friendship of short duration with young women. His timidity and the just-described penchant for flight had hardly impressed his partners and only deepened his frightfulness. A date was often equated with an execution and cancelled.

I commented: "And even the speech here is like an ejaculation immediately followed by silence."

"As soon as I'm able to express a thought, I've got to—"

"Plug it."

"After blurting it out. Even in the term: instead of a steady stream of ideas—"

"—or flow, speaking fluently—"

"I certainly never could characterize my talking here that way!"

**Excerpt 2: "Not Having the Right to Have Something Good"**

After the summer break he returned determined again to break off the analysis because it had not fulfilled his expectations. He started looking into alternate possibilities. I decided that any encouragement by me of his continued stay would only be counterproductive. After the third consecutive hour of his deprecations about what analysis had done and could do for him, I concurred and said that it would be pointless for him and for me to continue if he felt that way: "We have heard this feeling expressed with increasing insistence for the past year, and there is no reason not to listen to your decision." Later I added that the power to repeat the past was at this time stronger than the power of insight, and that it was what prevented him from experiencing anything good, from accepting any help or love or warmth [851/852].

My statement had a most powerful impact: *"Not having the right to have something good?"* Really, why not? He was not harming *me* by breaking off now, but himself. It reminded him of his *wish to run away* from home, as an aggressive fantasy of punishing his mother, but one only falling back on him now, as his *fear of traveling*. Thus, it was a specific threat, one that was especially upsetting for his mother (and very effective in this sense) when he went, at age 16, away to college, and that was now being repeated with me: *"I leave, and you will be sorry."*

"And what made me finally realize this was when you displayed a kind of indifference: 'When I leave it doesn't make all that much of a difference to him. I don't injure him. He simply finds someone else, and I'm left out in the cold and have not accomplished the minimum: to have injured the authority,' you. I've only deprived myself again of success. And when I thought over the weekened: 'He doesn't even seem to show a sense of caring,' so was that a cover for my saying: 'If he only showed that I had an effect, that I was hurting him! That I've succeeded in hurting him!'" That is, that I would react like his mother who got hysterical when he came late to dinner [853].

So it was, after all, the fulfillment of his aggressive wishes, in the sense of his well-tested power over mother (as example), that necessitated the stringency of his self-punishment, namely in the form of not allowing himself anything good.

I said: "So far so good, but I think there is a deeper dimension: that the concern about these certain aggressive wishes had to shield you against the deeper fears of love, closeness, surrendering." I implied here obviously that I considered aggression not to be the primary element, but itself motivated and in need of further explanation—a momentous decision, by the way, in regard to daily technique as well as overarching theory (see Mitchell 1993).

He immediately agreed: "So that those wishes to attack that are so frightening are in themselves a substitute for the even more frightening feeling of love."

"And I base it upon this: that you have become relatively able to talk here about hatred and anger, but never about love. And not only to talk about it, but also to feel it."

"That's a very strong coincidence, because last night I was singing the words of a song: 'My love is . . . ' and I told myself with it: 'This is ridiculous! You don't feel any love toward anybody anyway!' It's irrelevant to me. It doesn't exist."

"And so nothing good can come from anything because life is without love."

"That is very true, and even with some momentary pleasure like going to a concert or climbing a mountain, it's tempered by this—the overriding issue of the *absence of love*. I cannot put it aside. Nothing can compensate for it."

"And all the solving of things like anger cannot do a damned bit of good because of this issue."

He mentioned Oedipus Rex and the implications of that myth and said he himself certainly had not grown up without love at home.

I countered with pointing to the inner conflict: "*Love was present, but dangerous. You haven't grown up without love, but to fear love.*"

"And all the attributes of coldness were there: I had to block it out."

"Its absence is a protection."

"It's avoidance, a running away from it. And I've certainly shown a talent for *crowding out feelings of love by supplanting them by intense feelings of hate.*"

"The fulfillment of loving wishes was even more terrifying than that of angry and vengeful wishes." Yet what was really the danger that required such drastic and general *defense by aggression*?

"I want to go back to the sexual excitement I felt toward my brother. That is well documented. And the fear of losing control, of wetting the bed. *Wherever there is excitement about love there is always the fear of some form of shame of losing control not only over urination, but also emotionally*" [855].

Stated in theoretical terms: Excitement, and perhaps feelings in general, become overwhelming; they quickly get out of control. They appear in sexualized form, as one way of archaic defense set up to regulate affect. As we saw, the result of such severe *disturbance of affect regulation* is the archaic equation of (1) *overwhelming feelings, overstimulation, the sense of bursting, "I cannot stand it anymore," the traumatic state* = (2) *sexual excitement* = (3) *violence, aggressive fantasies*. At that time this archaic equation was not yet clear to me, but it leaps out from the material.

I inquired though: "Why would the anxiety be so particularly strong with women?"

"All the hostility and venom and rage against my mother. The other side of the coin: the intense love feelings for her."

"Moreover, that all the hostility was borne out by the observation: the woman is without a penis; she seems mutilated."

"That my wish was enacted: the shock to discover that the girls had no penis. Cause and effect: I wish bad things on women, and then at a certain point the discovery that it *had* happened."

"And that point seems to have been at camp—at least as far as we have the evidence; the shock was there. And also the conviction confirmed: if you did bad things you would be sent away and lose love and lose the penis. And we also know how deeply engrained the magic view was at home, with all their superstitions" [857].

After that he spoke about how his feelings of fear and isolation seemed to dissolve, and how the sense of freedom was becoming the dominant feeling. He felt closer to me, trying to reach out, "a wish for greater intimacy without fear."

I commented "that the power that always says: 'You don't deserve anything good,' is weakened."

He felt much freer talking; the silences had shrunk very much: "The greater freedom in the sessions leads to the danger of sexual intimacy—seems to lead—to the loss of control."

"That is not the danger itself," I objected, probably incorrectly, "to lose control; but rather what would *happen* if you *did* lose control."

Today I would say that losing control over the affects, the *collapse of affect regulation*, and the *conflict between global but opposing affects* is indeed a *primary danger*, evoking a most profound sense of helplessness, and does not require resorting to fears of abandonment, rejection, castration, or self-condemnation, as I assumed.

But he complied with my implied suggestion: "The fear of *losing the penis.*"

I tied it together with what we had found: "And there the camp experience served as a symbol: 'It *can* happen, I could become a girl if I allow these things with my brother.' This is one danger. And another one we know pretty well too." [silence]

He: "I tie it in with not allowing myself anything—that *I don't deserve anything good.*"

"The self-punishment. That is the second. And when you think of your fear of traveling specifically, and what you said yesterday?" Here I referred to a dream the session before about homelessness after a hurricane.

He: "The fear of disaster."

I: "Specifically: homelessness! They [the parents] die—in response to: 'I leave, and you will be sorry.' This is the third anxiety, as expressed in the travel fear; that you *lose* the people you are close to. And the fourth we have known from the beginning: *ridicule*."

I summarized this *hierarchy of anxieties*: "The *castration anxiety*, repeated in the fear of women; the *fear of ridicule*, probably in the episodes with your brother, with tickling, erection, and feared urination, repeated in the social withdrawal and the fear of humiliation everywhere; the *fear of losing your parents* as expressed by the threat of 'flying in a handbasket to heaven' or to hell, repeated in the fear of traveling; and the *fear of the inner condemnation*, of the self-punishment, repeated in all the acts of 'I don't deserve anything good.' And the *claustrophobia* is the old anxiety itself concretely experienced. So all the forms of the original anxiety we have discovered are repeated in the various symptoms of the neurosis. And every anxiety had its reality, its confirmation, *then*, necessitating this need for self-punishment and constraint *now* from within. Everything was *real*: your mother injured herself [when trying to beat up the brother], your father was severely ill [his heart disease]; the brother was harshly castigated; the penis can be absent, as shown by the girls, hence taken away; ridicule was heaped on you [because of his timidity and withdrawal]" [859]. This reality foundation of his anxieties, as well as of the related vindictive wishes, is at least one reason, I believe, for the sense of reality about guilt, murder, and death that he had been bringing up earlier on ("I must have done something!").

One thing added two sessions later in the given sequence [861] was the specific wish to deprive me of success with him = of power = of penis—the wish to *castrate* me, the feared retribution, now all internalized, as reflected in a dream. But this hypothesis found little response, and cannot be seen as confirmed.

Another reality factor added later on was the family tradition and mythology: "It is very dangerous to separate; separation, leaving, is bad" [927]. The reality aspects providing these anxieties with their virulence were the aggressive events in the family: fights between the parents with threats to leave, sadistic punishments meted out or threatened, the sadistic quality of the sexual play with his brother ("excitement coupled with pain"), followed by his own sadistic wishes toward the brother.

The patient was amazed about "the drastic turnaround," the sense of much-increased freedom. He began dating a woman: "It all fits in so well. It just seems as if there is a real kind of growth taking place. These lessons are not only learned in the abstract. They can be seen in actual practice, with increasingly positive results. Things seem to be moving toward a greatly increased capacity to act and say and do what needs to be said and done. And here too I find a much greater freedom to say things."

And yet, something was missing, a crucial practical aspect was lacking. The patient had indeed made great progress in his analytic work although it did remain still somewhat intellectual. He appeared, however, completely unable to break the stranglehold the anxieties had on him. His outer life appeared nearly as constricted and deprived as when he had started the analysis. After he again had to cancel a bigger trip abroad at the last moment out of extreme panic, he felt so overpowered by despair that he seriously contemplated killing himself. Then he himself suggested, after about 950 hours of analysis, entering a phobia program that also included some adjunct drug therapy. To his surprise he found that I not only did not object, but, in the light of the severity and recalcitrance of the manifest pathology and the deep discouragement of the patient, welcomed and encouraged such a combination treatment.

### Excerpt 3: Other Archaic Equations and Sequences

There were, however, further factors and aspects of "drives"[4] that specified the hierarchy of anxieties further. The fear of separation hid his *conflict of jealousy*, specifically and most accessibly toward his brother: he wanted to own him exclusively: "There is the total jealousy in the sense of betrayal . . . when I was sent away by him [when he, the older brother, wanted to play with his friends]" [1047].

We could discern, or "reconstruct" in an egopsychological sense (A. Freud 1936, Gray 1973, 1982, 1986, 1987), several sequences leading up to the massive self-punishment, the masochistic end state, and the "negative therapeutic reaction":

One is: sexual *excitement* with the brother → fear of losing control, for example in the form of erection → exposure and shame; the second is: wishes for *revenge* on his brother for his assaults and his belittling → quasi-magical implementation of those wishes by mother (the beating of the evil-doer) → vicarious sadistic enjoyment → guilt  turning of these wishes against the self; the third is: sole *possession* of the brother → jealousy → wish to get rid of the rival and spurning of the treacherous beloved, as manifested by his own attempts "to go away" (running away, traveling) → self-punishment in the form of being lonely, of being unable to lead an independent life, and of the thwarting of all his larger ambitions.

The relationship to the brother, which has been central in the reconstruction presented up to now, covers a deeper and similarly structured one toward his father, and that one in turn a similar one toward his mother: "*The company of the two men was a protection against mother*, but fraught with jealousy" [1049].

The mother was, as mentioned, a profoundly anxious woman and prone to sudden "hysterical rage" and panic. From early on he had felt compelled to cling to her in a kind of *hostile dependency*, as in the form of his great fear of separating from her when he had to go to school. "The clinging was not out of loyalty but out of desperately trying to protest—to deny hate—the murderous wishes" [1054].

Every *success* would mean, besides the more superficial triumph in the conflict of jealousy and the murder of the rival, a *separation from his mother*, and with that not only her angry withdrawal from him, but also the *murderous equation of separation and death*, an equation that lay in the family's superstition never far beneath the surface. By dependency and inability to leave her he protected himself against the murderous anger at her. Thus he also remained "loyal to her by not betraying her by a relationship to a woman."

On the one side, each act of success and step toward *independence*, equated with the intent of *rebellion and triumph*, meant: "I hurt my mother = it is a killing rejection," or "I get rid of the rival." Thus it had to lead by necessity to *guilt*.

On the other side, by *passivity* and submission he defended himself against the jealous rage toward brother or father, and by *dependency* he shielded himself against the equally deep and dangerous anger against his mother; yet each act of failure, brought about by these symptoms of dependency and retreat, had to lead with equal necessity to *shame*.

All these strands were abundantly relived and observed in the transference.

It was more and more likely, though not conclusively confirmed, that the unifying link for all these separate strands lay in early childhood *masturbation* that was accompanied by sadistic fantasies and may have gotten vigorously suppressed by his intrusive grandmother or mother.

He suspected that both the severe separation anxiety and the equally deep fear of rejection and humiliation, the shame anxiety, were used as a defensive shield against the recognition and experience of *castration anxiety* as central to the neurotogenic conflict. In his own words: "The real issue is not separation itself but the fear about sexual freedom. The wavering whether I should go away or not is a screen for the underlying conflict—*the wish for sexual freedom against the fear of castration*" [1056].

I am myself today more inclined to see a profound interaction between these various forms of anxiety. One form stands in for the other, defends against the other, is intertwined on many levels with the other. The intensity of the general anxiety about separating from his mother and equally of the general "social" anxiety about exposure and ridicule had to serve as defense against the very specific castration anxiety with brother and father, and probably also in reverse; one did not have necessarily to be developmentally older than the other. And in turn, the very intensity of this struggle served the masochistic "payment of dues": "To set up the no-win situation is itself a very self-punishing act" [1056].

To repeat just one piece of evidence for the centrality of the castration anxiety: ". . . basically the anxiety about intimacy with women—and there it is the absence of the penis that is very disturbing—and also the homosexual wishes that have to do with the confirmation that the penis is still there" [1057].

**Excerpt 4: Resolution and Farewell**

The patient was, as result of the deep changes brought about (after session 1068), able to go on his long-planned and never before accomplished trip to England. This permitted him the rounding out of many of the insights gained earlier.

An important addition consisted in the uncovering of the following connection in regard to the travel phobia. When the parents traveled in his early childhood and left him and his brother with the grandparents whom he feared and disparaged, he wished his parents very ill: "They leave me in order to punish me because I have been such a bad boy. In turn, I wish for them to be killed on the trip; I hope they will never return."

However, their leaving also meant that he would be left alone with his brother, and while that entailed some forbidden excitement and sexual play, it also led to a deep resentment about having been exploited, of feeling vulnerable and weak. There was guilt engendered by his anger, his vengefulness and his envy against his brother, and shame about his weakness and inferiority in front of the big one [1083].

This conflict about his parents' leaving was now being turned around to form one of the lead phobias: "Now I go away in order to punish my family, but this time I will be killed." Leaving was seen as an aggressive statement and would evoke aggression in response—the magical retribution by equalizing fate [1069].

With these insights it had become possible for him to state now with confidence, not out of spite and despair anymore, as so often before: "I can terminate now. I've gained enough that I can go on from here and be able to deal with things on my own" [1071].

The insights about leaving applied to the termination of the analysis as well. Leaving me meant punishing me and killing me; hence again it had to be followed by the turning against himself, and with that came paralyzing guilt. Yet now it had all been recognized and worked through and did not lead anymore into the vicious circle of rebellion, despair, and self-destruction.

Another dynamic connection was now newly taken up in this context: "I have heard that the molested child tends to accuse himself. That hits home: I feel guilty for having been excited and engaged in those plays with my brother; it's my fault. The greater the excitement, the greater the blame and the fear." This was especially so since he also had loved his brother: he had been the only source of love in the loneliness and coldness, the fear and the strife prevailing at home, and present also after the parents had left. "Whom would I have when the parents were gone?" [1074].

Now that this conflict about the brother had been solved, the anger freed and expressed, and the guilt for it become unnecessary, he felt: "I'm not going to be bound and constricted by it anymore" [1075]. "I really feel transformed. The forces of progress have gained the upper hand over the 'reactionary' forces, that fascistic drill sergeant within" [1080].

That early sexual excitement with his brother had a clearly sadomasochistic nature and pointed back to the one form of sexual connection with his mother that had eluded our attention nearly totally and could only be caught before the gates closed: the importance of the *enemas* in that relationship. Therewith the *woman* had become the *repository of anal excitement*, and it was that form of excitement that had turned to fright and to the large-scale "analising" of the image of woman (which, of course, had been well-known to us for a long time). It was the *projection of his own anal excitement* with his mother and the fusion with punishment in such *anal-masochistic love* for her. This was repeated in the spanking episodes; the allegedly experienced punishment had to serve as a screen memory for the real event of the frequent enemas, and the equation of *excitement and success* felt with it. The brother's factual thrashing, which he witnessed, was a symbolic fulfillment of his revenge, the magical implementation of his wishes. It was a symbol for that *double resentment*: the resentment in regard to his own helplessness and entailing his thirst for revenge, and the resentment dwelling in the inner punishing angel and drill sergeant. How much of the latter might have been taken from the outer judging authority? Certainly a lot. Inwardly he thus reiterated the anal-masochistic "lust and pain" experienced in the enema episodes.

About the nature of the effectiveness of treatment he added: "There was the insight I had derived from a certain situation, then a little later from another situation; gradually it becomes apparent: this is more than just conjecture. When I'm in a situation and anxious, I cannot consciously recite: this is just an example of whatever. It's similar to reading words; you cannot break them down into individual letters. It has become part of you. One cannot take the situation and break it down into the components, but the insight becomes part of you."

I said: "The wrong connections fall by the wayside, and the right ones stand out more and more."

And he responded, "When they are not correct they don't come up, and the right ones come again and again" [1071].[5]

He looks back in the last session [1092]: "The key difficulty was that progress was unbalanced. The insights were there, but they were not accompanied by any visible change. They were rooted in the intellect instead of being felt. They seemed to fit the facts and seemed to make sense, but more as an intellectual abstraction. . . . Without dreams it would have been virtually impossible to get to the unconscious factors. The insights seemed to fall into place and take hold once they were given this little behavioral push. After the trip it became clear that I had this strength within. There was no arguing about it, that was such rock-solid evidence that I could be on my own in a foreign country. I had to give in to the evidence that I had overcome certain obstacles. And no one else did it. I did it on my own. It was irrefutable. I finally was convinced of the real validity of the insights and that the change had taken place."

These were his last words in the analysis. In a subsequent letter a month later he confirmed that he was doing fine and that the gains had been retained.


## SUMMARY OF DYNAMICS

As is the case in most severe neuroses I present in these books, it was also only possible here, thanks to a combination of several treatment modalities, to attain the therapeutic transformation desired by the patient. The lifting of the repressions by analysis was combined with a disciplined learning to face up to the phobic anxiety and to overcome it step by step, and with the temporary dampening of the overwhelming unpleasurable affects with the antidepressant Doxepin.

In this context, it seems to me that the behavioral therapy carries out what Freud, in *Lines of Advance in Psycho-Analytic Therapy* (1918), had to assign to the "demand by the physician," that is, of the analyst himself—actively to induce patients to stop the phobic avoidance. The division of labor possible in this case appears to be more advantageous and for me attained paradigmatic value; when necessary it became a resource in other treatments as well.

The major focus throughout the analysis was on the anxieties and the defenses; among the latter it was mostly on repression and several types of drive reversals: turning from passive to active, especially in the form of role reversals, turning against the self, and, with that turning active into passive, as well as reaction formation and isolation.

One defensive tactic however, a favorite, if not typical, for depressive persons, is that which consists in *making the other feel as guilty and as humiliated* as he feels himself. This is brought about by overt or covert *blaming*. It is a move of turning the tables that encompasses the defense mechanisms of projection, turning passive into active, and a shift from identification with the victim to identification with the accuser. It also amounts to a very powerful form of transference resistance. I believe much of the *negative therapeutic reaction* can actually be ascribed to such a *turning of the tables* by *blame*. It means: "Now it is you who finally gets to feel the full force of my superego that has tormented me all my life."

This very important and frequent form of transference of defense by turning the tables entails that the analyst feel absolutely impotent, a total failure, one who did worse than no treatment at all. In this way, Jacob undertook to place his heavy burden of guilt, shame, and resentment squarely on my shoulders, and he did this, following a solid family tradition, with considerable success. It is therefore extremely important to understand this transference-countertransference pattern in its specificity and to analyze it. Success and failures of the treatment of cases like this depend very much upon its recognition, understanding, and toleration.

Perhaps most important, we dealt with two opposite sets of *identifications*: on the one side the deprecated, dependent, castrated, passive, and anal identity, largely patterned after the mother; on the other side the aggressive, sadistic, competitive/competent identity, one of defiant triumph and revenge, largely patterned after the punishing figure of the father (who used to implement mother's penalties) and the sexually attacking and successful brother. The first identification was mostly shame-laden, the second fraught with guilt.

Shame and guilt were leading factors both in the formation of the symptoms (dynamically) and in the eventual compromise formations (phenomenologically).

Most prominently any form of success, any kind of triumph had become equated with guilt: *triumph = guilt*. These identifications were more or less conscious, but all the in-between factors linking these two parts of the equation had become unconscious. They were, as we saw: (1) his love for his brother and the sexual quality, mostly of a sadomasochistic nature, of that love, contradicted by the wishes for taking revenge on his brother and the sadistic fantasies connected with this; then (2) the implementation of these sadistic, vindictive desires in reality by his mother—as it were, their success or triumph—namely in form of severe physical punishment of the brother; and (3) the ensuing guilt and the turning of all sadism against the self, in the form of (feared) castration first, humiliation second, and total abandonment third, as a kind of *regressive spiral of chastisement*.

Perhaps the original sin in this was the separation from mother. For this possessive woman and in the entire family mythology, separation and individuation were acts of revolt, and ultimately of murderous rage. The deepest equation was, as we have seen: *self-assertion = separation = killing*. And this was the main spirit guiding the inner judge.

A second equation parallel to the first one: *excitement = shame* has been described in detail. The intervening links were: ejaculation, loss of control, urination, exposure, ridicule, and expulsion. Tickling was the paramount example for his equating pleasure with pain, passivity, and inferiority. "All excitement rapidly turns from what I would *do* to what could *happen* to me" [1067].

Passive submission and dependency changed from being sexually pleasurable into being a source of fright and shame. The equation is now: *love = pleasure and excitement = passive submission = defeat = being tied down and locked in*. And this basic equation can be traced farther back than just to the events with the brother (wrestling and tickling), namely to the enemas his mother gave him and kept threatening to give him—signs of loving affection and attention, but also of intrusion, humiliation, and passive submission. They came to be seen as a kind of symbol for this deep ambivalence vis-à-vis her.

Yet I wonder if there was not a still deeper equation underlying that pervasive sense of shame, which would be analogous to the one found in regard to guilt. Perhaps it could be found in this: *being flooded by feelings = loss of power = self-loss = dependence = being unworthy to be loved and respected*. Why this equation of love, dependency, passivity, and shame would have become so intensely repressed is probably to be explained not only by the hierarchy of anxieties I have already described in detail, but to that deeper, properly *traumatic* equation of *overstimulation = sexual excitement = violence*. I think it is, as Gedö (1979) rightly stated, Freud's "actual neurotic" core of the neurosis, a quantitative element. Evidence for this could be amply retrieved from the case material although such an encompassing formulation had not been made during the treatment itself. On that level with its preverbal influences (as in the case of Vera), both the masochism and the implacable inner judge, and consequently also the phobic constriction of his personality, would all serve some kind of *affect regulation*, a kind of structure that was to stop the overwhelming feelings and to give him a foothold in the frightening flood.

This makes it more understandable that for this man, as for many other patients suffering from severe forms of neurosis, a judicious combination of treatment methods became more likely to be successful than analysis alone. In this case, the three methods of *insight + behavior modification + antidepressant medication* worked synergistically and in concert, not antithetically. Thus, the lifting of the repressions by analysis was combined with a training in braving and conquering phobic anxiety by action (in behavior modification), and with a temporary quieting by drugs of the overwhelming unpleasurable affects.

## THE TRAGIC DILEMMA

I now would like to review the main elements from a more general vantage point:

1. There existed a deep ambivalence, above all toward the mother, whereby *separation* was equated with *crime, murder, and death.* A. H. Modell (1984) spoke in a similar context about *separation guilt:* "The right to a separate life is perhaps invariably [with narcissistic patients] accompanied by an unconscious fantasy that separation will lead to the death or damage of the other . . . They were possessed of a basic belief that they had no right to a better life" (pp. 56–57).

The basic phobic attitude itself expressed his dread of separating himself from the fear-filled and angry mother. Every success represented *eo ipso* a symbolic separation and was prohibited. He was suffering from an extremely intense, yet consciously unexplainable sense of guilt—"as if I really had committed a murder." The feared retribution had to be correspondingly massive and omnipresent.

2. The counterpart to his inability to achieve any separation and individuation on any developmental level was the sense of *powerlessness*, the state of helpless exposure, which went far beyond that of any infantile dependency and passivity. This was not simply a regression, but in itself already

a pathological phenomenon. Because every self-assertion was profoundly dangerous, it had to come to a "nothingness" of his self-esteem, and to extreme self-contempt. This itself already caused deep *shame*.

To this perceived weakness and exposure there was another occasionally hinted-at motive—the wish and also the fear to become like the other by means of *seeing*, to merge with the other by perceiving—the motive of a kind of *"primary" identification*. It played a role both in his phobia about women and in his wish for the male partner, but also in his anxiety about all human contact and love: love is closeness, and closeness is merger and union, and with that extinction of the self. Since it was in particular the processes of seeing and being seen (and, more generally of perception altogether) in whose medium merger as well as overpowering and annihilation would occur, these processes of perception had to be largely blocked—by the way shown also in very many dreams where his view of a theater play, a sports event, or a concert was blocked. *Shame* is the specific protection mechanism against the dangers in the domain of perceiving and being perceived.

3. The *spite and negativism* and similar "anal" attributes assuming such an eminent role in his character are derivatives of the original wishes for self-assertion, remnants of the effort to protect himself against total exposure and shameful nothingness, the healthy self-defense of the child.

It is evident that the phobic core of his neurosis (see Sandler and A. Freud 1985) comprised in addition to the just-mentioned elements all the later layers of rivality conflicts. In this regard, the competition for the love of his brother against father and mother, and second, the competition for the love of his father against mother and brother, were much more pronounced than the triangle of the "positive" Oedipus conflict and the rivality for the love of his mother.

However, these three elements, (1) of separation guilt, (2) of deep shame for helpless dependence, for the primitive merger fantasies, and for the flooding by affect, and (3) of defiance as an attempt to reassert control, are clearly of a dyadic nature and originally refer entirely to his mother. His *conscience* has become entirely the executor of that guilt and shame and with that has itself become *dramatically split*. Whereas in later life it is often the case that guilt and shame are synergistic—the same behavior, the same actions or intentions may trigger both emotions at the same time, depending upon the vantage point from which the inner judgment occurs—originally they are antithetical: shame refers to weakness and powerlessness, and guilt refers to strength and power. *Separation guilt* and *dependency shame* are in contradiction to each other. This causes the very important and deep *split of the superego*, which we already met for similar reasons in Vera. And it is this *duality of guilt and shame in their extreme form* which transcends the configuration I have described in Chapter 4.

The *guilt–shame dilemma* is generally of greatest importance. In a weakened form it is nearly ubiquitous. In the severe neuroses its strongly pronounced version is hardly ever to be missed.

As already illustrated, quite generally for many of these individuals, many of their affects are overwhelming, their needs and wishes seem all-encompassing, and specifically, the ideals and values sought quickly assume the character of absoluteness. And it is this last element, the absoluteness of their ideals (hence the categorical nature of their self-judgment, and with that the extreme versions of guilt and of shame) that leads over to a final observation that may be of a more general interest.

If the essence of the "tragic phenomenon" consists in setting some *value absolute* and pursuing it at all costs, at the (near-) exclusion of other values, yet in inevitable conflict with such other values, then the extreme version of these, at least originally, opposite affects of guilt and shame would indicate something of great philosophical importance as well. The fascination of the *guilt–shame dilemma* goes beyond its clinical importance for severe neuroses: it forms the core of most of the tragedies. In especially clear form one can discover it in the Athenian tragedies where every one of the heroic figures insists upon not being viewed as weak (treacherous, faithless, without honor, giving in), is therefore unable to yield, and must, by such obstinate insistence upon an absolutely maintained value, violate the rights of the others, of the state, or of nature—the order of the gods.Thus, inviolable limits are transgressed, and such transgression has to be punished, the culprit must be destroyed. There are other elements in the "tragic phenomenon": overwhelming, global affects and with that the tragic pathos, the irresistible compulsiveness of action and occurrence, the conflict between high values, whereby any solution of the conflict is precluded because of the totality of the exaggeration and idealization of such values, and finally hubris as aggression in the service of such exaggerated ideals. Yet all these can without difficulties be seen as parts or consequences of that basic dilemma.

The Ananke of the fate of these "tragic patients" corresponds to the implacability of the repetition compulsion; in the words of Aeschylus in *Prometheus Bound*: "Art is so much weaker than compulsion" (τέχνη δ᾽ ἀνάγκης ἀσθενεστέρα μακρῷ).

## "CORRECT COMPREHENSION AND MISUNDERSTANDING OF THE SAME DON'T EXCLUDE EACH OTHER" —COMMENTS ON KAFKA'S *TRIAL*

As a literary prototype for this configuration I propose, however, a modern example: Kafka's *The Trial.*

All of Kafka's works, because of their extreme introspective density, suggest a psychoanalytic approach. Yet they are, in their ambiguity and multilayered character, anything but easily interpretable. Any facile approach to them, any quick application to them of any theory, is contradicted by this complexity.

In addition, most of his major works are fragments, with additions and crossed-out paragraphs appended, which increases the tentativeness of the work, and hence the provisional nature of any interpretation.

Frederick Karl (1991) adds to this quandary by rightly stating that "Kafka's works are a gigantic mosaic, and each piece touches upon another, so that it is unwise and misleading to discuss one work as isolated from the rest" (p. 105); instead of such isolated analysis one has to observe "'cross-textuality' or, in more technical terms, 'contextuality'" (p. 105).

Still, it may prove interesting to take one major work, *The Trial,* and examine in it at least the one aspect elucidated by the study of the dynamics just presented. It is my conviction that what we find in the analysis of that one aspect would be applicable to the rest of Kafka's oeuvre—certainly not as a comprehensive understanding, but as *one* parameter for it.

Departing from Kafka's indebtedness to Nietzsche, Karl (1991) states:

> For Kafka, *amor fati* meant a brutal interplay between a destiny that the individual has already worked out for himself and that individual's own striving to transform the way in which that world can be perceived. Kafka's 'pain' resulted from his inability to bring together two seemingly conflicting ideas: that our destiny has been written for us, and yet that our inner urge, an obsessional need, rages to change our very perception of destiny. His many comments on paradise, on its loss and our efforts to regain it, nonetheless are aimed at how we have been predefined, even as we seek to break from that design into a transformation of the self. Nietzsche and Freud provide essential ingredients here, and Kafka made them representational ideas. [p. 108]

Put differently, it is the conflict that, on the one side, the individual wants to *submit* to what is given—as societal constraints, as outer and inner *authority,* as *limitations* of perception and permission—in order to gain a longed-for belonging and acceptance. On the other side, the individual wants to *defy* all those confining structures, in a revolt especially against a stifling, crushing, meaningless, corrupt form of authority. Ostensibly this authority that the protagonist tries to defy is on the outside; yet it still is one that can always appeal successfully to its parallel existence within.

In our metaphors we would say it is the conflict between the *compliance with an archaic, sadistically sexualized superego* and the endless, yet always doomed, effort to overthrow this inner authority, in order to achieve a *more authentic self.* Thus it would be a superego that is part of one's inner world, introjected, but not one with which one feels truly identified, one that very easily becomes reexternalized again. The ego, in its search for identity, for an authentic sense of inner unity and external appearance, cannot accept the dictates of that inner authority, yet neither can it survive in disowning them. The ego is caught in this battle between irrational command, whose validity is deeply in doubt but whose power is inescapable, and the drive to be true to oneself, in the sense of having one's own will and confirming one's autonomy, to master one's own fate, to return to Karl's reference.

I now would like to deepen this analysis.

As the title *The Trial* (*Prozeß*) already indicates, at its center it is an issue of accusation, hence of guilt (*Schuld*) or innocence (*Schuldlosigkeit*), the two terms forming the obvious axis of the drama. With increasing insistence, all the forces point to the shift toward the pole of guiltiness. All persons are seen as entering into some sort of collusion with the law and the largely secret judicial authorities to serve the accusation ("Everything belongs to the court" *Es gehört ja alles zum Gericht*) (Kafka 1935, p. 161), while always indicating that if Joseph K. only did the right thing, then the accusation can be evaded, somehow, and they might be able to help him. Yet the ultimate condemnation approaches with the same inexorability as the word toward the end of the Letter to His Father: "everything one single great guilt" (*alles eine einzige große Schuld*) [translated as "liability"] (Kafka 1919, p. 121).

We can track this crescendo of "guiltiness" through the novel. Joseph K. identifies with accusation and guiltiness while simultaneously trying to defend himself against them. He refers to the disorder in Frl. Bürstner's room when he says: "it was done by others against my will and yet, as I've said, through my guilt; therefore I wanted to ask for forgiveness."[6] The very prosecution is already proof for this guilt, that is, "that the court is being attracted by the guilt."[7]

He protests his innocence again and again, "it belongs to this kind of judiciary that one is not only innocently being condemned, but also unknowingly."[8] Accordingly he wants to defy, to smash, to take revenge on this court, for example by taking away the seductive wife of the court servant (*Gerichtsdiener*).[9]

One notices here (and already at the beginning with Frl. Bürstner), and ever more strongly, how he falls in, again and again, with women who at first seem to want to help him, but betray him subsequently (the very same is the case in *The Castle*). The relationships are at the same time very erotic; greedily, thirstily, devouringly he falls over the woman like a beast of prey, and yet the relation appears thoroughly functional, impersonal, objectified. Is that part of his guilt, namely that he uses everybody with whom he associates, albeit to liberate himself from the smothering web of persecution? That the others, especially the women, are but tools, just as he himself is thoroughly depersonalized? And that sexualization is one way of dealing with such suffered dehumanization, one defense against the trauma of objectification?

Returning though to the theme of his revolt ("one always rebels"—[*man rebelliert eben immer*], says the servant of the court, p. 72): his brief acts of defiance against the accusation are followed by a sharpened sense of condemnation. But it is not, as we might expect, a deeper feeling of guilt because of such rebellion, but by expression of pervasive shame: "it was too embarrassing for him . . . the sudden weakness" (*es war ihm zu peinlich . . . die plötzliche Schwäche*) (p. 78), "the first unquestionable defeat" (*die erste zweifellose Niederlage*) (p. 68), "how humiliated these have to be" (*wie gedemütigt die sein müssen*) (p. 73). It culminates in his accepting the extreme shame of being completely depersonalized: "he tolerated it that those two were negotiating about him like about a thing; he liked it even most that way."[10] The "information giver" (*Auskunftgeber*) calls on him as a weakling to rise (*Also auf, Sie schwacher Mann*), and K. thanks him with joy and shame (p. 81 f.). Ever more he is the excluded one; the others whisper about him, and he is unable to understand them, but he feels the looks of their eyes lying heavily on him (*aber auf K. lagen diese Blicke doch schwer*, p. 92). It is all quite reminiscent of the statement in his Letter to His Father: "It is the general pressure of anxiety, of weakness, of self-contempt."[11] This episode is immediately followed by the sexualized whipping of the two guards—"we have to undress and be totally naked" (*wir werden uns ja ganz nackt ausziehen müssen*) (p. 95) by the spanker (*Prügler*), where one of them, Franz, says, kneeling, pleading, and crying: "I'm so awfully ashamed" (*ich schäme mich ja so erbärmlich*) (p. 96). Certainly, it is not K. here who is speaking; to the contrary, he is the one who is beseeched. But if we take the whole novel as an inner "process," almost like a dream, the sequence should not be irrelevant in showing the ever more insistent *shift from guilt to shame.*

And this is the point I am driving at: while the novel seems to revolve around that axis of guilt and innocence, it turns ever more into one of the polarity or *axis of dignity and self-respect versus shame, humiliation, degradation*: "Up to now you were our honor; you are not permitted to become our disgrace.[12] The whole family would be completely debased,[13] says the uncle.

More and more the women turn from being instruments of deliverance and lust into those of submission, degrading self-loss, and humiliation: "Now you belong to me" "You crawl away with a little dirty thing";[14] it is said first by, then about, Leni.

A new act of defiance and asserted innocence, again along the first axis of guilt and innocence ensues: "Above all, it was necessary, if anything was to be attained, to refuse a priori any thought of possible guilt. There was no guilt."[15] Joseph K. had to dismiss his advocate. This bravely spiteful resolution is again immediately followed by a stream of memories of shame and embarrassment, and a renewed decisiveness: "Today, K. did not know anything anymore about shame."[16] He is determined to take over his own defense, to reassert his autonomy and will, and to show what Karl (1991) calls (in regard to Spinoza) "the need to preserve the self, to maintain one's pride of being, the power of what one stands for" (p. 110). It is *an anti-shame heroism of liberation from submission to the forces on the outside*: "his complete and final deliverance" (*seine vollständige und endgültige Befreiung*, p. 142 f.). Yet this too ends in oppressiveness and fainting when he is faced with the outlook that, no matter what, the court will "bring up from somewhere the great guilt [of the accused] where there had originally been nothing."[17] Not one real acquittal has been known to him,[18] says the painter, known under the pseudonym "Titorelli."

The guilt never ends; even at the time of acquittal the new arrest is already planned.[19] No sign of guilt is ever forgotten, no lasting forgiveness ever possible: "No document gets lost; with the court there is no forgetting" (= amnesty).[20] On K.'s lips are the signs of condemnation,[21] claims the ultimate victim of the process, merchant Block. Here again the axis shifts: from signals of guilt and final judgment to images of abasement, of humiliation, of shame. Any autonomous action is counterproductive: "Waiting is not useless . . . only independent action is useless."[22] Block reports the mixture of self-praise and "doglike self-abasement" in the lawyer's submission to the court (Eingabe).[23] Block himself presents the picture of total, abject dependency and self-surrender, "distracted by shame."[24] Immediately following the executed revolt of K. against the lawyer, the images of degradation of Block, a kind of alter ego of K., cascade. The lawyer calls Block "this miserable worm" (*dieser elende Wurm*, p. 195), addresses him with the familiar *Du*, instead of the proper *Sie* (in contrast to his talking to Joseph K.): "You have been called, still you are unwelcome."[25] The merchant does not dare look at his defender, as if the view would blind him (*zu blendend, als daß er ihn ertragen könnte*) (p. 202), again a clear act of "blinding shame." Accordingly, K. expresses his contempt of Block: "Kneel or crawl on arms and legs, do whatever you want."[26] It ends with the merchant's total degradation: "This was no client anymore, this was the dog of the advocate."[27] Accusation and defense have become absolute powers on the outside now; the person's self has lost the last shred of sovereignty, and with that of dignity. It is a state of absolute shame: "Shame on you, in front of my client!" (*Schäme dich hier vor meinem Klienten!*) (p. 208). It anticipates Joseph K.'s own end: *not guilt, but shame*, due to the surrender of his consciousness of *truly being himself* to the *dehumanizing forces on the outside*, a state of ultimate *passivity, dependency, and self-loss.*

In the penultimate chapter this shift is first marked by his loss of memory and comprehension, then by the nightlike darkness at midday, and finally in the wonderful midrash given by the preacher, "Before the Law." The call goes out to him, Joseph K., as the central person, with his name, somewhat like God's call to Adam after the fall: *Ayekka?* "Where are you?" (something K. had originally done himself, in front of Fräulein Bürstner, p. 38). His guilt is looked at as proven; the process itself is gradually passing over into judgment.[28] But the decisive statement is: "You are seeking too much help from others, especially women."[29]

The deception in K.'s views about the court lies, says the priest, in that a guardian irrevocably blocks the entrance; that he, K., allows these forces of outer authority (of "duty", *Pflicht*) ultimate power over himself, and that he abdicates his own personal autonomy to these forces of condemnation from within and without. The watchman says: "Try anyway to enter, in spite of my prohibition."[30] K. accepts totalitarian authority (the watchman as "duty," *Pflicht*, p. 227), instead of free, personal decision. By identifying and complying with what Nietzsche called the "worm of conscience" (*Gewissenswurm*), personal dignity, every right to self-respect, is shredded, and real life doomed. The preacher repeats: "Don't accept the meaning of others without examination" (*Übernimm nicht die fremde Meinung ungeprüft*) (p. 226), and again, a little later: "You should not care too much about the opinions" (*Du mußt nicht zuviel auf Meinungen achten*) (p. 229). In reality, the watchman is subordinate to the seeker, but he is, wrongly, treated as if *he* were absolute power. All the compulsion comes from within, not from without.[31]

Is he totally blind about the real question? The priest screams down to him: "Don't you see two steps ahead of you?" (*Siehst du denn nicht zwei Schritte weit?*), (p. 223). So much deals with not seeing, not knowing, with darkness, but also with a blinding light, connected with his own metamorphosis (p. 260)—all interpretable as phenomena of shame. The recurrent image of the blinding light is reminiscent of Nietzsche's words: "That feeling: 'I am the center of the world!' occurs very intensely when one is suddenly attacked by disgrace. One stands there as if dumbfounded by the surf and feels blinded as though stared at by *one* big eye that looks at him and through him from all sides."[32]

What do we make of the priest's quote of the "explainers" (*die Erklärer*, the *dorshim*): "Correct comprehension of something and misunderstanding of the same don't exclude each other completely?"[33] This paradoxical statement refers to the guardian's view of his own power and of the immense power of the other guardians who are closer to the Law and their intolerable sight (*unerträglichen Anblick*). "All these utterances may in themselves be correct,"[34] yet the way he presents them to the seeker "is clouded by simplicity and arrogance" (*durch Einfalt und Überhebung getrübt*) (p. 228). I understand this paradox so: "Yes, the powers of inner and outer authority (the superego) are great, are huge, may even be immense, yet the power of the person assuming the responsibility for himself can vanquish them. As big as the might of the inner judge is, the assertion of one's identity as a responsible self is still greater."

Related to this, the preacher says: "'. . . one does not have to hold everything for true; one has only to hold it for necessary.' 'A gloomy opinion' said K. 'The lie is being turned into the world order.'"[35]

What irony: the priest preaching from the pulpit of the St. Vitus cathedral pronounces, bowed and in darkness, first a classical midrash, with all the pilpulistic exegesis, and ends with the statement that practical necessity overrules the truth, leading K. to respond with a quote from the posthumous work of Nietzsche about the supreme rule of the lie. As I understand this: where instrumentalism and pragmatism (the powers of duty, convention, and authority) rule supreme, the end is untruth and darkness. And this is exactly the judgment about K.'s life. His own will and judgment, with that, have merged with the court's: "The court doesn't want anything from you. It accepts you when you come, and it dismisses you when you go."[36] The outer authority and the execution are merely a reflection of the rigid inner authority and the self-loss.

Thus K. becomes a unity with the two executioners who walk him to the quarry. Facing again the woman whom at the beginning he had used or tried to use, Frl. Bürstner, his resistance collapses; he follows her. Finally, he sees it as his duty to bore the butcher knife into his own body, but even that act is shifted to the outside; again he is too weak to take the responsibility. His last vision is that of a human being opening a window and reaching out, as if offering his help, and K.'s own last gesture is that of a desperate plea, without address; the other is impersonal, dehumanized is he himself.

The very ending of the novel is therefore: "Where was the judge he had never seen? Where was the high court he had never reached? . . . 'Like a dog!' he said; it was as if the shame should survive him."[37]

Thus, behind the ostensible "process" dealing with guilt or innocence, with accusation and defiance, with judgment and execution, appears more and more insistently the issue of humiliation, degradation, shame, along with that of the autonomous self, the core of the person responsible for himself, his authenticity.

Yet, what is the important issue of guilt about, what is the more important issue of shame about? I believe the answer is in short this. K. himself is guilty that he has treated everybody else as well as himself as if they were things to be used. His guilt consists in the *instrumentalization and exploitation of human beings*, himself included. This is somewhat akin to what we see in Ibsen's *John Gabriel Borkman*, a crime for which there is no forgiveness: the murder of love, "soul murder," but more broadly: the blindness to everything individual, the dehumanization, the "soul blindness." For doing this to others he is guilty.

In turn, we notice that he seems strangely *unable to take responsibility* for himself, his life, for his fate, for his right to become the center of action. He is not so much irresponsible—in a conventional sense he is, to the contrary, a thoroughly responsible citizen—but in a deep sense when it is a question of the meaning of his life and of his behavior, when he engages in reflection about himself, he does not recognize responsibility. And this is a profound weakness, a shameful failure, not an act of guilt and sin. I believe it is this inability which is referred to both by the darkness ("Don't you see two steps ahead of you?") and by the blinding light of uncovering.

But the situation is even more complex: the entire world in which K. lives and is successful obeys this *principle of dehumanization*, of treating the other as a thing, or as we see in *The Castle*, as a stranger, and with that not really as somebody to be respected in his individuality. In that book, the ostensible polarity is "foreignness" or "strangeness" versus "belonging," yet with the same issue of dehumanization both inflicted and suffered by the other K. As a stranger "one" is merely part of a category. To be treated in this way, however, is ultimate contempt in action, with the result of total shame in the "object." Joseph K.'s shame, is, I believe, rooted in this utter dehumanization as a basic existential experience.

In this way I see the work as a great presentation of the tragic dialectic between shame and guilt—opposites of abused power in guilt and of weakness and failing in shame—between which the person may be inescapably caught, a walk along abysses that yawn on both sides of a narrow path—a crushing conflict that drives its victim into death.

## ENDNOTES

1. In the treatment of this case my regular consultations with Paul Gray proved to be of invaluable help. Moreover, he saw the patient a few times during acute crises of threatened breaking off of treatment and thus made possible the eventually successful therapy.

2. One of the descriptions of Edith Dombey: "Entrenched in her pride and power, and with all the obduracy of her spirit summoned about her . . ." (p. 544). That novel abounds with striking drawings of what we would call "clinical narcissism": narcissism as a term aptly summarizing descriptive details, but not as a purported explanatory device, at it has often been used.

3. Here I was taking up a valuable distinction made first by Nietzsche and elaborated by Erich Fromm and Isaiah Berlin.

4. I use the drive concept here as a pragmatically very useful abstraction for bundles of recurring, mostly unconscious wishes, needs, and impulses without subscribing to the metapsychological drive theory.

5. This is his own version of what Grünbaum (1984) has dubbed Freud's "tally argument."

6. (*Es geschah durch fremde Leute gegen meinen Willen und doch, wie gesagt, durch meine Schuld; dafür wollte ich um Entschuldigung bitten*) (p. 34).

I quote and translate directly from the German text, edited by Max Brod (1935, 1946).

7. (*Daß das Gericht von der Schuld angezogen werde*) (p. 45).

8. (*und es gehört zu der Art dieses Gerichtswesens, daß man nicht nur unschuldig, sondern auch unwissend verurteilt wird*) (p. 59).

9. (*Daß er das ganze Gericht . . . sofort zerschlagen konnte, . . . es gab vielleicht keine bessere Rache an dem Untersuchungsrichter und seinem Anhang, als daß er ihnen diese Frau entzog und an sich nahm*) (p. 66).

10. (*Er duldete es, daß die zwei über ihn wie über eine Sache verhandelten, es war ihm sogar am liebsten*) (p. 81).

11. (*Es ist der allgemeine Druck der Angst, der Schwäche, der Selbstmissachtung*) (p. 112 f.).

12. *Du warst bisher unsere Ehre, du darfst nicht unsere Schande werden* (p. 104).

13. (*Und daß die ganze Verwandtschaft mitgerissen oder wenigstens bis auf den Boden gedemütigt wird*) (p. 107).

14. (*Jetzt gehörst du mir . . . Verkriechst dich mit einem kleinen, schmutzigen Ding . . .*) (p. 121).

15. (*Vor allem war es, wenn etwas erreicht werden sollte, notwendig, jeden Gedanken an eine mögliche Schuld von vornherein abzulehnen. Es gab keine Schuld*) (p. 136).

16. (*Heute wußte K. nichts mehr von Scham*) (p. 138).

17. (*Zum Schluß aber zieht es von irgendwoher, wo ursprünglich gar nichts gewesen ist, eine große Schuld hervor*) (p. 160).

18. ([*Ich habe*] *nicht einen einzigen wirklichen Freispruch erlebt*) (p. 165).

19. (*Die Richter haben ja schon beim Freispruch diese Verhaftung vorgesehen*) (p. 170).

20. (*Es geht kein Akt verloren, es gibt bei Gericht kein Vergessen*) (p. 170).

21. (*Sie würden, nach Ihren Lippen zu schließen, gewiß und bald verurteilt werden*) (p. 185).

22. (*Das Warten ist nicht nutzlos. . .nutzlos ist nur das selbständige Eingreifen*) (p. 186).

23. (*Wobei er sich auf gerade hündische Weise vor dem Gericht demütigte*) (p. 188).

24. ([*Dieser . . . sagte*] . . . *zerstreut vor Beschämung: "Ja, man wird später sehr abhängig von seinem Advokaten"*) (p. 193).

25. (*Du wurdest gerufen . . . trotzdem kommst du ungelegen*) (p. 202).

26. (*Knie nieder oder krieche auf allen vieren, tu, was du willst*) (p. 203).

27. (*Das war kein Klient mehr, das war der Hund des Advokaten*) (p. 205).

28. (*Man hält wenigstens vorläufig deine Schuld für erwiesen . . . das Urteil kommt nicht mit einemmal, das Verfahren geht allmählich ins Urteil über*) (p. 222).

29. (*Du suchst zuviel fremde Hilfe, . . . und besonders bei Frauen*) (p. 223).

30. (*Versuche es doch, trotz meinem Verbot hineinzugehen*) (p. 225).

31. (*Vor allem ist der Freie dem Gebundenen übergeordnet. Nun ist der Mann tatsächlich frei . . . die Geschichte erzählt von keinem Zwang*) (p. 230).

32. (*Jenes Gefühl; "Ich bin der Mittelpunkt der Welt!" tritt sehr stark auf, wenn man plötzlich von der Schande überfallen wird; man steht dann da wie betäubt inmitten einer Brandung und fühlt sich geblendet wie von* einem *großen Auge, das von allen Seiten auf uns und durch uns blickt*) (Nietzsche [1886], *Morgenröte*, Book 4, 352; p. 234).

33. (*Richtiges Auffassen einer Sache und Mißverstehen der gleichen Sache schließen einander nicht vollständig aus*) (p. 228).

34. (*Wenn auch alle diese Äußerungen an sich richtig sein mögen*) (p. 228).

35. (*"Nein," sagte der Geistliche, "man muß nicht alles für wahr halten, man muß es nur für notwendig halten." "Trübselige Meinung," sagte K. "Die Lüge wird zur Weltordnung gemacht"*) (p. 232).

36. (*Das Gericht will nichts von dir. Es nimmt dich auf, wenn du kommst, und es entläßt dich, wenn du gehst*) (p. 233).

37. (*Wo war der Richter, den er nie gesehen hatte? Wo war das hohe Gericht, bis zu dem er nie gekommen war? . . . "Wie ein Hund!" sagte er, es war, als sollte die Scham ihn überleben*) (p. 239).

# 6

## Global Affects and the Problem of Absoluteness

Qin'at sofrim tarbeh chochma—קנאת סופרים תרבה חכמה
(The competition of writers increases wisdom)
—Talmud *Bava Batra* 21a

## "DESIGNS" (*ENTWÜRFE*)

Of course, the findings presented in these chapters as well as in the parallel work (*Flight from Conscience*), whose major findings are used in these two concluding chapters—i.e., psychodynamics that had been hidden behind compulsively repeated impulsive actions, one of the main forms of what is experienced as so "demonic"—were in a sense "accidental," insofar as I had to rely upon what I could learn from the intensive work with my patients during a specific period of time. Their selection is to some extent contingent. While this is a very restricted field of a dozen cases, though one investigated into great depth and well-documented, comparisons with other patients and with those I have been following in supervision allow the assumption that they are pretty typical for large numbers of patients with severe neuroses in the United States and Europe.

Something similar can be said about the literary and philosophical considerations in my book *Broken Reality* (Wurmser 1993): These too represent an "accidental" selection, encounters with certain works and authors that could have occurred somewhat differently as well. With that I just want to say that I simply describe here a series of encounters that have been important for me and that share certain attributes—meetings with patients, with writers and philosophers, with cultures and books—and that any claim for completeness and hence for an encompassing and categorical schema would be premature, even arrogant. The profound yearning for theoretical closure clashes with the sense of multiform, often self-contradictory, that is, paradoxical truth.

With that I mean also that again and again the clinical observations break open the comprehensive and closed theoretical models. Therefore I find that offering different outlines (*Entwürfe*), even sketches or drafts, is pragmatically more satisfying than a well-rounded theory. Such designs are in-

251

tertwined with each other, not necessarily sharply delimited. Actually, they are extended metaphors which I have described as configurations; the sequences and equations also often consist of metaphorical transitions (Wurmser 1977a). They form part of a large whole, as the summarizing outline will show, but of a whole that we still glimpse only in parts.

It seems to me also that Freud himself quite freely used his explanatory models as *drafts* and as *metaphorical constructions* that could relatively easily be shifted, discarded, and replaced. A good example is the coexistence of his topographic and structural models, which can be largely but not fully brought to congruence with each other. The later model does not replace the former, although such complete congruence has repeatedly been attempted (e.g., by Arlow and Brenner [1964]).

In theorizing there always exists the great *danger of all too bold extrapolations*. Yet encompassing conceptual designs are indispensable, and with them it is inevitable that we rely on such extrapolations. The commandment is then that we remain open toward new insights and acknowledge the speculations as such. Before I turn to a deepening of these thoughts, I give a summary of what we have found clinically, albeit in a theoretically deepened reformulation.

## THE SHIFTING OF THE BOUNDARIES:
## SOME PRINCIPAL RESERVATIONS ABOUT
## THE CONCEPT OF "BORDERLINE" PATHOLOGY

Various types of neurosis select certain parts from those metaphorical models, prefer very different forms of defense, arrive at different configurations, and rely upon different equations or sequences. Therefore also my deep unease about the collective "borderline" diagnosis. More generally speaking, with others—Beres (1974), Calef and Weinshel (1979), and more recently Abend and colleagues (1983)—I have been disturbed by the ever more widespread and cavalier use of terms indicating severe psychopathology: psychosis, borderline, ego or superego defects, unanalyzability, manipulativeness, and so on. The effects of such sloppy and pejorative-judgmental diagnostic terms on what we do and how we approach our patients can be drastically detrimental.

Denial is, as Basch (1974) wisely remarked, one example of this tendency, where a ubiquitous defense against some aspects of perception has been almost automatically regarded as primitive and diagnostically ominous. In truth, it can be part of the psychopathology of everyday life; it is a typical part of the neurotic process; it may be widespread even in well-analyzable cases, severe or not so severe though they may be, or it may, in certain specific forms, be one part of the profound psychotic decathexis (or rather: of the psychotic form of compromise formation). The same holds true for the ubiquitous phenomena of ambivalence ("splitting"), of projection and turning passive into active ("projective identification"), and of "narcissistic" and "masochistic" fantasies.

The "borderline" diagnosis has, in spite of all the valiant efforts at definition and dynamic description, become both a wastebasket category and, clinically, an excuse: Beres (quoted by Abend et al. [1983]) suggested "that 'borderline' is such a poor term that it be discarded altogether, since it designates merely a loosely linked group of patients with severe character pathology" (p. 25). In Michels' (1983) formulation "Borderline was called a patient who seemed at first analyzable but then did not turn out to be." Abend et al. (1983) come to the conclusion "that a description does not constitute a definition. Nor a diagnosis. Far from supplying the hoped-for enduring definition and clearcut diagnostic criteria, we were forced to say that 'borderline' *is not a diagnostic entity, or a discrete recognizable syndrome;* it is at best *a loose supraclassification*" (p. 242).

What can be observed in the more severe forms of neurosis (Freud speaks of "severe neuroses," e.g. 1940b, p. 180)—now usually classified as "borderline," and with their specific differences according to type of neurosis—is not principally and qualitatively different from what can be seen in the milder forms. It seems to me very important to emphasize this *continuity,* and not to work out a sharp and principal difference between the lighter and the more severe forms.

On the other side, I believe it is more consonant with clinical experience to assume such a *break in continuity* between the neuroses and the main forms of psychosis. Even though the mental contents may be the same, current knowledge makes it more likely that we can assume that some basic mental processes in the psychoses are radically different from those encountered in the neuroses and in need of other principles of explanation.

By blurring the boundaries to the psychoses the biological nature of some processes in the latter tends to be overlooked. Because of such an inexact diagnostic, disparate clinical phenomena are falsely equated and wrong claims are being made about cures of psychoses by psychotherapy (I do not mean that these might not occur, I only refer to the sloppiness of many such claims). Certainly there are commonalities insofar as what is biological is always reshaped by what is meaningful and derives from the life history. The contents of even quite complex constellations may be interpretable, yet there exists always a break within, that appears to be beyond meaningfulness—at least as far as our comprehension reaches today.

Another questionable consequence consists in that three separate types of phenomena are automatically equated: emotional illness = regression to earlier ontogenetic levels of development = preexisting fixations to normal, albeit extremely early phases. Thus illness is viewed as the repetition of normal phenomena, and early development is being entirely seen and interpreted through the lens of later pathology. That view proved to be of the greatest heuristic fruitfulness with the neuroses but it is extremely dubious in regard to the psychoses. All those extrapolations about early infancy and the regression theory of the psychoses have been severely shaken by the new infant research (see Fraiberg 1982, Lichtenberg 1983, 1986, 1989, Stern 1985, and others). I believe it is a matter of scientific modesty not to explain the psychoses with introspective methods alone. For that we need other approaches, at least as auxiliary methods.

The attempt to explain what is neurotic by what is psychotic—the unknown by something that is even more enigmatic—is also absurd. We also do not need a grammar of Chinese to clear up a linguistic problem in Russian; at most it can help us by analogy in its description.

In contrast to the descriptions usually given of the treatment of such patients, my experience, as stated in Chapter 1, has been that most of those severely ill neurotic patients, the so-called borderline cases, respond well to a classical approach, if this treatment method is not restricted to "insight" but rather used as it was originally devised—as a method combining the shared exploration with some auxiliary measures of suggestion, of behavioral approaches, and even occasionally of medication, while retaining the central importance given to the careful understanding of conflict: of the defenses, of superego configurations and superego-induced affects like guilt, shame, and depression, and of the vast range of other affects, and all this preferentially within the transference, moment by moment. Decisively, the difference is only an issue of *more or less, not of either-or.*

If it is the major thesis of "borderline" pathology phenomenologically that there exists a deep disturbance about the feeling of identity, then the main experience in the analytic work, instead of adducing a separate mechanism of "splitting," is, as I have stated before, rather the issues of superego pathology, which lead to the phenomena of identity splits and splits in the experience of the object world. Especially the exploration of the absoluteness of these patients' ideals, hence the categorical nature of their self-judgment, and with that the extreme versions of guilt and of shame, offers a promising access to a deeper understanding of their profound and massive conflicts.

The leading question is: What should be the *focus* of the analyst's activity in every individual case so as to obtain the optimal *long-range change?* Such an optimal way of focusing has to be specific for every case. That means, there is not *one* analytic technique, but each patient requires his or her own optimal form, a technique that entails a wide spectrum of interventions, which are set up so that both the *rational alliance* and the *reliving of irrationality* are permitted, facilitated, and protected.

The question then arises, to what extent the *technique determines the theory*, with the theory then secondarily being used to justify the technique, rather than the other way around. Of course, we deal in this with a circular process, not with some unilinear causality. Still, the primacy of the technical approach could determine the clinical findings, which then in turn are ordered according to what is viewed as explanatory for those observations; the theory is then again used, in a circular process, to dictate the nature of interpretations and other interventions. It is one form of what Gadamer (1975) called the "hermeneutic circle." A different technique—in my case the emphasis on the forms of anxiety and other affects of unpleasure, the defenses employed, and the superego aspects evoked during the analysis of inner conflict—would have to lead to different experiences, to different ways of explaining, and hence to different kinds of theoretical understanding (meaning ordering the data) from Kernberg's (1984) or Kohut's (1971, 1977) approach. It is not so much a question of right or wrong, as it is one of greater or lesser help as to long-range intention. The emphasis on "active confrontation of contradictions," hence of the primacy of "splitting," the pursuing of the negative transference, hence the stress on direct interpretation of aggression and its view as primary, the neglect of superego interpretations, and more generally "a prepatterned technical approach," all tend to create an atmosphere of strong exertion of authority, if not of provocation, which cannot help but intensely color the reactions of the patient— mostly in the sense that the patient feels humiliated and judged, and thus confirmed in his abysmally low self-esteem. *Much of the "borderline" pathology in treatment can be viewed as an artefact of a technique that is implicitly or explicitly not morally neutral, but judgmental.* By assuming such a non-neutral stance, one creates a *real* relationship with strongly sadomasochistic features and thus blocks the opportunity to *analyze* the superego conflicts, the superego transference, and the problems of masochism. Instead of helping the patient to learn to observe himself and the workings of his mind, one suggests to him to adapt, and one provokes the aggression and submission going with such educational imposition. *The beating fantasy is enacted, not analyzed.* In particular, the consistent neglect of the enormous shame sensitivity of most of these patients seems to me a gross error in technique and itself entails a basic violation of neutrality (cf. also Nathanson [1992]).

Still, these approaches reveal themselves not so much as wrong, but as more narrowly useful than they claim: They are valuable tactics of short-range, mostly behavioral change; they override by authority and by the over-ruling of guilt and shame the deeply hidden, largely unconscious conflicts, on behalf of immediate exigencies. Such interventions can indeed be life-saving—as *crisis intervention*, but *not as long-term treatment*. It seems to me that they require to be complemented by other approaches of understanding and treatment if deep, long-range changes and at least partial resolution of unconscious conflict are to be attained.

I myself have found the technical precepts, for example, of confrontation of contradictions or drive interpretations, very useful in an emergency, yet counterproductive and eventually detrimental in the psychoanalysis or psychoanalytically oriented treatment of such cases. It blocks above all careful superego analysis, which is anyway in these cases often already impeded by the life-protective measures necessary.

And there is yet another argument against the indiscriminate use of this concept. "Borderline" has become, like narcissism, one more category used to condemn someone else, and to justify aggressive behavior under the guise of health care, as have the terms going with it, terms like "defect" or "split-ting," but also "projective identification" and "denial"; these have turned into an arsenal of weapons. When we remember how it was one of Freud's most important insights that we all have many of the same problems as our patients, that we all share in those conflicts, that we use the same defenses and suffer from the same anxieties and attain the same conflict solutions, and that it is all a matter of degree rather than of an either-or, then it must strike us that these new dichotomies and the judgmental attitudes promoted by them are a lamentable retrogression, not a progression, a regression, in fact, in terms and spirit to Janet and to Charcot.

Our paramount task is not that of being the outer authority, of confront-ing, limit setting, moralistically intervening, dramatically and authoritatively interpreting, or pointing to reality, even with these patients. Rather we may do best in the long run by helping our patients to *examine* their superego precisely in the transference, instead of having them obey or overthrow it.

Impulsivity is, as we have seen, after all an attempt to break out of the confinement of the superego—an attempt doomed by its very nature to failure. As I commented earlier (Wurmser, 1988), the superego is still the sleeping giant of psychoanalysis. Having said all this, I do not suggest that we discard the term "borderline" altogether, but, for all the reasons given,

I consider it better to use it only when we really are uncertain: Is this now a residual state after a psychotic episode? Or do we have strong indications for the imminence of a psychosis? Yet even then it is indispensable to go on specifying what type of psychosis approaching from beyond that border we refer to: manic-depressive, schizophrenic, epileptic, or an organic disturbance of the limbic system? Many could, in fact, simply be seen as neurotic decompensations into dissociative states ("hysterical psychosis," as for example with Vera).

*Border* and *borderline* mean something specific; they do not connote a huge gray area, an in-between *terra certaminis* that encompasses an enormous domain of psychopathology. No country would be happy if much of its territory, including its capital, were suddenly designated "a borderline area."

## AN ENCOMPASSING DESIGN

The question I posed at the beginning was this: How can we explain something we regularly encounter in our patients, which strikes us as a demonic compulsion to act periodically, again and again, in ways that are extremely detrimental to their interests in the long run and that impress both them and outsiders as something uncannily strange, different, bizarre? Is this *fate-determining repetition compulsion* a supraordinate, metapsychologically basic power, perhaps a manifestation of the "death instinct," or the "force of inertia" inherent in the id? Or is it rather an expression of the attempt to master actively in the repetition a passively experienced psychological situation, namely a wish for mastery inherent in the ego? Or is it, as Waelder (1930) suspected, a special factor of inner life, on a par with the three main structures of the mind—ego, id, and superego? Certainly this compulsion to repeat can be ascertained in *all* neurotic disturbances, yet with particularly dramatic and fateful force in those I have called the severe neuroses.

As I put together the notes of the cases that struck me as the most impressive ones of the last decades and surveyed them in toto, this demonically compelling force to repeat self-destructive behavior, usually in impulsive fashion, was indeed a prominent feature, but there was much more to it. It proved to be a thoroughly complex formation.

### The Doubleness

I would like now to give a summary of the dynamics that goes beyond those observed in the individual cases and has more general validity.

Of course, there were the well-known main conflicts: the common or positive oedipal triangular situation with the double conflict of a sexual and aggressive nature, the counterversion of the negative Oedipus complex, and the competition with the siblings for the parents' attention, typically entailing wishes to eliminate those unbidden intruders. Already less-known was what has been ascribed to the separation and individuation phase—the conflict between the wish to detach oneself from the overpowering mother and to assert oneself and the countering need to keep her protection and remain sheltered under her wing. With that come closely allied conflicts in regard to body control, saying No, and complying, retaining and giving away, purity and dirtiness, and all those other "anal" conflicts. Then there were conflicts about wishes for dependency—if not complete merger—versus those for independence and isolation, between limitless gratification and total renunciation, that is, more or less distant derivatives of "oral" strivings.

As I let the material "speak" to me, certain images emerged, bright patterns that began to contrast against the dark background. I now very briefly repeat these patterns, which partly overlap but keep their shape as images. They have fuzzy borders and cannot be pressed into a schema but rather are kept something artful, in the nature of comprehensive metaphors of an almost mythical character, in a way that it may be comparable to what Einstein described as the attainment of scientific insight, namely the emerging of certain images in the series of impressions, images that repeat themselves (*Motiv des Forschens* [1918]).

Here we find at first, and at the core, the *anxiety* about certain objects or situations that begins and continues with certain variations from very early on through life. Opposite to it stands a *protective* system. Both are tightly joined: they are clearly derived from the one ambivalently experienced parental, sibling, or caretaker figure, or from several overlapping figures. In it, the hated part is being seen and dreaded in some menacing shape, and the beloved part is sought as protector. The hated and feared part is also chosen as the carrier of all the hateful attributes of one's own personality—jealousy, malice, vengefulness.

Real brisance is reached only then when these two aspects are perpetuated in the superego—when the phobic separation of the evil from the good side is followed by a similar severance into an anxiety figure and a protective figure as inner authorities. This evil inner voice that consistently condemns, that does not let anything good remain in the self (*das keinen guten Faden läßt*: "it does not leave any good thread"), a kind of *sulphurous conscience*, cannot be borne forever. Either it comes to suicide, which promises an escape from this angrily judging voice, or it comes to certain impulsive actions on the outside, thought to be redemptive.

In these actions one bonds with a figure that should unite within itself those two contrasting superego figures, and thus reconcile the opposites and solve the tension, namely in the form of a change or transition: "By submitting, even subjugating myself, I can transform a condemning, accusing figure into one that forgives, accepts, approves, and protects me. Then I can also absolve myself and finally reconcile myself with my self." In form of the masochistic-impulsive action sequence, forgiveness is hoped and striven for, and yet, after a fleeting union, it is lost again and replaced by renewed punishment and debasement. It is, however, very much part of this sequence that stubbornness, spite, rebellious rage also show up, and that the partner is called upon to put a stop to these wild feelings and wishes and to prove his power precisely by binding the patient and tying her down and forcing her to the ground (or the same with reversed gender roles)—in reality, in fantasy, or metaphorically. Only the one having this power of the No can affirm his value and his strength as a protector. And this means that he should be as cruel as the patient's own superego in order to be credible as a reconciling and defending counterforce.

What I have just described can be traced in the first fully presented case of Vera (Chapters 3 and 4). I have called this sequence as presented up to this point the Cassandra configuration; but it is still only one part of the dynamic and does not offer the full answer.

It does not explain why it comes to that peculiar split of the entire existence, to this juxtaposition of an ability to function that, although emotionally barren, is still adaptive and effective, and to those wildly demoniacal actions where life itself is put at risk. Something is still missing here.

## Global Identification and the Shame of Being Oneself

If we picture the case once more to ourselves, one thing towers up like an erratic block out of the debris of her fate: the huge theme of not-believing and of not being believed, that is, the listening, but not hearing, the looking, but not seeing—and the not-being-seen, that is, not being allowed to be herself.

The first thing that needs therefore to be added is the great and pervasive significance of *denial,* the form of defense that consists in that one does not want to perceive the emotional meaning of certain parts of reality, that one makes inoperative and invalid what one knows to be the case, and that one ignores what one has perceived. Yet why is this? Why this disbelief? And in reverse: Why do one's own parents seem to be equally blind toward the reality of their children? (See "Being Blinded by Images," p. 318.)

Something decisive has to be added: If we think of the prevalence of this defense by denial not only in the patients but also in the parents, it becomes clear that acceptance has been made dependent upon one thing: that the child *identifies* in a *global* way with a dominant and basic attitude of the family, whatever this may be. One ought not to be oneself—and this from a very early time on—and it can be tracked from then until the observable present. The child's own impulses, needs, and feelings are systematically bracketed out, have to be overlooked and made unreal, whether they are those of self-assertion or anger, sexual and tender desires or hunger, or imagination, the creative side, in what is in its essence most independent. The denial of large parts of one's own individuality is the precondition for the acceptance by the parents; failing it, there is rejection: being a stranger in one's own home and in the world at large.

Being oneself, that cannot be: then one is not seen, not recognized. One's self has to be hidden. Yet what else is this than the feeling of shame—the *shame of being oneself.* This is the paradox: While it is valid for most people that they have to develop themselves and assert themselves, that they should therefore be successful, in order to be proud of themselves and not be ashamed, here the premise is reversed: "If you dare to show yourself, you will be expelled, you won't be part of ourselves, but dwell as a foreigner amongst us, as one with whom we don't want to have anything to do. If you want to belong to us you have to submit and hide, or better still: give up altogether what is essential, your core, as something worthless. Only total conformity and submission is acceptable. Being yourself is a kind of self-exposure, an indignity, and brings shame. Most particularly *you should not show any of your feelings*; they are what is most personal and thus most suspect and most secret. They are the *dangerous core of being oneself.* All the genuine strong feelings have to be hidden and veiled, best by a cold façade of rejection or by a friendly smile of agreement and obsequiousness."

"It's more than the right of having one's own life that matters," we learned from Elazar (in *Flight from Conscience*); "What means even more to me is having the right to feel my own feelings and to trust my own feelings, to live them out, and to accept myself in those feelings. That is at the core of the neurosis: that those feelings are wrong, bad, and destructive."

Nietzsche means just that when he states:

Many know how to muddy and abuse their own memory in order to take revenge at least on the only one who also knows: —shame is inventive. It is not the worst things one is most deeply ashamed of: there is not only evil scheming behind a mask, —there is so much kindness [goodness] within guile. I could imagine that a person who has to keep something precious and vulnerable would roll rudely and roundly like a green, old, heavily plated wine barrel through life: the keenness of his shame would want it that way. A human being who has depth in his shame also encounters his experiences and tender decisions in ways only few others reach and of whose existence those nearest to him and most familiar with him should not know: his life's danger hides from their eyes and also his reconquered life's safety. Such a hidden one who instinctively uses speech for silence and concealment and is indefatigable in the escape from communication, *does want* and promote it that a mask of himself walks around in the hearts and minds of his friends; and in case he does not want this, one day his eyes will be opened to it that there is a mask of him anyway in those others—and that this is good. Every deep mind needs a mask: more still, around every deep mind a mask is continually growing, because of the always wrong, namely *shallow* interpretation of every word, of every step, of every life sign he gives.[1]

A young physician who comes into analysis because of severe depression, depersonalization, and social isolation describes in very impressive words this atmosphere at home: "When I just say No to my mother I already feel guilty. Or by being me it means: I don't want to be like you." To be his own person, to have his own will, to show his own feelings, means for his mother, a very intrusive woman, who always deployed her son as an ally in her lasting strife with her husband, that he is betraying her absolutely. It is viewed as rebellion and punished as such. "Often I think it is not permitted to me to feel that I'm doing well, but that I have to feel guilty for it. I think now of my mother how she always was depressed, and I was depressed with her." As if it meant: "How can you be so callous not to suffer with her?" He had completely identified with her in order to be accepted by her. His father is being described as a cynical, mocking man who has no good word for his son. "Sexuality too means a break with her. It is not right to be a man or heterosexual." Or to be successful. Depersonalization has here again the meaning: "I don't want to be identical with this sick and possessive woman, but I also cannot be myself; this is not permitted." Thus, like most of these patients, he has also developed a kind of pseudoidentity.

## Tragic Dilemma

Of course, the family attitude of *global denial* is by no means the only dynamically important factor. I only pick it out here because it has such a significant and manifold influence.

Another important factor consists precisely in those feelings and intentions that are warded off in the family as a whole—what should not be there but what is being communicated in glances and gestures and involuntary actions: their hatred, their resentment, their anxiety (Vera as well as Ingmar, Victor, Marcus, and Sonya in *Flight from Conscience*). Yet, how much is this communicated, how much of what the others feel is felt, how contagious is this! And since it cannot be put into words, since it is therefore not grasped as reality, how can one deal with it? How can one solve the conflict between the feelings one is not allowed to have and cannot put into words, and the façade that has to be maintained at all costs? How can one manage those overpowering storms of feelings that already in themselves threaten the power of words? How is it if those affective storms also swirl around on the outside and unite with the inner ones into a hurricane in which the self is being helplessly tossed around? It is just these uncannily mighty feelings that from so early on imperil the ego, as demons and frightening figures, seemingly from the outside.

This is yet deepened when outer catatrophes confirm these overwhelming anxieties, in particular massive fights between the parents (Regula, Reuven, Elazar, Victor, Peter, Jacob, Anne, Sonya), alcoholism of the parents (Marcus, Victor, Regula), and especially what has been experienced as cruelty against the child (Jacob, Vera, Thomas, and Anne, as well as Ingmar and Regula), or serious physical disease (Elazar). Then it is clearly experienced as if it were the fault of the child, and its guilt—whatever the disaster has been that has happened—is itself a turning passive into active. If the child holds itself to be the guilty one it must after all have the power to repair it or even to prevent it in the future. As we see in Sonya, helplessness leads to the phantasized and almost delusional *omnipotence of responsibility*, hence to the pervasiveness of guilt, as if to say: "*Better totally guilty than absolutely impotent.*"

As the 5-year-old child of one of my patients said at the time of the parents' divorce: "I know why Daddy went away: it was because Toby had cried too much."

Thus one has to be particularly strongly ashamed about the core of one's personality, about everything that does not fit into that *global identification* with the parental figures, and especially about the feelings that are the inmost of our identity. Denial is being followed by *radical repression*. Whatever contradicts this adaptation to the dominant basic attitude, which demands the denial and the repression of what is most essential to one's being, has to be rejected as something evil and defiant. It becomes a source of greatest anxiety.

Yet how long is it possible to suppress this elementary drive to be one-self, this *drive for psychic self-preservation*, even when such submission to op-pression is demanded precisely by the *drive for physical self-preservation?* In brief episodes of being bad, of defiant revolt, that other side, that rejected part-self, eventually breaks through, in spite! One stands by oneself and says: "Why should I be ashamed to own up to myself?" Yet with that, all the wishes and feelings, so long suppressed, of power and rivalry—of jealousy, envy, hate, in short, of gnawing resentment—break through in murderous rage. But how can the issue then be anything else but that one feels overwhelmingly *guilty*: "How can you do such a thing to those who have always meant so well toward you? How can you be so vile and want to do such terrible things to others?"

Thus, along with the global identification and the radicality of denial and repression goes an equally radical condemnation of self and others: on the one side in the form of shame: about being "weak" because one has shown one's own feelings and neediness; on the other in the form of guilt if one has revealed some wishes for self-assertion, for victory in competition, let alone revenge or envy, or if one has dared to give expression to resentment (above all visible in the patients Thomas, Vera, and Jacob, as well as Regula and Dilecta). Perhaps oversimplifying, I have summarized them as *dependency shame* and as *separation guilt.*

Thus it comes to the dilemma: either one withdraws, is again passive and dependent, and admits one's hopeless inferiority (Anne and Jacob, as well as Sonya, Reuven, Elazar, and Ingmar). Here, the patient becomes a little wheel in the family's giant machine, and yet is very deeply ashamed for being such a nothing. The *betrayal of oneself is a lifelong source of shame.* Or he (or she) takes it upon himself to burst the set boundaries; indignantly he wants to tear away from others what has been withheld from him (Vera, Regula, Victor, Jason). The child defies the superior power of the big ones and tries to remove the little ones; it wants to seize the secrets lurking behind closed doors and walls, and it tries to shrug off the guilt brought about by such actions or even just words of rebellion (Dilecta). I have called this *extreme conflict between shame and guilt the tragic dilemma.*

## Polarization

This massive self-condemnation, however, is only possible if the *introjection* of those figures that have been experienced as so extremely contemptuous and blaming has actually happened, namely that they have become inter-nalized as necessary restraints. Constantly the attempt is undertaken to identify totally with this imago of the cruel superego—to become oneself just as ruthless, inconsiderately brutal, and implacable as the inner judge is toward the self. Yet, this attempt has to be squashed at once because it contradicts the commandment of submission and passivity. Here again denial and repression triumph at first. All aggression directed outward is being turned back onto the self (Vera and Jacob, as well as Elazar, Regula, Ingmar, and Reuven) and experienced as if it broke in from within and without, from the inner and outer representatives of authority, and not from one's own uprising. Thus, projection joins introjection.

A typical sequence is the one Vera again and again lived through vis-à-vis her parents: "I would like to blame you—I blame myself—you blame me." It is the *projection of the condemnation.* Just as is the case in the phobic process, here too what threatens from the outside can be more easily evaded than the inner danger that in this instance comes from the superego. The illusion is that she may be better able to escape from the outer judge than from the inner, perhaps also to cajole and bribe him more effectively.

But this also entails the *polarization into absolute opposites* of the entire self- and world-experience. Protector and enemy, the two sides of the ambivalently experienced other ("splitting of the object"), are extended to entire systems of protection and worlds of menace—although they are usually concentrated ("condensed") in specific things or persons. The opposite poles become highly erotized, and the split into good and evil affects not only power and aggression, not only curiosity and self-assertion, but it also and very essentially pulls what is sexual and sensual away from the love and the wishes for union. "Bad" sexuality is now seen as irreconcilable with the highly touted love and the craving for dependency and unity.

Another big defensive effort that joins with the denial and repression (which almost necessarily follows the denial): the *reversal* of feelings and wishes—the effort to find something pleasurable in the anxiety and the pain, as Elazar had done, and to transform the images, so that terrifying violence becomes strength, and arbitrariness becomes admirable power. With such power he has to identify in order to become strong and untouchable himself (Elazar; see also Vera and Regula). In many, the "splitting" of the inner and outer authority into good and bad is followed by the *reversal into the opposite* (of affect and drive), and with that the tearing apart of what belongs together, the defense by *isolation*; for example, in Elazar an attempt to assure himself of the protection of the good power figure by merging with her and to make the counterforce ineffective by declaring it nonexistent. It is therefore a combination of the defense by reversal operating on affect and drive with the defense by denial that brings about what we know as *reaction formation*.

At the same time, the *ideal* of an impermeable armor is developed, a self-protection by *emotional untouchability*; its realization should assist him (or her) to become immune against these overwhelming feelings that assault the self from within and without. This peculiar ideal strengthens the voice of judgment: everything that contradicts this ideal must be disdained, stamped out, and eradicated; all weakness is contemptible and utterly ridiculous (Vera, Regula). That part of the self that is vulnerable and hurt becomes the inner executioner's victim. But this turns so easily again to externalization: the tormentor and executioner is sought on the outside, as a spurner and scorner who thus becomes the carrier of that ideal and the mouthpiece of that inner contemptuous condemnation—and the victim is the self. Or the reverse happens: in the fantasy the other is made into the powerless victim and extirpated so that the self may celebrate himself (or herself) as the omnipotent triumphator (Dilecta, Marcus, Peter). This is a line of dynamics we were able to follow time and again.

Another form of this important affect and drive reversal is, as we kept noting, the *turning from passive to active*, and with it the closely related ego-process of the *identification with the aggressor*, and, resulting from both, a "turning of the tables," the *role exchange* (all more or less synonymous with "projective identification"). Just as in the case of denial, these processes of reversal are known to be forms of defense that are operating early and at first mostly against the outside world, only secondarily against inner forces (Vera and Jacob, as well as Jason).

If the main stress is ostensibly not put on the introjection of that executioner-like conscience and thus on the aggression turned against the self, more value is placed on the aggression turned outward. With that the turning from passive to active becomes more and more a basic principle of the whole character (Dilecta). An instance of this is the transient *overthrow of outer authority* and the insiduous effort also to invalidate the inner one: by lying, by external rebellion, or with drugs (Jason, as well as Sonya, Marcus, Victor, Peter). I have spoken in this connection about the Prometheus–Pandora sequence. Yet, as we recognized in the follow-up on Dilecta, that triumph is not only Pyrrhic, it is just the opener for the crushing defeat. The aggression boomerangs; the executioner within is hale and well, the seeming sadism is but a camouflaged masochism: "*countermasochism*" is a bold protest that resembles the scorpion that stings itself.

A further form of especially *regressive* defense in overwhelming conflict, resulting from the conscience's claims for absoluteness, may be found in the radical turning away from the outside and the retreat into a passive-dependent state, a withdrawal into a highly erotized, yet at the same time frightening inner world (Reuven, Elazar, to a certain degree also Vera and Regula).

## Two Attempted Solutions

The final result of these complex processes may be very varied. Frequently though, an essential element is the pervasive sense of *inauthenticity,* of the "false me," as Regula once called it (cf. Fromm's [1941] "pseudoself," Winnicott's [1965] "false self," Jung's "persona"); she opposes this "fake ego identity" (Erikson 1946, p. 372) or "pseudo identity" (Brodey 1965) to the other "me," the "self-berating part." Her entire adult existence was thus divided into an *ungenuine* and a *tormented* part. This was her double identity—analogous to Vera's identity split into a depersonalized and a masochistic part. One is a life under the dictate of the "inner judge" who seeks to punish her incessantly and mercilessly for all the forbidden impulses; the other is a life of concealment, of masking, of global denial.

Her double existence expressed, as we saw, the *ego split between the two attempted solutions* of the same conflict, the one attempt by depersonalization, adaptation, and occasional rebellion, and the other, more archaic attempt at solution by global identification, massive introjection, turning of the aggression against the own person, and by denial and repression of all the competitive, sexual, and destructive wishes.

The *splitting of identity* means a doubleness of two *ways of being:* one *way of being where the conflict is denied* versus one where this *conflict is newly reenacted* and of *menacing intensity.*

## AN IDEAL SEQUENCE

If we now try to represent all this schematically by distilling from all the sequences that we have observed, either as individual examples or as typical for various pictures of illness, an encompassing abstract version of such a progress, we obtain the following *comprehensive sequence,* a kind of "*ideal sequence*" that I present here only in a cautious approximation:

1. It starts off from the *main conflicts* of early childhood which clearly do not all begin at the same time, but by and large occur in parallel ways and in ever-new variants—the attempts and failures at affect and drive regulation, the conflicts in regard to perception and expression, to dependency

and individuation (original ambivalence), to power, control, and submission, and to competition and rivalry (especially those subsumed under the concept of the Oedipus complex). The earlier and the more severe the traumata or the disturbances of regulation, the more the affects will be of a *global and absolute* nature and the more severe the conflicts.

2. The first attempt at solution is that of *global identification*, which, as described, is accompanied by just as *global processes of denial and repression*, by *introjection* of the condemning figure (the inner "judge," "executioner," or "dwarf," just to mention some of the major metaphors), and with that by the *turning of the aggression against the self*. This attempt entails the formation of an *archaic superego* with its *claims for absoluteness* and exaggerated ("narcissistic") ideals and the corresponding need for a "*pseudo-identity*," a "false self": "I find security only in adjusting and assimilating myself entirely to the other and in renouncing my own feelings. But I pay for this by seeing myself as a miserable wimp and can have only contempt for myself." (One patient divided the world into "wads" and "wimps.")

3. The next attempt at solution is, corresponding to the global identification and global denial, the *splitting of the superego figure*, that is, of the inner and outer authority, into a hated and feared one and one that is longed for as protective and beloved. This means that both imagoes, the protective and the dangerous one, have issued from projection, condensation, and displacement. Thus it comes, as we saw especially in the chapters on the addictions, to the *doubleness of anxiety objects and protective persons or systems.* Part of this doubleness is that one's own dangerous wishes, especially the aggressive ones, are experienced as being vested in, and as now coming from, the phobic object, whereas the protective object approves of them, though in distorted form: "I find protection from the merciless inner authority by seeking approval from someone on the outside—someone who, though threatening violence or degradation, can still be reconciled and thus is in the privileged position of unburdening me from all my guilt and shame. In my merging with this person I feel myself again to be whole and good. In opposition to this figure, others are arrayed who withhold such approval, are irreconcilable, and reject me unconditionally. I want to eliminate these just as much as all those who are weaklings like myself, but I dread their revenge."

4. The next solution undertaken consists in the *turning from passive to active* and in the *externalization* of the inner conflicts. A turning outward of the aggression in the form of defiance, lying, breaking the law, and violence takes the place of the anxiety. Very importantly with this, it comes to a role exchange: the various parts of the superego as well as the self-representations

of the "weak child," of the "victim," of the "vulnerable one," or of the "guilty one" might be sought and fought in the outside world: "I am fed up always being the good child and the victim. I want finally also to get my rights and my satisfaction. I have suffered enough, performed enough—enough is enough! Now I am the person who finally seizes the power and the possibility of pleasure." Particularly often it comes to the reversal of the triangular relationship: "Not I am the excluded third, but you are!"

5. The relations to the polarized figures are *sexualized* as well as regressively entwined with *anal-sadistic* and *oral fantasies*. The condemnation of such desires reflects the *absoluteness of the superego commandments*: only an ideal of sexual innocence and purity in the detachment from the body's needs can fulfill them. Repression and denial cover everything that has to do with sexual wishes. Everything sexual either appears disgusting or is equated with torture and violence—the regressive defense of the sexual drive by aggressive, and in particular anal-masochistic fantasies. "Only in the complete submission and bondage to the tormentor do I have a chance of finding access to power and approval and absolution. But the rage about the self-debasement necessarily involved in this can become overwhelming and erupts in fury against the other and against myself. For we are after all one and merged with each other."

6. These overblown superego claims and the deep anxieties, determined by the recurrent traumatization, are directed against the quality of the affects and drive wishes themselves: by *reaction formation* they are being reversed into their opposite—whether this refers to forbidden wishes (of competition, of revenge, or of anal or genital sexuality [especially those that can be traced back to early masturbation], but also wishes for self-assertion, for self-exposure, and curiosity)—or to the affects of anxiety, pain, depression, or shame. "The craving to be united with the other and to find shelter and love with the powerful authority is much too dangerous. I better withdraw and seek help and sustenance within myself, by renouncing those wishes completely, and reassure myself that help can be coming my way only from those fantasy figures within; these endow me with strength to resist the inner dangers. Thus I can even transform anxiety and suffering into pleasure, vengefulness into compassion, pride and vanity into humility and bashfulness and dirtiness into purity. If I foresake in this way all selfish desire I shall eventually be accepted after all—by my conscience as well as by the outer authorities."

7. If all these attempts prove insufficient, there always remains the opportunity to get away from those claims of absoluteness and from the ensuing conflicts by trying to cut oneself off from the world and conflicts gener-

ated by the interaction with it and to find solace in "*splendid isolation*": "The world consists only of disappointment. I feel like a locomotive that runs under full steam but whose brakes are fully throttled; it stands in place. Will and counterwill stand in full battle gear against each other, and I cannot do anything else but forgo the world and withdraw entirely upon myself. Although this does not bring me any peace, it diminishes at least my sense of shame in front of a sneering environment." Yet the mask of contempt and desinterest necessary for such turning away does not succeed for long.

8. Usually, the end result is that more or less *global defense against the inner life* that can reach from affect blocking and states of depersonalization to extensive psychophobia, the denial of the significance of the entire inner life, and connected with that a sense of the inner split—that sensation I have described as pseudo-identity and as *ego- and identity split*: "I live an inauthentic life; everything is phoney and without reality."

As befits such sequences, the end of the "ideal sequence" leads to its beginning: one faces the same unsolved conflict again. The most frequent endpoint is that of the regression to global denial.

In most of the patients studied here we recognize in the course of their impulse sequences parts of this abstracted encompassing "ideal sequence," hardly all eight steps, yet commonly a majority of them. Yet they usually also show a predilection for one of these attempts at solution, which then provides the respective diagnosis. However, one effect of the multiplicity of factually existing solution attempts is that the superficial diagnosis arrived at is often not very satisfying. The correspondence with the diagnosis of the neurosis can be derived without much ado from the seven forms of solution. The sequential series shows the masochistic-depressive, phobic, impulse-neurotic "sociopathic" (or "character perversion"), hysterical, obsessive-compulsive, narcissistic, and finally depersonalizing conflict solution. All seven may be either symptomatic or characterological.

Yet it is also evident that most patients, although preferring *one* solution attempt, have part of the others as well, which is what brings about those larger configurations. In spite of all these solution attempts, the patients are of course unable to get rid of the underlying conflict, and the affect storms and anxieties threaten to break through. Therefore on each step it can come to an ego split—to the seeming break between the main state and a leaping over to the state of another solution attempt, mostly by regression. Often we also can observe during this impulse sequence a rapid progression of an entire series of such attempted conflict solutions.

Although developed in the severe neuroses, the schema is applicable also to the somewhat milder forms (like Thomas, Anne, and Elazar). Here the differences are of a quantitative, not of a principal nature; in the severer forms, the regression is stronger, the danger that the ego is being overwhelmed greater, and the affects of unpleasure are more intensive. But it is also true that in these the main processes and connections are clearer and more impressive, and that they can teach us very much about the nature of the neuroses.

The transition to a psychotic state is conceivable at several points along this scale of the "ideal sequence," but what would cause such a crossing of this boundary is really unknown. Is it the radicalness of the family disorder? Is it the massivness of the "family superego" that brings about such absolute, yet mutually contradictory introjections, and thus leads to such an excess of precipitated emotional contagion and affects, but also to a correspondingly severe suppression of the most essential needs and massive conflicts? Or might it rather be decisively a primarily biological factor that *must* intervene? How do, during development, acute, and more decisively, chronic traumatogenic affects interact with brain physiology and alter it?

In addition to those inferred configurations and sequences, certain unconscious *equations* recur that lead to the characteristic phobic core symptoms, above all the equation of the claustrum with closeness, anxiety, and commitment, the equation of passivity and dependency with self-loss, falling, and floating down, and then those basic equations of affective flooding with violence and with sexual excitement, of separation with killing. They lead to specific counteractions: wanting to break out, burst, and flee in regard to the first and third, or to the fantasy of flying and frantic workaholism in the second, or to fantasies of merger and total dependency, of "selflessness" in the fourth.

These deep and recurrent *equations, sequences, and metaphors* only gradually emerged in the course of the current writeup and became valuable technical tools, along with those I gave in Chapter 2 as methodological presuppositions. They can be followed just as well microscopically, within single sessions, as macroscopically, in the life history and the development of the neurosis as a whole.

Neither the ideal sequence nor the other schematically described factors should be understood as closed systems. There certainly are other steps and configurations that eluded my examination of this restricted field of observation, or variants of, or different perspectives on, those circular processes.

The further treatment of the question of the repetition compulsion requires a brief digression to the closely related issues of narcissism, masochism, and splitting.

## THE LEAP FROM DESCRIPTION TO EXPLANATION

The greater the conflict, the severer the anxiety and the more pronounced the so-called narcissistic phenomena. Why is that so? Because unsolved conflicts represent inner dangers, dangers are accompanied by anxiety, the anxiety is an affect, intensive affects overwhelm the system from the beginning, and narcissism is characterized by absoluteness and the dissolution of boundaries, the "too-muchness" of whatever goes on within.

All the fantasies that, in form of configurations and sequences, change into clinical reality entail in their essence boundary violations, and can thus be called in the widest sense "narcissistic"; not only are the affects overwhelming, but also the claims by the drives are exaggerated, particularly those having to do with *power demands*—whether in fantasy or in reality, and whether in externalized form or turned back onto the self. To what extent these *boundary transgressions* within the described configurations *serve defensive purposes* should be evident from the clinical cases. These violations of limits decisively disturb and disrupt the surroundings. The result in most of the cases is either a withdrawal from all relationships that have to do with closeness, or an exploitation of such relations: the others become two-dimensional cardboard figures. These patients really make their companions into "objects," things, taking seriously indeed and implementing the dehumanization entailed in our cliché of "object relations." Or they are so vulnerable that their resentment seems unquenchable. The image created by the term "narcissism" is therefore a summary metaphor of extraordinary breadth. Its span encompasses self-esteem altogether, as well as the overestimation of the others or of one's own person, the appearance of invulnerability and the rebuff of others, joined with the hidden sense of deep vulnerability; contempt coupled with great sensitivity, the need for power and fear of powerlessness, the fantasy that everything is permitted and allowed to him (or her), enormous expectations posed to the self and the corresponding abyssmal sense of total failure, and finally even the perversion of treating oneself as a sexual object.

If everything metapsychological is peeled off and all the inferences and constructions bracketed, the term *narcissism* is understood, as far as I can see, as the *dissolution of certain boundaries in value, truth, and action*; or, putting it in slightly different words, a *transgression of limits in valuation, reality perception, and enactment.* If this understanding is correct, then it refers to a *too-much*, a too-much of power claimed or of self-regard, a too-much of love or hate, a too-much in valuing the other (idealization) or in self-admiration (grandiosity). This means we use this concept, at least implicitly, in a *quantitative* sense. The way it is practically employed, for example in case discussions and supervision, or in the literature, the concept of narcissism is a *judgment of measurement* and always refers to something that is *immoderate, excessive,* and *boundless.* All the cases presented in these two books can in this sense be considered "narcissistic."

At the same time it can also be said that all the patients expertly sabotage themselves, are self-destructive, and know how constantly to bring it about anew with their repeated actions that they are punished, degraded, and rejected. They suffer, and it often seems that they can enjoy happiness, joy, and pleasure only for brief moments and only concomitantly with suffering and pain. Thus they are of course also *masochistic.* The bonds they engage in, the relationship they have with their own conscience, are those of tormentor and victim, of judge and criminal, of sadist and masochist. Is therefore the repetition compulsion a manifestation of a *primary masochism?* Or also simultaneously expression of a *primary narcissism?* Does it therefore show both of the supposed elementary forces of the human being at work, of Eros in its most original form, and of Thanatos as death instinct? It surely fits wonderfully in the mythical painting of those two basic instinctual drives (*Urtriebe*). But does this also accord with our experience? I do not think so.

I am rather of the opinion that *repetition compulsion, narcissism, and masochism are excellent descriptive terms,* but that *they do not explain anything.* They describe in bold summaries and comparisons fantasies, subjective experiences, and objective attitudes. They represent the results of certain defensive strategies. And they refer to certain configurations, sequences, and equations of the kind we have time and again encountered in patients with severe neuroses.

If they are transformed, however, *from descriptive to explanatory concepts,* the analytic investigation of the motivational connection suffers some kind of short circuit. Instead of tracking the actual causes and motivating reasons in their complexity, we assume that we have done so already by using those beguiling terms: they are *pseudoexplanatory.*

Experience shows that it is, at least in wide areas, the showing up and resolution of inner and outer conflicts that leads to therapeutic change. Beyond this there are deep disruptions of the regulation of affects and drives that require correction and the lifting of which leads to clinical improvement. In all this it remains valid that the criterion for the comprehension of causality is *cessante causa cessat effectus* (if the cause is taken away the effect ceases).

This means, therefore, that those causes can only be found in inner and outer conflicts, probably in disorders of regulation that are independent from such conflicts, but that enter into them, and in the traumata causing those conflicts. Drives, repetition compulsion, affects, and defenses do not explain psychologically anything yet. They are part of the nexus of understanding, but do not give the *knowledge of causality* which, as Grünbaum (1984) has rightly stressed, was striven for by Freud and has to be the goal of all scientific comprehension (Wurmser 1989a,b).

What requires above all a deeper explanation is the central position of conflict in general for the understanding of the psyche. Yet such an explanation is of a philosophical nature, no longer a psychological one, and thus in a true sense "metapsychological." This means it would be broader, deeper, more fundamental than psychology alone.

Crucially, the confusion of *description* ("these attributes belong to those phenomena, and these phenomena belong together with those phenomena") with *explanation* ("with this cause that effect ensues, or this is the result of the acting together of those causes and reasons") stands in the way of the scientific inquiry of psychoanalysis and its theories.

This view has been taken up by Grossman (1986) specifically in regard to masochism:

> At present, it has become evident that masochism is a term of little precision and that its value is descriptive and evocative. . . . Masochism cannot be usefully invoked to explain complex clinical phenomena (p. 381). . . . "Masochism" designates a type of fantasy and those clinical phenomena based on those fantasies (p. 386). . . . The attachment to the painful aspects of the relationships, the equating of passivity with victimization, and the confusion of activity with aggression are emphases common to masochistic fantasies (p. 389). . . . The masochistic perversions are concrete enactments of such fantasies and *serve as prototypes* for clinical interpretation (p. 390). . . . The [pleasure-unpleasure] principle is [in contrast to the description of the conjunction of pleasure and unpleasure in the same acts] a principle concerning the process of resolving mental conflict and is not a term describing the affective characteristics of the outcome. This issue comes close to the fundamental questions of psychoanalytic explanation" (pp. 410/411).

Parallel considerations about *narcissism* were expressed by Rangell (1982). I believe this concept has by now acquired such a surfeit of meanings and is used in so manifold a way that it would be best to *restrict* it, like masochism, to the *description of fantasies and actions* and to *refrain from using it as a fundamental explanatory principle.*

The *narcissic fantasy* would then have as its content that one's own self-estimation, consciously or unconsciously, is increased "without measure" as to value and power, that the others have entirely to serve these excessive needs, that a particular form of pleasure consists in the transgression of boundaries or limitations, and that everything relative has to be rejected in favor of those absolute claims. The activities founded in this fantasy configuration relate to exploitation of the others, violation of the normative standards and barriers set by nature and culture, and unbounded rage when these demands are rebuffed or fail; occasionally they can also include a truly narcissistic perversion—sexual excitement by one's own mirror image or infatuation in oneself (cf. the cases of Reuven and Elazar).

Yet what is the explanation for such narcissistic fantasies and actions if we distance ourselves from the concept of an elementary drive of narcissism? Or do we have indications for such a basic force as cause, for example as part of a conflict? Clinical experience and direct observation both seem to argue for the first answer; the *narcissistic fantasies are nothing original, but something derivative, although something extremely important.* They stand always in a dynamic context that points beyond themselves to something that is deeper.

## SPLITTING

In this context of the premature explanation, it may also be rewarding to investigate the topic of "splitting" in the meaning given to it by Melanie Klein (1932), Kernberg (1975, 1976, 1984), Mahler et al. (1975), and many contemporary authors. I have used the term ego-split or splitting of identity throughout in a sense that has not much in common with the fashionable concept of "splitting," but goes back to Freud's notion of "splitting of the ego" (1927, 1940a,b). Again, I believe that something observable has here been shifted from describing into explaining. Splitting, the phenomenon of polarization in valuation, we see all the time; yet is this really a fundamental process, a basic element of explanation? I doubt this very much. What do I base this rejection of a theory upon, a theory so widely shared and also determining the practice more and more, even in the United States?

The phenomena are in fact clear, and we had many occasions to trace examples of them; one's own person or the important persons in the surroundings are being experienced either as absolutely good or as absolutely bad, although the assignment of such attributes may abruptly change. The absolute either-or is again and again being actively pursued. It is an essential part of the impulsive action sequences and with that of the repetition compulsion. In such social actions in particular—in families, groups, institutions, on wards, in administrative systems—the observation of such "splitting" is very valuable. It is also well known from mythical thinking how it has been forever a deep emotional need of man to separate out good and evil in an absolute way (Cassirer 1923b). Melanie Klein (1932) saw in this process an original defense. Correspondingly, Kernberg (1984) speaks about splitting as "an active defensive separation of such contradictory self and object images" (p. 112 f.).

However, the insights contributed recently by infant research cast a new light on these processes, which we are able to observe in all the cases described here as severe neuroses, and thus on the issue of "splitting" as a supposedly fundamental dynamic process and a special archaic defense.

It has become evident that those condensations into good versus bad self parts, into good versus bad objects, do not occur at the very early times postulated. Lichtenberg (1986) states unequivocally that

> in ordinary development the premise is not confirmed that a major integrative effort is required to overcome the persistent disruptive effects of aggressive drive tensions in order to approach unity of self and object experience. . . . The origins of these split groupings of self and object representations and the defensive use to which they are put derive from the organization they receive from symbolic processing. They are based on categorization (secondary process) combined with condensation and overgeneralization (primary process). This reconsideration of the theoretical conception assumed by myself (Lichtenberg and Slap 1973) and others (Klein 1952a, Mahler 1968, Kernberg 1975) is based on my belief that infant research has failed to support the inferences on which the theory stands.

(For very similar conclusions, see Stern 1985, pp. 245 f.)

It is crucial that, according to the evidence of today's infant research, the *original units of experience* consist of *action, perception, and affect,* bundled together; these units, originally and for a long time, *lack symbolic representation.* Images or hallucinatory reawakening of pleasure experiences, and with them also the concepts of part-self and part-objects, of inside and outside, and the processes postulated between them, are of a far later nature, and stem from a time when the ability to symbolize is clearly established.

These phenomena, subsumed under the descriptive term "splitting," are therefore relatively *late symbolic elaborations* (from the late second year on). We can readily detect examples of such "splitting" of good and bad, but they are part of the complex outcome of neurotic conflict, especially conflicts involving archaic superego structures, archaic identifications with the aggressor (mainly with the aggressor as accuser, as *blamer*), and overwhelming early affects. Such archaic superego and identification patterns are typically accompanied by those overwhelming, primitive, *global affects* that we have continued to encounter, above all anxiety and depression, but also rage, shame, and guilt.

As Waelder (1936) already noted, all these processes, which are now used to justify a special diagnostic, psychodynamically based grouping of "border-lines," are commonly observable, but they derive, at least in his view, from early oedipal conflicts, including the superego condemnation of fantasies of competition; they are but one band on a broad spectrum of dynamics, not their rock-bottom and origin.

The ubiquity of these observations is by the way a further reason to re-ject the postulate of a dynamically based, diagnostically separate group of "borderline" cases. It seems therefore more likely that the *deepest and preverbal strata*, as far as we can allow ourselves to draw any inferences, do not per-tain to such good–bad splits, but rather to *affective storms caused by primary misattunements and failures in regulatory interactions* between caregiver and infant. Gaensbauer (1985) writes about "the persistent influence of high intensity affective events on the child's emotional reactions to subsequent events" (p. 522). Those affects in the infant in turn generate affects in oth-ers; Gaensbauer calls it "transactional momentum"; Nathanson (1986) speaks in this context of "affect transmission" and the "empathic wall": *affects are highly contagious*.

Infant research has shown that this affect transmission from the mother and the other persons in the surroundings plays a big role in the emotional development of the baby. Already very early, the infant tries to protect itself against excessive intrusions by affects and moods of those around it—in a kind of *interpersonal affect defense* (Gaensbauer [1985], Nathanson [1986], Stern [1985]). It might well be that such early efforts at *affect reversal, turning from passive to active*, and other forms of affect defense are being simulta-neously used as defense against the drives. If the retrospective experiences with the severely traumatized patients allow us these conclusions, these *in-terpersonal* forms of affect and drive defense certainly play a crucial role in regard to the severe traumata of the first years of life.

It is such affect transmission and the interactional ways of dealing with it that later on contribute decisively to the affective patterns of the transfer-ence from the patient's side as well as to the effectiveness of the therapist's style.

Early forms of dealing with massive, traumatic interferences—a kind of protodefenses—are measures like gaze aversion (Beebe and Sloate 1982) and "walling off"—the emotional turning away, the timid withdrawal from the traumatically experienced person (Gaensbauer 1985). The latter, though somewhat ressembling what is commonly called "splitting," shows the "striking specificity of a 'cognitive-affective schema' based on a previous traumatic experience" (Gaensbauer 1985, pp. 528–529). I believe this is more akin to the phenomena of the "split identity" described here than to the supposed basic defense of "good–bad splitting."

Fraiberg (1982) gives a particularly helpful account of these early forms of defense. In sequence of appearance, she lists the following five proto-defenses: avoidance, freezing, fighting, transformations of affect, and reversal (turning of aggression against the self).

Thus the theory of early affects, of their great variability already during the first weeks and months, and of the abiding need for affect regulation, a theory independent from any drive theory, is one of the radical modifications made necessary by the new findings.

This then is a theoretical reformulation of the phenomena commonly now referred to by the mechanism of "splitting." *Splitting is a descriptive, not an explanatory concept.* Clinically we may use these phenomena as starting points; they are not the basic element for a mutative interpretation.

Here again it is the premature leap from description to explanation which deflects our look from what is central and informs a basic therapeutic attitude which is, *in the long run,* less beneficial for the inner growth of the patient than the patient exploration of the *complex dynamics behind the phenomena.*

## SPLIT IDENTITY AND ITS ORIGIN

In the continued pursuit of this train of thought, the question of the nature of the *splitting of identity* and *ego-split* poses itself even more insistently. I have used these two terms almost synonymously.

As to the former, it is striking how often with the severer forms of neurosis we may observe how it is as if another personality took over. Kernberg (1984) is quite justified in putting this at the center of his description of these cases; many of our patients describe it that way too. And as to the latter term, I understood it in the same way as Freud (1940a,b): the side-by-side existence of acknowledgment and denial of certain perceptions felt to be traumatic threats, and hence a *functional tearing asunder of essential ego-functions* (see Chapter 2). I consider the term purely descriptive: "I know this already, but I ignore what you tell me, and I arrange my life the way I wish," proclaims Regula's chronically alcoholic sister (*Flight from Conscience*). Vera confessed she was aware how degrading, how damaging, and how dangerous her liaison to the "slug" was, but that she had to ignore this knowledge over and over again and believe and hope that things would at the end still turn out all right and that ultimately she could be happy with him.

Evidently, this *doubleness of knowing and ignoring* is accompanied by *two ways of being, two forms of identity*. On the one hand, Vera is impelled by her keen insight and perspicacity to sever her tie with the man, is ashamed, even alienated and depersonalized from what has occurred. On the other, she makes light of her knowledge, runs after him again, humiliates herself in front of him, and experiences wild ecstasies of submission and union. She feels herself like two persons. This is what I (again descriptively) mean by "identity split"; in such doubleness of personality, a kind of *splitting of the self* occurs, each *part-identity* comprising a combination of id, ego, and superego aspects in pretty regular and understandable combinations, without there having to be amnesia (cf. Lichtenberg and Slap 1973). The concept is an abstraction out of many descriptions and does not represent any particular form of "defense by splitting."

In those observable sequences, the *avowal* of one *part-identity* necessarily means the *disavowal* of the other—hence the great importance of narrowing down or falsifying the perception by *denial*.

These concepts of the *denial of one's identity*, the assumption of a *part-identity*, the *conflict* between such part-identities, and all this under the sway of *opposite parts of the superego,* are of much greater significance than is generally appreciated. Living such a part-identity, an "adopted or imposed identity," as one of my patients called it, arouses an uneasiness that one is not in touch with one's feelings. This *pseudo-identity* is particularly pronounced as the surface manifestation of severe shame conflicts but the entire duality of such part-identities, which splits much of life asunder, can often be understood as that of massive conflicts between the shame part of the superego and its guilt part.

Thus the duality of denial and countervailing fantasy has less clinical relevance than the duality in which two alternate part-identities, two part-personalities of great complexity, stand in sharp conflict with each other and use denial as their main weapon against each other. In both versions of duality, the sense of *depersonalization* accompanying such large-scale denial is very marked.

Yet what does this all mean, how can we explain this really—especially if we forsake the concept of "splitting" as an elementary explanatory device?

If "the ego's object-identifications . . . obtain the upper hand and become too numerous, unduly powerful and incompatible with one another, a pathological outcome will not be far off," writes Freud in "The Ego and the Id" (1923, p. 30).

> It may come to a disruption of the ego in consequence of the different identifications becoming cut off from one another by resistances; perhaps the secret of the cases of what is described as "multiple personality" is that the different identifications seize hold of consciousness in turn. Even when things do not go so far as this, there remains the question of *conflicts between the various identifications into which the ego comes apart* [emphasis added], conflicts which cannot after all be described as entirely pathological. [pp. 30/31]

I suggest that what Freud here refers to as identifications also and prominently encompasses introjections into the superego, this agency being regarded by him at that time as "a differentiation within the ego" (Freud 1923, p. 28).

Usually one part-identity is primarily experienced in the form of a storm of intensive, "global" affects, moreover of affects that are mutually contradictory, whereas the second part-identity is marked by reasonableness and adaptedness, but also by flatness and affective impoverishment. It is also evident that this phenomenon of pseudo-identity and split identity results from complex processes and shows many transitions, in sequences characteristic for the individual. In fact, those contradictory part-identities are only the extremes within the multiform sequences, as we have been actually able to observe in our cases. Also, these inner figures that oppose each other in the various versions of conflict (one example has been presented from Regula's analysis; I could do something similar for most of my patients) are not simply "inner objects," which would be understandable as introjections of "external objects." Rather, they are results of complex processes: they are themselves compromise formations.

"Yet how can this form of dissociation be *explained?*" one may impatiently ask. Does it suffice merely to speak of overwhelming affects to understand this "split"? What does this "split" of the self and of the other really consist of?

Clinical experience does now give us an unequivocal answer: *every act of defense leads to a split in the self-experience, and the more pronounced this defense is, the more radical the experience of the split turns out to be.* But where does this defense come from; when and how does it begin? This is perhaps the most fascinating question of the entire psychoanalytic theory of mental life. I believe nobody can as yet answer it. Here I restrict myself to the sharpened question concerning the nature and origin of those radical forms of "split-ting" as they can be observed in these severe neuroses and as they are by many today, especially Kernberg (1975, 1976, 1984), explained by a special and elementary defense mechanism.

I do not believe that we deal here with a particular form of defense, but rather with the logical result of the *absoluteness* and the *global quality*, not only of the affects, but of the identifications and the introjections, and with that of the other defensive processes, especially repression and denial. This means, however, that *the phenomena of "splitting" are due to the absoluteness and global quality of the conflicts entailed.* What is absolute does not tolerate some-thing else that also claims absoluteness; global claims are mutually exclu-sive. Most decisively from all the factors at play, it is *the absolute and categori-cal demands raised by the conscience, the global either-or judgments,* which, above all and again and again, can be observed to engender such intense conflicts, such global affects, and consequently these processes of "splitting." "Noble sentiments pushed to extremes produce results very like those of the worst vices" (Balzac, *La Cousine Bette,* p. 124).[2]

To use the political analogy: if the "regulator" himself becomes *categori-cal* and proffers demands of an absolute nature, if the power representing law and order tries to assume total power, it is bad enough. If, however, the police and the military struggle with each other for such absolute power, then we get a division of the state and a kind of "anarchy from above." Or, shifting the analogy somewhat, in Joseph Conrad's (1911) prophetic words about Czarist Russia:

> The ferocity and imbecility of an autocratic rule rejecting all legality and in fact basing itself upon complete moral anarchism provokes the no less imbe-cile and atrocious answer of a purely Utopian revolutionism encompassing destruction by the first means to hand, in the strange conviction that a funda-mental change of hearts must follow the downfall of any given human institu-tions. [p. 51]

*Kategorein,* or κατηγορεῖν in Greek, means "to accuse." Thus in Jewish mys-ticism the devil is often called with the Greek loanword *Katigor,* the Accuser (the same meaning, by the way, as the other Greek word *Diabolos* or devil, and the Hebrew Satan). Just so is the child's early morality: absolute, cat-egorical, "all or nothing."

And that is what usually happens in these identity splits: one superego-part that is allied with the outside world and constantly urges adaptation and conformity is being attacked and overthrown by another superego-part which insists for example upon its own more autonomous values and proudly, even arrogantly clamors to be honored and given all the rights. This second (usually regressive) superego-part is manifested in narcissistic fantasies and in archaic ideal images of the self; it entails massive self-condemnation for all signs of vulnerability or weakness. However, in this struggle between the "adapted" and the "regressive" parts of the superego, there are often interim steps, intermediate attempts at conflict solution, a blending of both superego antagonists.

## LOYALTY AND VALUE CONFLICTS

Obviously, one particularly clear example for this polarization within the superego is derived from profound and often lifelong *loyalty conflicts*. In most of the cases, the loyalty conflict cannot be as clearly elaborated as with Regula or Jason, where it was above all a matter of completely irreconcilable loyalty ties and loyalty claims of divorced parents, or as with Anne, Elazar, and Reuven, where the parents were strongly at loggerheads. This is the simplest paradigm for loyalty conflicts: the one between massively hostile parents.

Another much more insidious form of loyalty conflict exists between the overt values and ideals in a family versus the more hidden ones—a kind of *value split*. In Ingmar's case it pertained, for example, to the overt attitude of piety, peacefulness, and benevolence, opposed by absolute demands for obedience that were enforced with unpredictability, brutality, and a silent judgmentalness that doomed all individuality to shame. Then there is the loyalty toward the brother who had committed incest against the loyalty toward the sisters who had been raped. Moreover, there is the façade of righteousness of the family that has to be shown as an example to the community, versus all the secrets no one can touch upon, a conflict between fealty to the family and the value of honesty. Behind all this there hides a "family demon" of killing.

A similar value split can be found in Vera's life, where the Christian message, coupled with a deep ethos of responsibility and the obligation to protect others from harm, is opposed by a virulent resentment that wants to embitter all pleasure and joy and to suppress all autonomy; together they seem, as *value conflict,* to determine the family milieu—not necessarily objectively so, but at least as it had been experienced by Vera. More deeply, in her family it is the unsolved conflict between ambitious striving, thus competitiveness, and the required humbling of all pride and the renunciation of all such self-centered wanting. In her own words: "I can see it in two different ways, on two different levels: On the one hand, I show my loyalty by identifying with the good mother, and also by my identification with the bad mother. On the other hand, I show my loyalty towards my parents by staying forever a little child and do not dare to compete with them" [962].

In the case of Jacob, it was again more personal: the loyalty toward the brother who, though repeatedly punished, always knew how to assert himself personally, and the loyalty toward the mother who, though exerting power over the children, had to hide from the world in the shelter of her home and spread her timidity like a fog. Then we suspected also a conflict between the need to keep the masturbatory plays with his brother and similar games a secret; this stood against the threat: If you lie you will go in a handbasket to heaven (if not yet farther away and down). There were also the often very loud and severe fights between the parents with threats of leaving that aroused such loyalty conflicts.

Dilecta's loyalty conflicts consisted less of those between mother and father, although this played a certain role—the mother being out for money and social success, the father happier to gamble and to drink. Far more important, it was a third type of loyalty conflict, the conflict between the loyalty toward her family that was peculiar, versus the wish to belong to the "normal" surrounding, the *loyalty conflict between family and the outside world*, an evil world that is much in discordance with the values within the family. Altogether this seems to be an important type of conflict—of conscience and value—that has a lot to do with loyalty (see also Regula, Thomas, Victor): "My family is different from the others; I am ashamed for them, and yet I feel bound to them and have to remain loyal to them." One result is the obligation to keep everything confidential that goes on at home; any and every revelation, including the revelations inherent in being in therapy (and this especially!), is experienced as betrayal.

Reuven's mother, whom he feels duty-bound to love, looks with contempt at the evil ways of the world, and with much bitterness and resentment she assails pleasure-seeking men. Reuven's father is described as an old lecher. Thus, Reuven's deep bond to her, his identification with her, and the loyalty toward her, set him in sharp opposition to the ways of the "evil world" from which he scornfully distances himself—and yet he looks jealously and enviously to his happier peers who rub the details of their sexual exploits under his nose.

A fourth type is one also already mentioned: the commitment toward a person on the outside and the wish to protect one's own values, the core of one's own identity (*self-loyalty*): it is the internalization of such loyalty relationships with outer persons. Keeping the loyalty toward oneself means honor, violating it means deepest shame. There is probably nothing that evokes in the adolescent and the adult as much shame as when one feels forced to violate this need for self-loyalty, and must "betray oneself," usually on behalf of another overriding obligation. In the loyalty conflict between two parents, the loyalty toward oneself is the first to be sacrificed. How can "the little real me" be anything but bewildered and concealed?

Another outcome of this type of loyalty conflict is the often perceived need to establish a kind of *counter-identity*; here, in an important segment of activity and feeling, the expected loyalty is being refused and one attempts at all costs to become the opposite—one tries to *disidentify*, often against a most intense pull of wanting to identify and thus preserve the loyalty. Again it is a conflict that has largely become unconscious.

This can be demonstrated in each of the cases: Regula is honest and abstinent in a family of alcoholics where truth was seen only as what was of advantage. Reuven is miles apart from the alleged lechery of his father, but also from his mother's ambitiousness and her blaming. Vera was for a while demonstratively promiscuous (against her mother) and vulgar (against her father). Victor tried to be capable and generous in helping, and Ingmar considered himself absolutely unable to be successful and to defend his own rights, but with the help of lying, drinking, and cocaine he felt, although only for the moment, in charge of his destiny. Such a counter-identity is in itself a breach of loyalty and has to be guilt- and shame-laden. Sexuality and aggressions are then deployed in a defiant assertion of one's own "real self" (Vera and Ingmar).

Loyalty conflicts are ubiquitous. It is their severe, broad, and deep presence from early childhood on that is bound to lead to a split identity. I do not stress the role of this type of conflicts to slight the role of other types of inner conflict. Rather, it pertains to *one* side of many, if not most competitive and ambivalence conflicts, one that has not had much attention paid to it: the involvement of the superego not merely as a punishing agency but also as one that demands faithfulness and obeisance towards an outer figure or an inner value or ideal.

In short now: *absolute, but contradictory superego demands*, in the form of *loyalty conflicts* and the *shame–guilt antithesis, global but opposing affects and wishes; global identifications, global denial and repression*; and *massive introjection of traumata* work together (synergistically) on many layers of genesis and dynamics to lead to the phenomena of split identity and split experience of others. *Ego split and split identity are results, not causes.*

Moreover, the *demand for absoluteness* stands in direct contradiction to the *need for inner unity*. More specifically expressed, the total claims shown by the superego and by many of the affects and impulses contradict the drive for psychic self-preservation, that is, the deep need for synthesis. Both needs belong to what is most essential in the human soul and can probably be traced back to the origins of mental life. The question of how they get into such opposition and strife against each other belongs among the problems whose resolution may have been prematurely claimed on sociological or biological grounds, but that require further empirical inquiry.

## THE ORIGIN OF CONSCIENCE IN A SPLITTING OF THE SELF AND AS PRINCIPLE OF INDIVIDUATION

We have noted how the conscience presents one version of self-reflection: as self-observation, as measuring of one's own person against a measuring rod of valuation, with the image of the ideal self as well as a code of ideal actions serving as yardsticks, as self-criticism, as self-condemnation (in form of the inward sense of guilt and shame), as self-punishment, and eventually as reconciliation with oneself, as one's inner reacceptance. All these acts of conscience—the superego functions—are rooted in a splitting up of the self into a subject and an object. Class (1964) writes about the Greek concept of συνειδέναι ἑαυτῷ—knowing in (with/by) oneself, the Latin *con-scientia*, hence conscience:

> This "knowing with oneself" determines that the human ego is, as it were, split up into two separate half-persons whereby the higher "positioned" one observes the "inferior" one and "shares in the knowing" of all its acts. The knowing issues from the ego and at the same time refers to the ego; subject becomes at the same time object, yet both are not united, but fractured, divided from each other. When the bad conscience stirs, one of these "ego layers" vehemently resists; it defends against this knowing. [Class 1964, p. 7, quoted by Cancrini 1970, p. 32][3]

Snell (1930) talks similarly about a "splitting of consciousness" that only then becomes an impulse of conscience (*Gewissensregung*, stirring of conscience) when one "is conscious of an action (*sich einer Tat bewußt*, p. 14).

Cancrini (1970) objects to Class's (1964) and Snell's (1930) views by stating that it is *privacy* that underlies the Greek concept of conscience, not inner conflict. When indeed συνειδέναι ἑαυτῷ above all means the private sharing of knowledge of the ego with itself and therefore corresponds to the necessity to express a knowledge which, based upon the perception of an individual *privacy*, can be characterized only as a knowing of the ego with itself, then it cannot be that the aspect of inner conflict has any importance for its formation.[4]

In my view, both of these understandings, derived from historical and semantic investigation, are correlated to very important psychological observations: those of individuation as self-delimitation, as privacy, and as inner unity ("*Selbsteinheit*") (in Cancrini's terms: "[*la*] *privata esclusività della conoscenza stessa*"), and those of self-division in inner conflict ("*la scissione dell'io in due parti*"); both accompany the primary, if ever so rudimentary stirrings of conscience, whatever the time might be we assume for these basic processes, whether we postulate with Stern (1985) that individuation is a basic process of psychic life, at least with the emergence of the "core-self" at the end of the second month of life, and also presume with him that the process of self-division already exists toward the end of the first year of life (with the "intersubjective self," with those observations that might refer to inner conflict), or whether we follow above all Mahler (1968, Mahler et al. 1975) and assume the beginning of both only during the second half of the second year of life. Psychologically, both basic observations are valid and important: Conscience (and with that its supraordinate agency, the superego) brings with it an inner splitting into opposite parts of the self, while reaffirming and defending the sharp demarcation of the self against its surroundings. It stands in the service both of relations with others and of what I have earlier called psychic self-preservation: the defiant affirmation of wanting to be oneself. It is what George Eliot (1876) so perceptively called conscience (already quoted in Chapter 4): "a fear which is the shadow of justice, a pity which is the shadow of love" (p. 455). Separation guilt and dependency shame are two basic structures of the superego.

If, with Kant, we understand the conscience as an autonomous inner value structure (Cancrini [1970]: "*una concezione della coscienza kantianamente intesa come autonoma formazione di valori*," p. 37), that is, if with Hartmann and Loewenstein (1962) we see in the superego a structure of secondary autonomy, then it may be justified to put its beginning only after the "destruction of the Oedipus complex" (*Untergang des Ödipuskomplexes*) (Freud 1924a): [the superego] "which is only now being formed" (p. 177).

However, if we see in conscience, and therefore also in the theoretical structure of the superego, an inner formation that exists in constant conflicts, that originates in conflicts (Brenner 1982), and that often disintegrates under the blows of such conflicts, then it makes more sense to assume its origin at the time when we encounter the first manifestations of shame, of caring for the other, of remorse, and of the expressions of guilt, although they are by no means really internalized as yet—most likely during the second year of life. Its precursors may lie in the very early glance aversion, later on the stranger anxiety, and eventually the turning of aggression against the self (Fraiberg 1982).

## THE AFFECTIVE CORE OF IDENTITY AND THE QUESTION OF GLOBAL AFFECTS

It is the affects that give the psychic life its richness. Our identity has an affective core that goes back in its origins to the first weeks and months (Emde [1983], Gaensbauer [1985], Rangell [1982]). Our dreams provide us with an affective immediacy of experience that often cannot be put into words or described; they give us a part of that deep affective continuity our identity is really rooted in.

Also, the affects at issue go far beyond those of love and hate, and this from the very earliest times on. Interest, surprise, joy, depression, sadness, contempt, astonishment, disgust, shame, rage, anger, dread, anxiety, and doubt are observable from very early on and in subtle gradations. By "early" I mean partly the first few months, partly the first one and a half years, that is, before the often presumed starting point of the ability to symbolize.

Yet why would overwhelming global affects or drive tensions be experienced as unpleasure, and why would they be dealt with in such a futile manner, namely in the form of these continually repetitive and idle attempts? Is it even correct to state that global affects would have to be unpleasurable? Clearly that is not the case.

The affects described here as global are by no means in and by themselves pathological or dangerous or disagreeable. In fact, the very richness of creativity is founded in the plenitude of such global emotions. Art, and probably most of all and earliest of all music, endows the affects with symbolic form (Klausmeier 1978; Langer 1953), including those of such global quality. And more: on many hierarchical levels, art gives the *conflicts between affects, and thus between values and ideals, between wishes and ideas* symbolic expression.

What is decisive with such global feelings, and the absolute valuations based on them, is the degree to which the ego is capable of steering these intensive ("fulfilling") emotions, or how far it is being inundated by them, overrun, put out of function (as we saw perhaps most eloquently stated by Sonya). There are affective states of such a global nature—ecstasy, consuming interests, joy, lust—that by no means, in spite of their want of moderation, have to be unpleasurable, nor would need to be warded off, provided that the ego, that is, the feeling of one's own power of will and decision, can declare its agreement and alliance with them. Again, the answer lies in the factor of conflict, not in that of the absoluteness or globality of the affect per se (or of the motivational system or drive joined with such affect).

Too much affect may be attributable to overstimulation from without, to traumatization more generally, or to understimulation, to constitutional factors. Each of these factors may disrupt the affective balance, but which affect or affect groups and affective discordances are at issue in this, probably depends upon the kind of disruption and the individual's disposition, not only upon the developmental phase in which such a misattunement occurs (Stern 1985).

In a sense, these global affects have mostly missed the connection to their proper time: they are disjoined from the past of conscious remembrances and from the future of planned intentions and willpower. Instead, they determine the present by their flooding force. Symbols, or more accurately the processes of symbolization, are powers that build a bridge from the past into the future. Affects that have been severed from symbolization or have never linked up with it are detached from the ego's control, and thus from rational decision and correction by the perception of reality. It is the attempt at synthesis, the striving of the ego for *psychic self-preservation* that ever again demands for the unsolvable conflict to be once and for all dealt with, yet which has to fail in this task because of the detachment from symbolization (Kubie 1978). This leads to constantly recurrent sequences of compromise formations and attempts at control.

And with that we have returned to the question of the repetition compulsion.

## ENDNOTES

1. (*Mancher versteht sich darauf, das eigne Gedächtnis zu trüben und zu mißhandeln, um wenigstens an diesem einzigen Mitwisser seine Rache zu haben: —die Scham ist erfinderisch. Es sind nicht die schlimmsten Dinge, deren man sich am schlimmsten schämt: es ist nicht nur Arglist hinter einer Maske, —es gibt soviel Güte in der List. Ich könnte mir denken, daß ein Mensch, der etwas Kostbares und Verletzliches zu bergen hätte, grob und rund wie ein grünes, altes, schwerbeschlagenes Weinfaß durchs Leben rollte: die Feinheit*

*seiner Scham will es so. Einem Menschen, der Tiefe in der Scham hat, begegnen auch seine Schicksale und zarten Entscheidungen auf Wegen, zu denen wenige je gelangen, und um deren Vorhandensein seine Nächsten und Vertrautesten nicht wissen dürfen: seine Lebensgefahr verbirgt sich ihren Augen und ebenso seine wiedereroberte Lebens-Sicherheit. Ein solcher Verborgener, der aus Instinkt das Reden zum Schweigen und Verschweigen braucht und unerschöpflich ist in der Ausflucht vor Mitteilung,* will *es und fördert es, daß eine Maske von ihm an seiner Statt in den Herzen und Köpfen seiner Freunde herumwandelt; und gesetzt, er will es nicht, so werden ihm eines Tages die Augen darüber aufgehn, daß es trotzdem dort eine Maske von ihm gibt, — und daß es gut so ist. Jeder tiefe Geist braucht eine Maske: mehr noch, um jeden tiefen Geist wächst fortwährend eine Maske,* dank *der beständig falschen, nämlich* flachen *Auslegung jedes Wortes, jedes Schrittes, jedes Lebenszeichens, das er gibt.*) (Neitzsche 1885, p. 51).

2. (*Les sentiments nobles poussés à l'absolu produisent des résultats semblables à ceux des plus grands vices.*)

3. (*Dieses "Mitwissen mit sich selbst" bedingt, dass das Ich des Menschen gleichsam in zwei getrennte Personenhälften aufgespalten ist, wobei die "höhergestellte" die "niedere" beobachtet und alle ihre Handlungen "mitweiss." Das Wissen geht vom Ich aus und betrifft zugleich das Ich; Subjekt wird zugleich Objekt, aber beide sind nicht einheitlich, sondern gebrochen, voneinander abgeteilt. — Wenn sich das böse Gewissen regt, leistet die eine der "Ich-Schichten" heftigen Widerstand, sie wehrt sich gegen dieses Wissen.*)

4. ([*Il "consapere con se stessi" espresso dalla formula* συνειδέναι ἑαυτῷ, *così come dalle formule di struttura analoga, si determina perciò, secondo il Class, mediante un processo riflessivo, che presuppone un contrasto all'interno dell'io.* . . . ]. *Se, infatti,* συνεδέναι ἑαυτῷ *significa innanzi tutto il 'consapere' privato dell'io con se stesso, e risponde quindi all'esigenza di esprimere un sapere che, basato sulla constatazione di una* privacy individuale, *si caratterizza come un "con-sapere" dell'io soltanto con se medesimo, non può avere importanza, nella sua formazione, il momento del dissidio interiore.*)

# 7

## The Repetition Compulsion

γένοι᾽ οἷος ἐσσὶ μαθών
Learning, become who you are
—Pindar, *Pythia*, 2.72

*Sinnig und schwer gehoben also war Jaakobs Seele in den Tagen, da er mit dem Bruder den Vater begrub, denn alle Geschichten standen vor ihm auf und wurden Gegenwart in seinem Geist, wie sie einst wieder Gegenwart geworden waren im Fleisch nach geprägtem Urbild, und ihm war, als wandelte er auf durchsichtigem Grunde, der aus unendlich vielen, ins Unergründliche hinabführenden Kristallschichten bestand, durchhellt von Lampen, die zwischen ihnen brannten.*

—Thomas Mann, *Joseph und seine Brüder*[1]

## COMPULSIVENESS AS ESSENCE OF THE NEUROTIC PROCESS

Let us take up once more the central question about the nature of the repetition compulsion. It was held by Kubie (1954, see also Wurmser 1978), and has been at least the implicit tenor of the clinical work presented here, that the *decisive criterion marking the neurotic process* is precisely this character of stereotypical, compulsive repetition, the seemingly irresistible force of certain feelings, thoughts, and actions, that pushes itself through, compellingly, undeterred by the rational wish and choice of the personality's core: "The essence of illness is the freezing of behavior into unalterable and insatiable patterns" (Kubie 1958, p. 21).[2]

We may now add, the more severe the neurotic conflicts are, the deeper is this subjective sense of compulsion and the more drastic also are the objective manifestations of compulsiveness.

As mentioned before, in a daring leap from description to explanation, this seemingly compelling "drive" to repeat certain mental processes in an old, stereotypical fashion was metapsychologically transformed into a primary force of the psyche—"repetition compulsion" as manifestation of a supposed "death instinct" and of "primary masochism" (Freud 1924c), or as an elementary power of its own (Waelder 1930).

If we refrain, however, from large generalizations and theoretical presuppositions and stay entirely within the realm of what is psychological, we recognize that this repetition compulsion aims at the resolution of inner conflicts that are largely unconscious and therefore not solvable. Because the attempt fails it has to be renewed time and again, and this manifests itself, as we just have seen, in characteristic sequences of attempted solutions; they all fail and yet have to be repeated in vicious circles specific for the various syndromes. The reason for this is that their real goal, the removal of the original conflicts and of the traumata connected with them, is not reachable, since the affects battling each other are themselves unknown; their qualities are cut off from consciousness. This is roughly the answer given by Kubie (1954, 1958):

> At the other end of our spectrum [as opposed to the realistic form of symbolic thinking] is the symbolic process in which the relationship between the symbol and what it represents has been either distorted or completely ruptured by an active process of dissociation in time and place between affect and its occasion, which results in that dissociation between symbol and its root, which leads to what is called "repression." As a consequence, the symbol here is a disguised and disguising representative of unconscious levels of psychological processes. In this area the function of the symbolic process is not to communicate but to hide, not deliberately but automatically, and not only from others but even more urgently from ourselves. [Kubie 1958, p. 30])

We may however persist in asking: Why are those connections torn? Why should there be repression at all, or defense more generally? I believe that the answer has to be seen in the *absolute, overwhelming, and hence traumatic* nature of what assaults the self at first from the outside, afterward from within, urgently requiring working-through and adequate response—whether those outer traumatizations come in the form of condemnation and brutality, or complete misrecognition or overstimulation (that is, soul blindness and soul murder), or whether the problem lies in those inner reactions of a global and total nature that try to deal with those dangers and damages. In other words, the defense directed against the trauma or the chronically traumatic environment is just as radical and uncompromising as the traumatization itself. The result is an inability of the ego to integrate these affects symbolically. Thus the provisional answer is: *what is absolute cannot be reconciled; the unsolvable conflict requires the defensive tearing-apart of connections.*

## REPETITION COMPULSION AS
## A SEQUENCE OF CONFLICT SOLUTIONS

Yet why this compulsion to repeat? The answer, on the basis of what just has been developed, is that when a problem is unconscious, it cannot be solved;

it remains unfinished business. The greater such a conflict, the stronger the need to solve it, yet this need must be met by failure, and hence the need to repeat the attempt to solve it.

What is the purpose of such compulsive repetition? Is it conflict resolution as an end in itself? Pleasure gain and avoidance of unpleasure? Mastery and self-assertion? Integration and synthesis? And does not something in this last question about synthesis lie that is teleological: the attainment of what is fitting to oneself, what fulfills one's essence—that one reaches, in Aristotelian terms, the personally best "form," the entelecheia? All this has then more to do with value philosophy than with psychology.

The answer obviously depends on what we postulate as the meaning of what goes on in the mind. Whatever the answer given by any metapsychology, it has to be of a philosophical nature and is only partly founded in experience. On the other side, such a philosophical foundation can thus only be avoided if we restrict ourselves to the parts, the individual aspects, and ignore the larger context. And yet, mutatis mutandis, it is the aim of every science to reach what Holton (1986) called the aim of physics: "a unified perception of all physical events, causes and effects" (p. 88). It is true, in psychology we are still far away from the point where we could attain such a synthetic comprehension of the whole, yet each one of us who is dedicated to the theoretical inquiry of pathology and its resolution is moved to lift single explanations from what is individual and concrete to a level of generality. This aim stands in dialectical opposition to what I quoted in the Introduction from Isaiah Berlin. The two value orientations are complementary.

This, however, means that we have to ask ourselves what the background for these generalizations is. And with that we are compelled to give at least an outline of the whole context in which both one's own observations and the theoretical conclusions find their place. But then we cannot get around the obligation to rethink the fundamental terms like repetition compulsion, narcissism, the model of instinctual drives, and the conflict concept. What do we really mean with them? Where do not-clarified presuppositions creep into the concepts themselves? What is explanation, and what is description?

It is clear that Freud (1930) saw the repetition compulsion linked to the "conservative character of instinctual life" (p. 118):

> For it is possible to recognize the dominance in the unconscious mind of a "compulsion to repeat" proceeding from the instinctual impulses and probably inherent in the very nature of the instincts—a compulsion powerful enough to overrule the pleasure principle, lending to certain aspects of the mind their daemonic character, and still very clearly expressed in the impulses of small children; a compulsion, too, which is responsible for a part of the course taken

by the analyses of neurotic patients. All these considerations prepare us for the discovery that whatever reminds us of this inner "compulsion to repeat" is perceived as uncanny. [Freud 1919b, p. 238]

"... the compulsion to repeat must be ascribed to the unconscious repressed" (Freud 1920, p. 20). He then asks, "How is the predicate of being 'instinctual' related to the compulsion to repeat?" (*Auf welche Art hängt aber das Triebhafte mit dem Zwang zur Wiederholung zusammen?*) (p. 36), implying already their partial congruence. He replies: "*It seems, then, that an instinct is an urge inherent in organic life to restore an earlier state of things* which the living entity has been obliged to abandon under the pressure of external disturbing forces; that is, it is a kind of organic elasticity, or, to put it another way, the expression of the inertia inherent in organic life" (Freud 1920, p. 36).

In 1926 he adds, "The fixating factor in repression, then, is the unconscious id's compulsion to repeat—a compulsion which in normal circumstances is only done away with by the freely mobile function of the ego" (p. 153). The "endeavour to undo a traumatic experience" can be seen at work in this compulsion to repeat (p. 120). The power of the compulsion to repeat is then called "the resistance of the unconscious" (pp. 161–162).

Schur found to the contrary that it was not necessary to have recourse to an overarching regulatory principle "beyond the pleasure principle." The repetition compulsion relates to "the ego's unconscious wish to *undo* the traumatic situation" (p. 178) and can be fully explained within the framework of the pleasure and unpleasure principles (p. 181), namely above all as a process of "repeating actively what he had undergone passively" (p. 189). This means that this compulsion to repeat should be counted not only to the id processes but to the unconscious ego processes.

It will have been noticed that I by and large concur with this reformulation. Yet this poses in turn a number of other problems.

Just for starters, the entire drive theory lies under a dark cloud of doubts. Some try to get rid of the drive model altogether because the duality of libido and aggression (or of Eros and Death Instinct, alias Thanatos) postulated by Freud, albeit of grand simplicity, does not do justice to many clinical observations. Moreover, a lot of resistance has been stirred up by that aspect of the drive model that deals with the supposed discharge of some hypothetical amount of energy, with the equation of pleasure with discharge and unpleasure with tension, and by the clinical recommendations derived from it, for example that of abstinence and the frustration indispensable for therapy.

Thomä and Kächele (1985) stress in their textbook, for example, that "the analytic method and the language of theory do not lie on the same plane"

(p. 15), and that especially the emphasis on the economic-energetic viewpoint and on the drive model has led to the current crisis in theory. Together with Gill (1976) (and many others, like Holt [1976], Klein [1976], and Schafer [1976a,b]), they assume that "metapsychology is full of images that betray their origin from infantile sexual ideas" (p. 24). They go as far as to claim that the reason for the crisis should be seen in the metapsychological confusion of biology and psychology (p. 25).

Their rejection of the drive model means among other things that aggressiveness and destructivity are considered reactive and determined by "their linkage to conscious and unconscious fantasy systems" (p. 133); these are declared to be correlates of self-preservation.

However, the complete discarding of the drive theory and of all quantitative aspects seems to me just as questionable as its one-sided and unquestioning acceptance as foundation for much of classical theory. I still see in both points of view—the economic and the drive models—metaphors and constructs that can claim a certain usefulness and with that validity without being able to be explanatory (Wurmser 1977a,b). *Metaphors give order, but not yet any causal connections.*

The drive model, understood as a dynamic model of opposite forces—enduring forms of fundamental wishes—is for me an indispensable resort in the daily work. Understood as a quasiphysical discharge system, it is for me as useless as it is for the other critics.

Quantitative considerations, both in regard to traumatizations (e.g., overstimulation) and to their correlates in inner conflicts, cannot be left out in my attempts to understand a patient. On the other side, I find the economic theory, the doctrine of "psychic energy," of "cathexes," and their "neutralization" and "deneutralization" as basic explanatory principles, as advocated especially by the New York school of ego-psychology, both unusable and principally unacceptable.

Yet both ways of contemplation—forms of dynamic and energetic thinking—seem to be immanent to human experience and reflection and can be traced in Chinese philosophy as well as in the thought tradition of the Occident, from Plato and Aristotle onward. Their psychological importance is one thing, their dogmatic fixation is something else, and their alleged explanatory potency something third.

As stated earlier, I am also convinced that the derivation of aggression from some motivational system, some "drive," for the preservation of the self and of its power, makes more sense than considering its autonomy as a separate drive form. Clinically, it has been more valuable for me to look at it in this way.

I do not think that any psychology can get by without any concepts and models of drives, but that the narrowing down to two basic drives of aggression and libido is unsatisfactory clinically in the treatment of the severe neuroses as well as in infant research. Rather, there are autonomous motivational systems, bundles of recurrent impulses and later on of wishes that, at least clinically, do not appear reducible to each other, such as sexual motives in the widest sense, claims for separateness, self-assertion and power, curiosity and the wishes for mastery of tasks, needs for attachment and also perhaps of destruction, although the latter might very well be reducible to thwarted wishes of other kinds, especially of self-preservation.

Fascinatingly, Lichtenberg (1989) brings the worlds of experience of psychoanalysis and infant research together in a bold synthesis. In particular, he suggests five motivational, functional systems that should replace the model of the dual drives. These new motivational systems that would better correspond to experience are the following five pairs, as given in a recent summary: "We took into account fundamental needs for the psychic regulation of physiological requirements, attachment and affiliation, assertion and exploration, sensual pleasure and sexual excitement, and the need to react aversively by using withdrawal or antagonism" (Lichtenberg et al. 1996, p. 7). Success in any one of these systems evokes a kind of pleasure specific for that system; failure brings about shame. The danger inherent to each system triggers the corresponding anxiety.

In the case of the severe disturbances studied here, the drives are just as extreme and manifest the same claims for absoluteness as the affects.

One result of the invalidation of metapsychology as a foundation for explanation is inevitably a far more differentiated way of looking at affects and affect signals as part of relational processes. The structure of any future basic theory will require a completely independent affect theory. Affects cannot be reduced to drives.

The reverse attempt, namely to derive drives from the affects, also appears to be an inadmissible simplification. The fact that the affects are visible long before the wishes does not yet allow this kind of reduction, a kind of "genetic fallacy" (Hartmann 1964). In my opinion, the large groupings of ostensibly primary motivational forces are too universal and evince too much of a neurobiological foundation for us to understand them merely as derivative.

If we turn again to the observations, they show us that the compulsion to repeat *consists of the sequences, equations, and encompassing configurations* described. This emphatically means that what is being experienced as *repetition compulsion* is *nothing simple*, but in actuality a *complex and sequential series of compromise formations*—a *sequence of attempted conflict solutions* that in turn consist of affects and drive impulses, of forms of defense and superego functions, of identifications and counteridentifications. In this sense we can even state that *the repetition compulsion is an attempt to solve conflicts.* Yet, while this statement is necessary, it is not sufficient.

Clinically we can also add at once that the obedience to the commandments of the archaic superego, the original form of the tragic dilemmas of extreme guilt and shame, plays in this a very prominent role, really a far more essential role than the drive components (*horribile dictu,* in the view of many with more traditional orientation). It is also to be noted, as emphasized by Schur (1966) and more recently by Gray (1994), that the ego processes, especially the defense mechanisms, are marked by such an automatic (mechanical) and stereotypically repetitive character, as we know from the impulses (the "instinctual drives," as they have become, rather fallaciously, known in the English translation from Freud's, or also from Nietzsche's, *Triebe*). These defensive activities have a seemingly irresistible "drive character." The same is true for the affects.

## THE NEED FOR SYNTHESIS

Why would it be so pervasively and persistently important to resolve conflicts and not to be deterred when these efforts falter? We do not have at once to go beyond psychology and resort to metapsychological explanations nor really against what we otherwise know from psychoanalysis, if we respond the way I have just done: chronically unsolved conflicts contradict the need for inner unity, that is, the ego's striving for synthesis. The repetition serves the conquest of the *inner* conflicts in order to enhance the synthesis of the inner world; it may also be used to resolve the conflict with the *outside* world in order to facilitate the reintegration into the community. Yet, as mentioned before, this attempt in the form of a series of compromise formations has to fail because the connections are torn and, in this form, cannot be tied together again.

Also, the more massive the polarities of affects and the higher the accompanying affective tensions are, the stronger is the necessity to find regulation with the help of a repetitive effort to reconcile what is irreconcilable and thus to restore inner unity. Thus, it is evident that the repetition compulsion very prominently serves not only the *resolution of conflict,* but also the *mastery and regulation of affect.*

Since the goal of a possible solution lies outside the realm of word representations and, with that, is usually barred from the symbolic process in general, the attempt at resolution by repetition keeps failing, as long as those polarities are not opened up to the symbolic processes.

The repetition compulsion would, therefore, have more to do with such *original, traumatically triggered, global affects and the defense against them* than with any postulated primitive quality of the drives or with a supraordinate regulatory principle of the id. We may postulate instead that the need for the unity of self and ego is indeed such a basic principle. The repetition compulsion does not have to express, in and by itself, a biological need for repetition, but rather it would correspond to an *original regulatory attempt to equalize intolerable affects and affect polarities, as part of the basic need for unity or integration of self and ego.* This attempt would be carried over into the later outer and inner conflicts, which are largely determined by these usually global affects.

With that, it could be the manifestation of an innate, that is, absolutely basic psychological and presumably also biological principle, one that would be *eo ipso* independent from experiences, to *equalize an excess of tension between opposites.* The postulate of such a principle—we could call it the *principle of binding what is beyond measure* (*das Prinzip der Bindung des Maßlosen*) in the interest of *inner unity or synthesis*—is speculative, and thus metapsychological in nature, like that of homeostasis, which is very much akin to it. The corresponding phenomena are explained by Freud (1920) by the unpleasure principle and the drive model: drive tensions that are too large manifest themselves as unpleasure and have to be warded off.

Repetition compulsion is based on the contradiction (again in fact a very basic conflict) between the *necessity for regulation of affects,* and hence the balancing out of opposite affective and drive states, and the *learned experiences,* that is, the interchange with the environment—when such an equalization, a balancing-out, has been blocked and thus the regulation becomes impossible. The connections between the felt affects and drive states on the one side, and the symbolic representations on the other have been sundered because of those experiences. The anxiety that is opposed to the reconnecting of what has been torn is the anxiety of repeating those experiences where regulation has been impossible. There exists therefore a *complementarity between affect regulation and inner conflict* (Lichtenberg 1986).

It is particularly important to stress that these *regulatory disturbances* ( *"deficits"*) *become part of the conflicts,* that they do not somehow run parallel to them, as something separate, and that they can be encountered in one or the other version pretty much in all the neuroses. I believe that disturbances of affect regulation are part of every neurosis, that it is not a matter of principal differences but of *quantitative* ones when we speak of milder or severer neuroses. The *qualitative* differences refer rather to the various types of neurosis that distinguish themselves by the preference for certain attempts at solution on the spectrum outlined in the "ideal sequence."

Thus I concur with Inderbitzin and Levy (1998) when they see "repetition compulsion" as descriptively useful, but criticize its use as an explanatory concept. They emphasize

> the detrimental technical legacy of the concept, which has cast a pessimistic aura of unanalyzability over a wide variety of repetitive phenomena, especially analyzable resistances related to aggressive conflicts. We conclude that the repetition compulsion is an anachronistic concept with detrimental technical implications and that it should be retired. [p. 32]

## SPECIFIC AND UNSPECIFIC EFFECTS OF PSYCHOANALYSIS

During psychoanalytic work, access occurs almost exclusively with the help of word symbols. And yet, there are all those *unspecific factors* that exert considerable, even indispensable influence upon affect regulation ("beyond interpretation" [Gedö, 1979])—the "holding environment" (Winnicott 1965), the active interest, the careful avoidance of criticism, the nonauthoritarian friendliness, the experiencing, feeling, and wishing in this new situation where it is permissible to feel, think, and say everything without translating it into action, and thus, as it were, without danger to let it romp to one's heart's content (*austoben lassen*). All these factors allow a bringing together of affective experiences—which have been severed from symbolization or have never been able to be led to such symbolization—with the experience of the world of symbols.

In this the personality of the analyst is of crucial significance, not so much, and not only, the correctness of his interpretations. We can refine this: if his interpretations are consistently beside the point, or if he communicates a critical, scornful basic attitude or an emotional coolness and distance, or, to the contrary, one of intrusiveness and of theoretical prejudice, then it means that the affect regulation side of analytic therapy is essentially missed, and again the possibility of bringing the opposites together as complementary values or needs has been thwarted: integration remains elusive. In this (frequent) case, analyzability is restricted to those patients who allegedly have no problems with affective storms, that is, either to those who pride themselves on a "successfully" obsessive-compulsive character, or to those who are professionally dependent upon this analysis (the candidates), or those who succeed in establishing such a severe masochistic transference that they speak of gain and progress just then and that is when and where they suffer most. I believe it is these *unspecific factors* that are subsumed under empathy or its lack.

## THE SUPEREGO AS HEIR TO THE EXPERIENCED ABSOLUTENESS OF TRAUMA

Used descriptively, phenomenologically, the *repetition compulsion* is, therefore, an *attempt to attain in symbolic ways regulation and conflict resolution* that proves *blocked because the affects and the drive needs* evoked by them and closely connected with them, the forms of *defense*, and the *superego demands* are all of a *global* quality and therefore *irreconcilable* with each other; therefore, the consistent endeavors to express them in symbols have to be defeated also. Narcissistic crises, loyalty conflicts, shame–guilt dilemmas, and concomitant aggressive impulses have a commanding position in the triggering of those sequences, of the ensuing impulsive actions, and of the splitting of consciousness and identity.

There appears to be *no repetition compulsion without the decisive participation of the superego.* This means, in regard to the patients discussed here, in the sense of *conflicts within the superego, specifically of loyalty conflicts or guilt–shame dilemmas.* The antithetical claims for absoluteness within the superego try to rule the inner life, and the compromises reached between them largely determine the affects, the forms of defense, and the admitted drive derivatives, and therewith also those interim steps, attempts at solution that can be encountered during the *sequences* of *impulsive actions.* Those single sequences and that abstraction in the form of the "ideal sequence" represent, therefore, a series of *compromise formations* in which *different aspects* of the *superego play a decisive role.*

*Repetition compulsion is a flight from conscience that fails, a revolt against the conscience and its ideals that founders, a reconciliation with the conscience that is hypocritical and at best transitory. It is a sequence of solutions for loyalty conflicts and other intrasystemic superego conflicts that mobilizes all the deep aggressions in the service of opposing loyalties, ideals, and values, and is being driven by resentment and affects connected with it (envy, jealousy, vengefulness, and above all profound shame).*

In spite of this recurrent defeat, the attempt cannot be given up, since it lies in the *nature of the ego to attain inner unity,* to overcome the inner rent, the inner contradictoriness, the doubleness of self and world experience. The *need for synthesis,* that is, for *psychical self preservation,* is so important and so preeminent, that, in intensity and penetrating power, it corresponds to an "instinctual drive,"[3] or can be formulated as a basic regulatory principle. (Both terms are looked at as psychological concepts; their possible biological significance is left open.)

As already considered by Freud (1920, 1930) and stated by Schur (1966), repetition compulsion turns out to be an attempt to repeat, actively and with reversed signature, the passively suffered trauma, with the aim of mastery. Unfortunately, the early trauma has led to *overwhelming affects* and hence, as described, to the *superego's demands for absoluteness*. With that, the intrapsychic conflicts have become principally insoluble and the affects and drive impulses (especially aggressions), stimulated ever again by them, have gotten insurmountably strong. Thus the trauma in a sense lives on; like a dragon in its cave, it broods safely and with tyrannical force in the conscience. In other words, *the superego more and more takes on in valence and symbols the representation of the experienced absoluteness of the trauma: its global vehemence and devouring, consuming character.*

Ultimately, the *conflict nature of the human being* is unresolvable; it belongs to human existence, to man's very essence, as we read in Plato's *Phaedrus*: "There is imposed on the soul pain and extreme conflict—ἔνθα δὴ πόνος τε καὶ ἀγὼν ἔσχατος ψυχῇ πρόκειται (entha de ponos te kai agon eschatos psyche prokeitai)."

## THE LAYERS OF PATHOGENESIS

This leads then to the following survey concerning the pathogenesis in all severer forms of neuroses, in the form of five critical factors:

1. The earliest disturbance, but one that remains observable throughout life, shows itself as *intolerance* toward affects, especially those having the nature of unpleasure (although not necessarily restricted to these): anxiety and sadness, their variants in form of shame, guilt, inferiority feelings, disappointment, and grief, and other related feelings of dysphoria, disgust, and tension. Not all of them can simply be subsumed under anxiety and depression. They may have to do with, on the one side, what Stern (1985) called "vitality affects," qualities of experience like "explosive," "rush," "fading away," "decrescendo," and, on the other side, the prevailing moods imparted to infant and child by the caregiver and later on the entire family, from very early on and more or less throughout growing up. Following Rangell (1967) (see also Kubie's [1963] similar concept of "central affective potential"), Emde (1983) speaks about the *affective core* that "guarantees our continuity

of experience across development" from the first weeks of infancy on (1983). "Broad based *failure in regulation*" (Lichtenberg 1986) in regard to those affects may underlie the later affect pathology we find in these patients.

2. Such massiveness and intolerability of affects, and especially of moods— the insufficiency, or defect, of affect defense, as I have described it earlier (Wurmser 1974, 1978), the breakdown in their regulation, as it could perhaps be more suitably called—is intertwined with a particular *severity of conflicts*, originally of outer conflicts (with the immediate environment, as for example the impressive studies of Fraiberg [1982] and of Gaensbauer [1985] showed), then, more and more of inner conflicts. "When regulatory disturbances become coded through the symbolic process," says Lichtenberg (1983), "the conflictual configurations that result take the symptomatic and characterological forms familiar to psychoanalysis" (p. 199).

In other words, the more severe the disregulation, the more extreme— archaic—the ensuing conflicts, and the more radical the affective judgments good–bad, safe–terrifying, pleasurable–unpleasurable, admirable–contemptible, shamefully weak–guiltfully strong, and so on; that is, some of the phenomena explained by many today as "splitting."

3. This entails that the *anxieties* engendered by those conflicts are particularly overwhelming, hence especially *disintegrating and fragmenting* (Rangell 1982). As Rangell stresses and we have witnessed in our case studies, all anxiety is fragmenting, all anxiety always affects the feeling of self, of self-value and self-integrity, and thus has a "narcissistic" aspect; the more intense the anxiety, the stronger the sense of going to pieces. In the past I have stated emphatically that there is no separate fragmentation anxiety due to narcissistic conflicts. Fragmentation is a result and cannot serve as a partial explanatory concept. We can state it somewhat more broadly—that it is intensive affects, like severe anxiety and rage, and especially the juxtaposition of several intensive affects—that have a severely fragmenting effect. The resulting *"narcissistic crises"* and the *narcissistic forms of restitution* form part and parcel of those conflicts.

Now I would correct this one-sided statement by adding that while the sense of fragmentation is very typically the result of anxiety, hence of conflict, we have to assume that the reverse is true as well, and that unsolvable outer and inner conflict means a breakdown of inner synthesis, hence fragmentation, and thus is itself an immediate source of anxiety expressing the danger of helplessness. The almost automatic equation of seemingly insoluble conflict with anxiety is a manifestation of this fact.

4. One important culmination point of such conflicts and opposite forms of dangers is the period in which there is a clear opposition between the

need to belong and the need to be oneself, that is, the separation and in-dividuation period (Mahler 1968, Mahler et al. 1975), with its convergence of early castration concerns (Roiphe and Galenson 1981), anal-sadistic in-vestments, and with them problems of autonomy and possibly some early oedipal strivings (Tabin 1985), the revolutionary acquisition of symbolization, and last but hardly least, the emergence of shame and other early superego manifestations. It appears that at that time some of the *massive and archaic identifications* occur that henceforth profoundly shape the entire character. These are of a typically *global* nature and later on necessitate equally large scale forms of *denial* (Müller-Pozzi 1985) and the mask of the "false self," ways of denial that determine most deeply the experience of self and world.

The "ideal sequence" outlined earlier and the observable impulse se-quences take their origin from this retrospectively inferrable first culmina-tion point and find their clearest shape in the oedipal phase proper, about one and a half to three years later.

5. The role of the superego in this pathogenetic layering is decisive, yet too often given short shrift. I shall come back to this shortly.

## THE BEGINNING OF INNER CONFLICT

It is uncertain how early we can talk about inner conflict. To answer this question, retrospective reconstructions are worthless and direct observations very difficult. Hints may exist in the phobias of early childhood and ambiva-lent behavior, for example in that described as "avoidantly attached," al-though even this has been strongly contested by others: Lichtenberg (1983), for example, considers it impossible to speak of inner conflict or neurotic processes before the ability of symbolization has been fully developed, that is, before the age of 18 months. It would indeed be extremely fascinating to set up research experiments so as to observe possible conflicts between opposite strivings or contradictory affects in early infancy and especially to examine the symptomatology of early disturbances specifically in this re-gard. The beginnings of such investigations exist (e.g., Fraiberg 1982, Emde 1983).

Grossman (1991) postulates such very early appearance of inner conflict:

> In the early cases, the issue seems to be self-control out of fear in conflict with the caretaker. . . . The early self-control generated out of fear and pain may perhaps be considered to be the precursor of inner conflict occurring at a presymbolic, sensorimotor level of development. It may not be conflict at the level of tripartite structure, but it may be conflict. [p. 45]

Similarly, Fraiberg (1982) writes, in regard to the first observable defense, avoidance (beginning at the age 3 months): ". . . perception itself can be caught up in conflict in the early months of life, so that registration appears to be closed off selectively" (p. 622).

I concur with this view.

## THE ESSENCE OF THE NEUROTIC PROCESS

What is it that we can, quite generally, observe as hallmarks of the neurotic process—in a less pronounced way in the milder forms of the neuroses, in much sharpened and more poignant ways in the severe forms of neuroses? What is, *descriptively* speaking, the *"essence of the neurotic process"*—in the widest sense (that is, if we also include, as I do on clinical grounds, those categories that are today often parcelled out as "borderlines," "perversions," and "narcissistic pathology")?

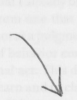

The first and major criterion is one that Kubie (1954) singled out and that I already briefly mentioned above, a quality that sets a normal act apart from one that is a manifestation of the neurotic process; he means this not as a judgment of value, but as a clinical description of that one attribute of behavior common to every neurotic action and absent from every normal act. His determining trait centers on the freedom and flexibility to learn and to change through experience, and to adjust to changing external circumstances.

> Thus the essence of normality is flexibility, in contrast to the freezing of behavior into patterns of unalterability that characterizes every manifestation of the neurotic process, whether in impulses, purposes, acts, thoughts, or feelings. Whether or not a behavioral event is free to change depends not upon the quality of the act itself, but upon the nature of the constellation of forces that has produced it. No moment of behavior can be looked upon as neurotic unless the processes that have set it in motion predetermine its automatic repetition irrespective of the situation, the utility, or the consequences of the act. [p. 182]

He gives this description an explanatory undergirding by claiming that whenever the unconscious system predominates, the resulting action must be repeated over and over, because its goals are largely unconscious symbols and unconscious symbolic goals can never be attained.

> Since the predominant forces are unconscious, they will not be responsive to the experience of pleasure or of pain, or to rewards and punishments, or to

logical argument—neither to the logic of events nor to any appeals to mind or heart. The behavior that results from a dominance of the unconscious system has *the insatiability, the automaticity, and the endless repetitiveness* that are the stamp of the *neurotic process*, whether this expresses itself through overt neurotic symptoms, or through art forms, or through subtle deformations of those general patterns of behavior that constitute the personality. [pp. 183/184, emphasis added]

I believe that with this Kubie has indeed stressed a necessary condition for the neurotic process (i.e., one criterion for calling a mental act "neurotic"—phenomenologically, not dynamically). I think however it is not a sufficient one. The second condition consists in the *polarization of the opposites*, the dichotomizing of the judgments of good and bad, of pure and impure, of sacred and demonic, or God and Devil—the extreme quality of love and hate, of trust and distrust.

Closely connected with that is a third criterion: the experience of *absoluteness and globality* of a value, an ideal, a commitment, a principle, the claim of totality for affective or cognitive comprehension (*Erfassung*) of self and world, and the equal totality and absoluteness of the denial and exclusion of that which does not seem to fit to this absolutely held principle. Most of all, the wishes and the affects have a particularly overwhelming, global, all-encompassing nature; they cannot be contained. Put in different words: there is an *overvaluation*, an overestimation of self or others; it is a transgressing of the limits, a dissolution of the boundaries, in value, truth, and action.

These three then are the criteria for *describing* the neurotic process, as it becomes glaringly obvious in the severely regressive patients. The important thing now is that each of these criteria has been selected not only as the major attribute, but also as the cornerstone to *explain* what was encountered in the severe neuroses. The first criterion, that of repetitiveness, was hypostatized in the form of the "repetition compulsion," or in somewhat different form, as the "primary masochism" or the "death instinct," alias Thanatos. What could not be successfully treated by analysis was ascribed to the intensity of that enigmatic, probably inborn force. The Ananke of the fate of these "tragic patients" corresponds to the implacability of the repetition compulsion.

Alternately, the second descriptively useful criterion of the polarities and radical dichotomies was taken and hypostatized in form of the concept of "*splitting*," which now was supposed to serve as a major tool of explanation: This pathology was thus pronounced because of the massiveness of such underlying "splitting" as an inferred basic defense mechanism. With that came the postulate of a special category of patients where this explanatory principle dictated decisive therapeutic action: the supposed cause had to be confronted and thus lifted. Of course, one notices right away the circular nature of that "explanation."

Taking the third criterion, again something universally observable in any neurosis, though much more pronounced in some than in others, it is very usefully, though descriptively labelled "*narcissistic*." Yet here again the valuable singling out of one aspect was being turned into a major claim of causality: the basic forms of such narcissism, of such globality, especially the wishes for omnipotence, grandiosity and entitlement, for idealization and merger, were declared the ultimate factors of explanation for the neurotic process, at least in a large group of severely ill patients. Deficiencies in the development of these basic needs led, so it is claimed, to characteristic defects, which had to be compensated for by the technique of empathic guidance and holding.

Another model of the use of this third criterion as cornerstone for explanation was the one profferred by ego psychology, notably Hartmann (1964): these phenomena are due to "deneutralization" of energy—the economic model of psychic energy becoming the primary system of causal explanation. Neurosogenesis was seen as a strictly "economic," that is, quantitative domain.

Clearly each of these explanatory models that we find scattered through much of our more recent literature, most notably represented by Melanie Klein (1932, 1952a,b), Kernberg (1975, 1984), Kohut (1971), and the adherents of ego psychology in the narrow sense (Hartmann [1964], Rapaport [1967], Jacobson [1964]) respectively, reflects an important part of the truth. I think where they go wrong is again in their *leap from description to explanation.* They give up where the work is supposed to begin. The patient, faced with any of these three criteria taken as basic and ultimate insights, answers: "I know all that. That is what I am suffering from. That is why I come to see you. And you simply tell me: this is what I should accept. The problem is that I cannot accept it, and I do not know why. Please, help me to find the reason why I am so *compelled*, why I do live in such *radical opposites* and feel so torn within, and why I am *overwhelmed* by these feelings that flood over everything like a storm surge."

George Eliot (1876) cautions us against such leaps from description to explanation, an acrobatic temptation our theoreticians have, as noted before, indulged in far too liberally. We find her sage warning after the unfolding of Gwendolen Harleth's contradictoriness of character:

> To her mamma and others her fits of timidity or terror were sufficiently accounted for by her "sensitiveness" or the "excitability of her nature"; but these

explanatory phrases required reconciliation with much that seemed to be blank indifference or rare self-mastery. Heat is a great agent and a useful word, but considered as a means of explaining the universe it requires an extensive knowledge of differences; and as means of explaining character "sensitiveness" is in much the same predicament. [p. 95]

We might put in words like "narcissism" and "overstimulation," perhaps even "deneutralized energy" for the two just cited by her, and we have not advanced from description to explanation even if some may claim so (death instinct, masochism, repetition compulsion, splitting are similar pseudo-explanatory concepts, though useful as description).

What is the answer to the question: What is truly explanatory in psycho-analytic work? Where do we need to stop in the exploratory quest for inner causality? And hence, What are the crucial, the mutative insights, meaning: the causally most effective interpretations?

Of course, as the references to the "leap" from description to explanation have already shown, the answers to these questions are extremely divergent, dependent on the theoretical orientation. What has been proposed in Chapter 4 emerges accordingly from the long (occasionally very long) intensive work with severely ill, but not psychotic patients—as simply the most helpful construct about the *specific unconscious causality* underlying those just described *core phenomena* of *compulsiveness, polarization, and globalization.*

The central concern for us as psychoanalysts is the consistent, systematic exploration of inner conflict, especially of unconscious inner conflict. No matter how we try to define our work, it always comes down to the fact that the focus, the center of our interest during our analytic work at its best, lies on inner conflict. Everything else moves to the periphery; it is not irrelevant, but our inner orientation is such that we notice it as part of the surrounding field, not as the beacon that guides us.

Thus psychoanalytic explanation rests in an understanding of *conflict causality*: the causes of what we observe are seen in many layers of inner conflict, in the way conflicts are the response to traumata, and the way the opposite forces in conflicts can become complementary. *Psychoanalysis is the study of the mind in conflict and complementarity.* Conflict does not simply refer to that between drives and ego, drives and superego, ego and outer reality, but also between opposite ego aspects, between discordant superego parts, as between different ideals and values, between sharply split loyalties, even between opposing drives, and between ideas and affects. Obviously conflict psychology is not synonymous with the exploration of oedipal issues or even with the structural model, as important as both are for conflict psychology; both of them deal with special forms of conflict.

The causality relevant for understanding and for effective intervention resides in the complexity and the intertwining of conflicts. Causality is relative to the goal intended by exploration or intervention—it is not absolute; it too is a pragmatic concept (though not exclusively so). What lies beyond conflict lies beyond psychoanalysis.

## SUPEREGO AND NARCISSISM

I think it is not an unwarranted generalization to state that throughout life, with the exception of the earliest period, inner conflict always involves the superego with some or all of its six major functions: (1) ego-ideal (above all the image of the ideal self and the code of ideal actions), (2) self-criticism and self-punishment, (3) stabilization of mood and affect, (4) self-observation, (5) holding guard over inner and outer boundaries and limitations, and (6) approval and protection of one's own person (the self). This means that the *superego becomes the main inner agency of regulation.*

Experience has shown that these functions, separately or conjointly, emerge long before the later oedipal periods. It is therefore not generally accepted anymore that the superego as a structure is simply the heir of the Oedipus complex, at least not in its late form. It is very conceivable that earlier forms of structure far precede the "dissolution of the Oedipus complex." This is another area where good empirical research could lead to new, as well as clinically promising insights. I leave the question open from when we can begin to talk with certainty about a structure called "superego"—whether only after the oedipal phase (however we measure it) or already much earlier—or if it is still justifiable today to speak in this sense about phases or periods, or whether it is not rather the case of lifelong issues possessing their own developmental lines. After all, we do see already from the very first weeks of life a clear differentiation of the relation to the mother, to the father, and to other people in the surroundings. When do the first observable triadic situations begin (see, e.g., Abelin 1975)? What form do they assume and when? Here too there could be exciting new possibilities for research This does not entail of course the adoption of the Kleinian constructs, but a suggestion to get help from direct observation where the retrospective inquiry has to fail in principle, and where indeed this approach has to be on the wrong track just because it tries a priori to equate psychotic phenomena with those of early childhood (see Reed and Baudry 1997). This presumption has been completely shattered by the new direct observations.

The later inner conflicts, as they become typically accessible by the analytic method, always involve the superego as a cardinal structure. The superego is itself, as Brenner (1982) emphasized, a compromise formation. Relations to others ("object relations"), drives, affects, and traumata are precipitated in it just like the defenses against them. These conflicts may re-evoke or reenlist those much earlier affects whose regulation had not been effective. But now everything, also those earlier affects, is being filtered and mediated through symbolic representations, hence through inner conflicts and fantasies—filtered through, but not restricted to them! And such symbolic representation occurs on many levels and may be conscious, preconscious, or unconscious (see Kubie 1954, 1958).

One corollary is that in these severe forms of neurosis we find a particular severity and even *polarization of the superego*—exaggerated ideals and expectations, and with that exaggerated condemnation of an all-or-nothing, black-or-white nature—and again this may cover the entire register from conscious to unconscious. From those devastating discrepancies follow equally exaggerated affects, primarily guilt, shame, and despair, secondarily rage, contempt, defiance, and envy defending against those affects. One effect of the intensity of such superego conflicts is, as we saw, the splitting of identity—in its extreme form to that of a multiple personality.

Another thing follows from this. The early conflicts and the global affects invested in them, which determine the superego formation, result in a clinical experience of paramount importance, which is that *"narcissistic" problems and disturbances always centrally involve superego conflicts*. It is far more helpful to treat *narcissistic conflicts as results of superego conflicts* than the other way around: to see narcissistic disturbances as more fundamental, as supraordinate to the structural ones.

If we turn to the *fantasies*, the largely narrative imagery and scenarios of self and objects and their symbols, they too partake in the radicalization of feelings and wishes, derivative compromise formations that they are. Just like the superego, they have become carriers of global affects, that is, they are very often of a "narcissistic" character, and have accordingly as their lead contents transgression of limits, merger and blurring of boundaries between inside and outside, omnipotence and omniscience, and immoderate claims. They show that hallmark of being without measure. And yet, it seems to me essential that, at least according to my experience, this is not a case of primary wishes that we ought to thwart or embitter for the patient (as has often been intimated to me), and that he should learn to renounce, "to learn as fool by suffering"; rather, these wishes for merger, omnipotence, and entitlement always serve as protection against anxiety, pain, loss, or shame, and therefore against affects usually of traumatic origin and overwhelming intensity. To say the same thing in other words: the so-called "symbiotic" fantasies and those of an alleged "primary narcissism" are not regressions to original drive wishes, but archaic, global forms of defense against global threats and sufferings. I stress this so much because the decision about the theoretical stance entails a very different therapeutic procedure: a confrontative, educational, and condemnatory stance on the one hand, an understanding of what seems deviant and grossly acted out as subjectively needed self-protection on the other. With the former approach most of the patients studied here, after the acute crisis situation, become untreatable, or at least unanalyzable. In such acute situations, this first approach may very well be indicated, indeed, it may be indispensable, even life-saving. If it is used, however, as the method of long-term therapy, it strengthens the narrowing down of the personality, the obedient (i.e., masochistic) submission to authority, and the phobic inclinations, and thus it often contributes to a deepening of what is already a painful sense of inferiority and shame and to an intensification of the aggressions resulting from this sense.

In turn, if we utilize a strictly analytic, interpretative approach at the time of severe crisis, like suicidality, other forms of self-endangerment or drug use, we run a risk that is just as serious: that we fail to stop the patient's self-destructive acting-out and thus do not give him the support he is crying for—"the wall to bounce off from," as Vera called it. The consequences of this can be fatal and, even if not, the therapy fails. This is the technical dilemma I shall shortly return to.

## SUMMARY OF THE MAIN CONFLICTS

With that we have arrived at a point where it becomes necessary to give an account of the main conflicts.

The notion of inner conflict did not originate with Freud; its systematic use as an explanatory device par excellence did. In his and even more so in our work, relevant *explanation* more and more moves away from the short-cut attempts at reducing our inner life to certain large factors, like trauma, stages of libido development, narcissism, masochism, repetition compulsion. To repeat: if these concepts are taken as explanations of causality, the clinician soon discovers that their usefulness stops precisely there, where the problem begins. They are the beginning, not the end of the search. Instead, the stopping point of such exploration is inner conflict, specifically inner preconscious conflict that stands for, and is derivative of, long-range unsolved unconscious inner conflict. Thus psychoanalytic explanation rests in an understanding of *conflict causality*. The causes of what we observe are seen in many layers of inner conflict:

> We seek not merely to describe and to classify phenomena, but to understand them as signs of an interplay of forces in the mind, as a manifestation of purposeful intentions working concurrently or in mutual opposition. We are concerned with a *dynamic view* of mental phenomena. In our view the phenomena that are perceived must yield in importance to trends which are only hypothetical. [Freud 1916/17, p. 67]

He continues, "It is important to begin in good time to reckon with the fact that mental life is the arena and battle-ground for mutually opposing purposes or, to put it non-dynamically, that it consists of contradictions and pairs of contraries" (pp. 76–77).

Such conflict causality is non-linear and of the greatest complexity (cf. my [1989a,b] discussion of Grünbaum 1984).

I give now a brief outline of the main groups of unconscious, pathogenic conflicts, which, with their infinite individual variations and in variable intensity, appear in the dynamics of the patients discussed here. It has proven pragmatically most accurate and useful to group these pathogenic conflicts under the following broad headings:

1. There is the preeminence of the problems of, and therewith the conflicts about, *affect regulation*. We noticed throughout a problem with an *intolerance* toward affects. I often have the impression that such affects are a kind of psychoanalytic bedrock, transcending the power of verbal mastery and both preceding and overwhelming the ability of symbolization. Although they certainly often seem to result from issues of later provenience, such as anal or oedipal problems, it still can be presumed that they antedate them.

*Conflicts about global affects* lead to mental phenomena that are typically viewed and descriptively encompassed as "oral" and as "narcissistic." Conflict exists *between clashing overwhelming affects that cannot be contained*, typically rage versus anxiety or guilt, love versus humiliation, pain and shame versus excitement. Moreover, there is the conflict between the often irresistible tendency to spiral down into *overwhelming affect* versus the desperate effort at controlling these affects and the shame about losing such *inner control*. Then there is the problem of being overrun or "infected," by the affect and the mood of the immediate environment, the collapse of the defense against affect transmission, from the outside the "empathic wall" (Nathanson 1986). It is a very archaic, the most archaic group of conflicts in fact (cf. the works of Krystal).

Yet these affects impart to all later conflicts their own intensity and radicalness. The fact that those archaic affects and moods now form such radical conflicts and extreme ("omnipotent") conflict solutions entails that the anxieties engendered by the conflicts are particularly overwhelming, hence especially fragmenting. If one of the characteristic features of "narcissism" is "the lack of measure," immoderation (hubris!), it is grounded in this globality of affect. The "narcissistic crises" and the narcissistic forms of restitution form part and parcel of the conflicts, are not beyond conflict nor rooted in some basic layer of self-pathology and fragmentation anxiety.

2. The second type of conflict is that between *wishes for self-expression and curiosity* on the one side, and on the other the fear of being overrun by the *intrusion* or *misattunement* (Stern 1985) of others and the need therefore to block them.

These very archaic conflicts, to which I have devoted considerable attention in my shame book (Wurmser 1981a), refer to the wish and also the fear to become like the other by means of *seeing,* to merge with the other by perceiving—the motive of a kind of *"primary" identification through perception and expression,* manifested for example as anxiety about all human contact and love because love is closeness, and closeness is merger and union, and with that extinction of the self. Since it is in particular in the processes of seeing and being seen (and, more generally of perception and expression altogether), in whose medium merger as well as overpowering and annihilation would occur, these processes of perception and expression are being interfered with or largely blocked.

3. One important culmination point of such conflicts (and of the opposite forms of dangers involved) is the period in which there is a clear opposition between the *need to belong and the need to be oneself,* the *conflicts about union and separateness.*

However, it needs to be maintained, as Stern (1985) so impressively argued, that issues (conflicts?) of individuation and separation versus belonging together and relatedness can be observed in primitive and external forms almost from the inception of infancy (cf. also the dramatic descriptions in Fraiberg [1982]). They may become interwined with anal and oedipal conflicts, and yet remain separable from them.

In many of these cases there exists a deep ambivalence, above all toward the mother, whereby *separation* is being equated with *crime, murder, and death* (Modell 1984, pp. 56–57), as we noticed in virtually all our case examples.

In some patients this manifests itself as a basic phobic attitude expressing the dread of separating from the fear-filled and angry mother. Every success represents a symbolic separation and has to be prohibited. Life is,

however, separateness. The patient therefore has to suffer from an gnawing, yet consciously unexplainable sense of guilt—"as if I really had committed a murder," as one patient (Jacob, in Chapter 5) expressed it. The
feared retribution has to be correspondingly massive and omnipresent. The
counterpart to the fear about such separation and individuation on any
developmental level is the sense of powerlessness, of utter passivity and
"masochistic" surrender, a state of helpless exposure. This is not simply a
regression to an earlier, normal state of development of supposedly "symbiotic" dependency, but in itself constitutes already a severely pathological
phenomenon and is very much part of that "delusion of omnipotence" rightly
emphasized by Novick and Novick (1991). Because every self-assertion is
looked at as profoundly dangerous, it has to come to a "nothingness" of self-
esteem and to extreme self-contempt.

4. *"Anal" conflicts about control of self and others*, about "autonomy" and
belonging, about "absolute power" (omnipotence), and the dyadic ambivalence conflicts, as well as those about the severe aggressions (rage, revenge,
envy, resentment) connected with those, appear to be particular forms of
these conflicts about *union and separateness*; but the more I study this problem of conflict causality and the hierarchy of such causes, the more I am
convinced that it won't do simply to keep them so subsumed. In patient after
patient the conscious and unconscious conflicts about *control* were inescapable. It was specifically the centrality of the inner and outer struggle for
power that convinced me to see in this a particularly important separate layer
of conflict: the struggle of defiantly asserting one's own control, especially
over one's "inner space" (the interior of body and mind), versus feeling
forced or induced to submit to such control from the outside, and all the
important sharp splits between inside and outside, between good and bad,
pure and dirty that ensue.

As stated already in the context of the globality of affects, I do not believe that these phenomena of *dichotomizing* all experience can simply be
reduced to one basic special mechanism ("splitting" as defense, "fragmentation anxiety" as one specific pathogenically central form of anxiety), but
that they rather represent the result of the *absoluteness* and the *globality*,
not only of the affects, but of the identifications and the introjections, and
with that of the other defense processes, especially the repression and
denial dictated by that global quality of underlying affects and moods.
These phenomena appear to be linked with particular severity of the anal
conflicts.

The main polarity is that of being weak, overwhelmed by feelings ("over-
stimulated"), mutilated, or shame-laden versus the ideal object's being pow-

erful, impenetrable, emotionally impervious, shame-proof, and phallic. Individuality becomes submerged by such rigorous categorizing according to an *axis of power and shame* (cf. my papers on "Nietzsche's war against shame": Wurmser 1990c, 1993, 1997a, 1999a). This *polarization* is prominently represented by anal qualities: messy versus orderly, stubborn withholding and defiant control versus submission and abject yielding. There is what Chasseguet-Smirgel (1991) and Grunberger (1979) describe as the "anal universe," where all boundaries separating genders and generations are being wiped out. *Spite and negativism* and similar "anal" attributes assume an important role in the character; they are derivatives of the original wishes for self-assertion, remnants of the individual's effort to protect himself or herself against total exposure and shameful nothingness, the healthy self-defense of the child.

5. Generally, *oedipal conflicts* are a series of *triangular conflicts* that very importantly also encompass the siblings; that is, not only Oedipus and Electra, but also Cain. As we noticed throughout this book, these various types flow into each other. The crucial importance of such triangular conflicts for all patients with severe neurosis—of competing for the love of one parent (or parental figure) and the wish to eliminate the rival—should not be diminished by the recognition of the other types of conflict. In this context I have not only found the affect of jealousy of great relevance, but also Oedipal envy; it is not correct to see in envy automatically a derivative of "oral" issues.

6. I think it is not an unwarranted generalization to state that throughout life, with the exception of the earliest period, inner conflict always involves the superego, in some or all of its major functions. As mentioned already, experience has shown that many superego aspects emerge long before the later oedipal period, and narcissistic problems and disturbances always centrally involve *superego conflicts*. The *conscience* becomes entirely the executor of the archaic versions of guilt and shame mentioned before and with that manifests itself as *dramatically split.*

The *guilt–shame dilemma* is generally of greatest importance. In a weakened form it is nearly ubiquitous. In the severe neuroses its strongly pronounced version is hardly ever to be missed. More generally, since many of the affects are overwhelming and the needs and wishes seem all-encompassing, the ideals and the quest for values also quickly assume this character of absoluteness. And it is especially this last element—the absoluteness of the ideal, hence the categorical nature of the self-judgment, and with that the extreme version of guilt and of shame—that is being controlled by the masochistic core fantasy (see *Flight from Conscience*). Thus the prominence of "moral masochism" is not merely due to the intersystemic conflict between superego and id, but reflects very centrally *intrasystemic superego conflicts* (Hartmann and Loewenstein 1962, Kris 1983a,b, 1985, 1987, 1988, Rangell 1963a,b).

We now turn to the question of loyalty and loyalty conflicts as intrasystemic superego conflicts (cf. also Böszörmenyi-Nagy 1973), where we have seen that loyalty is more than an ordinary bond; it sets up the other as a beloved authority over oneself, and specifically as an authority toward whom one has to keep faith. It is a kind of superego relationship and superego bond.

Thus it is the loyalty conflict that calls forth all the most intense affects. Basically the *superego-split and the resulting split identity* very often amount to *a sharp, largely unconscious loyalty conflict* that is recreated in new, preconscious, and therapeutically accessible versions, both within and without the transference relationship.

In the light of what has been found, the fascinating question imposes itself: *Is not the entire repetition compulsion, at least in many, an attempt to restore and resolve old loyalty conflicts?* And does this not also determine the nature of analysis or psychotherapy? This is such a new and so daring an assertion that it is certainly not generally valid. But that loyalty conflicts play a much greater role in the transference than commonly assumed—that I am inclined to think. How far is not every analysis already per se experienced as a disloyalty toward the parental home, and dreaded as a self-betrayal, as a breach of the loyalty toward the self? These are new lines of inquiry, which cannot be pursued here but are discussed elsewhere (Wurmser 1989a,c, 1993, 1999b).

All six types of conflict can regularly be encountered in severe and intolerable versions in the patients called "borderline," though with varying intensity. As so often, it is not a matter of an either-or, but of an as-well-as. Preoedipal and oedipal conflicts coexist and are intermeshed, and their relative proportions vary from patient to patient. All generalizations about their relative importance are specious. This is but another way of expressing what Abend et al. (1983) describe as "difficulties during *every phase of psychosexual and ego development*" (p. 207), and their statement that they had to conclude "that it is extremely difficult to separate the effects of preoedipal from oedipal trauma" (pp. 213–214).

Looking at it somewhat differently, we notice, as I have already mentioned, how these six layers are a hierarchy in which the lower levels are again all represented on the higher ones, and vice versa. Yet the sequence is at many places questionable. What is important is the series of conflicts that occur throughout life, but tend to emerge with special poignancy at certain stages of development. There may also be conflict between the different levels of conflict: "deeper" conflicts (e.g., union versus separateness) clash with more "progressive" developmental conflicts (oedipal ones): "A manifest conflict may well defend against a latent conflict" (Josephs 1997, p. 437). This refers not merely to the wishes, but also the forms of defense, the superego aspects and the affects (e.g., the "anal" superego versus the "genital" superego, as so beautifully developed in Lagerkvist's [1944] *Dvärgen*).

Concretely, the triangular (oedipal) conflicts centering around competition encompass now those of power and control, those of merger and separateness, those of exhibition and curiosity, and all the ancient affect storms. The superego conflicts reflect all the other conflicts that presumably emerged earlier, and these in turn, as we see them in the adult, are integrated in those later conflicts. Shame and guilt can be related to all the other five conflicts in very specific ways: shame about losing control over one's (overwhelming) affects or over the sphincters, shame about the exposure of feelings and extending to all self-expression, dependency shame, the shame of seeing oneself excluded from the intimacy of the parents; guilt about separation and the killing implicit in it, guilt about anal defiance and demand for control, guilt for the wish to exclude the rival and to be successful in competition (triumph = killing).

Superego formation and with it the area of loyalty conflicts are closely connected with (though not restricted to) early oedipal conflicts, insofar as they pertain to conflicts leading to the feeling of guilt. This is, however, not true at all as far as the shame side of the superego is concerned; shame develops largely independently from oedipal problems. It is the specific protection mechanism against the dangers in the domain of perceiving and being perceived, of self-expression and fascination (delophilia and theatophilia).

Global identifications, global introjections, and global denials and repressions have more to do with the basic attitudes in the family and the ruling value conflicts there than only with the Oedipus complex.

We could also say that it is certainly possible to subdivide those layers of conflict further; there are principally no limitations to the observation of further conflicts and hence to a finer differentiation of this hierarchy.

I am also uncomfortable about seeing them in a strictly chronological order. Conflicts of isolation versus union (separateness versus belonging) may antedate the specifically designated period, and they surely continue to be a very important issue. Oedipal conflicts in the sense of rivalry of a triangular nature may occur much earlier than the "oedipal phase" after the third year; they may in fact be concomitant with the "individuation and separation" phase, that is, simultaneous with conflicts around separateness. And when does the superego originate? Very strong superego elements are related to those conflicts about separation and about anal control. It appears artificial to assume that the superego as a system follows the end, the resolution, of the Oedipus conflicts.

Experience shows that the work on these unconscious conflicts is most fruitful if it occurs "at the surface," that is, if it begins with the preconscious (derivative) conflicts involving the most intense affects and explores their unconscious antecedents. With that it appears (at least to me, in contrast to many others today) to be not all that important whether one focuses on preconscious conflicts that refer to the current outside reality, to the transference, or to the past. Rather, what counts heavily is that they are "living," that they are experienced with affective intensity. The more broadly such preconscious conflicts can be explored, the more successful the outcome tends to be. Every one-sidedness, such as only focusing upon transference or upon genetic constructions, unduly restricts that breadth and is inimical to the solution of the conflicts. Here again we see the principle of complementarity at work.

I find it most useful to approach inner conflict through the gate of the superego, especially through the intrasystemic superego conflicts outlined before. But it is conceivable that entry could also occur through the other conflicts. However, if the access to one remains consistently blocked (e.g., by the acting out of the superego posture in the countertransference), the work has to remain seriously hampered.

It is really only the whole "concert" of the conflicts in their specific formulations, as recast in those fantasies and eventually manifested in the phenomenological features, that gives us the essential, psychoanalytically treatable *structure of causality*. What is decisive for us is that their fundament, the causality we need to get to, is those *core conflicts*. Their recognition, and the new attempt to resolve them, brings about the effective change, the recognition of their place in the inner chain of causal connection. Outer events, constitution, and biological factors are important causal factors, but they remain outside the domain of psychoanalytic exploration. Analysis deals with them insofar as they are filtered through the conflicts.

Beyond the conflicts we deal with *core affects* of a traumatic or physiologic origin, which often determine the severity of the conflicts we deal with. To what extent archaic affects of a global nature form part of inner conflict, to what extent they precede inner conflict, and to what extent they result from it, as well as the issue of the new dignity of affect theory, quite independent from drive theory—this has been a fascinating topic throughout the case presentations given. It is in fact likely that the patients' fantasies are specifically set up to deal with and to defend against *specific central affects of a pri-*

*mary and global nature*—respectively in regard to those major affects mentioned in the context of the core fantasies: pain, shame, resentment, grief, generalized anxiety, and disgust. This would enlarge the traditional anxiety theory and give a much broader canvas of affect pathology.

Although the transference of superego conflicts and with them of loyalty problems and the resentment connected with them is ubiquitous, it can only be accessible to analysis if its exploitation by use of authority is as much avoided as much as possible. Sometimes, we then encounter the objection that this kind of technique means: "You are acting out together with the patient because you do not confront (interpretatively) directly the aggressive impulses as they show up indirectly within the transference." The answer is that we can uncover those more or less still hidden aggressions better if we do not try to interpret them on the strength of our authority, but if we go out from the origins of these wishes (various threats to the self or suffered harm), from the anxiety about them, and the defense against them. With that we are least judgmental and find a way to deal analytically with the superego transference as part of conflicts, although, it is true, this approach is far more time-consuming. With the opposite method I have usually lost the patients, sooner or later, or the treatment changed into a clear and unanalyzable sadomasochistic relationship and had to be broken off in failure.

At times I noticed this on a smaller scale: When I was impressed by some works representing such a more brashly confrontational style, hints of a similar kind easily started slipping into my own remarks, occasionally with immediately catastrophic consequences for the treatment that could not always be repaired. As stated before, this kind of technique is invaluable for crisis intervention and perhaps also needed in hospitalized patients, especially nowadays where we are faced with the inexorable pressure to discharge patients after a few days. But it is an approach suited for short-term treatment, not for the long-term therapy of severely ill patients.


## "BEING BLINDED BY IMAGES" (*BLENDUNG DURCH BILDER*)

In all these cases it has to be acknowledged that there had been serious, sometimes very intensive psychic traumatization. To deny the reality factor in this, to ignore the trauma, would be tantamount to a confirmation and repetition of the pathogenetically essential basic attitude in the family and would make effective treatment impossible. And yet, here again the complementarity plays a crucial role: the recognition of the outer trauma does not diminish the significance of the inner conflicts, of the single affects, drives, and forms of defense, of the fantasies and part-identities. Inside and outside are equally important and complement each other. The traumata are, as said before, filtered through the lens of the conflicts. They become visible and accessible to therapeutic technique only through them.

The analytic inquiry of causality focuses on the conflicts, especially the inner conflicts. In this it finds its uniqueness and its value. Specificity and uniqueness of method do not mean one-sidedness or even exclusiveness in the understanding of the causes, however. Therefore it has become clear from the study of the genesis and maintenance of neurosis in the individual cases that the psychoanalytic understanding of the more massive pathology can be very much enriched by the parallel investigation of family transactions.

Loyalty conflicts in particular, which I have examined here from an intrapsychic vantage point, play a great role in family research, especially in the school of Böszörmenyi-Nagy (1973), for example with Helm Stierlin in Heidelberg (e.g., 1969, 1974).

The one cannot be reduced to the other, but the intrapsychic dynamic can be far better comprehended against the foil of the family dynamic, and the reverse is equally true. The complementarity of these two approaches— of psychoanalysis and family study (including the interactions between infants and their environment)—is just as promising for the deeper grasp and treatment of psychopathology as its analogon in physics for the mastery of the problems in quantum mechanics.

In this context, I think that the process described by the German analyst Felix Schottländer about forty years ago as "*blinding by images*" (*Blendung durch Bilder*) can be of particular interest precisely with the more severely ill neurotic patients. It refers to the *denial of the individuality of the child by the parents*—the inability to perceive the child's specific needs, wishes and fears, its individuality and autonomy, in favor of certain impersonal categories. I called the same process "soul blindness." The result of this severe pathology of the whole family consists (1) in a superego that evinces in itself a peculiar doubleness and split character; (2) a pervasive use of the defense by denial in the service of one or the other part of the superego, often in a massive and alternating way; (3) episodic breakthroughs in impulsive action precisely of that side of the personality that has fallen victim to that "blinding"; and (4) the feeling and impression of a "split identity."

The experience typical for many patients is just this: "My father and my mother have not seen me at all." "I was treated as invisible." As we have noticed repeatedly, this invisibility as an individual leads both to a radical form of shame about oneself and to that gnawing sense of resentment about the unfairness involved in such disregard for one's individuality. This stifling of self-expression and of its response to it means: "I have no right to my own feelings and thus to my own thoughts, my perceptions, and above all to the decision-making by my own will." If one feels robbed from the outside in this way of one's feelings and drives it is experienced as deep powerlessness, as an intrusion that cannot be fought off. The shame about it means: "I cannot even control my own inner life; what is innermost and most private in me cannot be protected against the intrusiveness of others." In particular it may be the other's feelings that are sensed as a dominant force raising its claims from without. Such shame and the deep resentment about this enforced self-loss and self-betrayal has to lead to wishes for revenge that should wipe out such helplessness—whether in the form of devaluation of and jeering at of the other (the reversal of the shame trauma), the reassertion of some drive wishes that have advanced to being symbols of autonomy (e.g., the power over eating), or in the form of outbursts of spite, rage, or hate. But behind all of those looms the profound anxiety about being passively exposed, losing oneself to the other, and being overrun by the other's affects and acts of will. We saw the equation: passivity = being penetrated = being flooded by affects = sexual intrusion = selfloss.

This blinding by images may be repeated in the present, both actively and passively, and the transference too shows the active blocking out of perception—whether with the help of drugs, by fantasies of idealization, or paranoid distortion. The patient reexperiences that particular family trauma, especially strongly as seen for example with Dilecta (*Flight from Conscience*), who kept accusing me that I could see her only through the lenses of my "little theories" and my "little rituals." Others expressed this more as persistent fear or interpreted every single remark by me as such an absolute, such a categorical condemnation that they wanted to break off our work at once.

More typically it remains the idealization of my person—which is of course one form of the "blinding by images." It repeats the family myths and goes along with the denial that has to facilitate the repression of massive rage and contempt and of the feelings of neediness. Such idealization is a superego transference that serves defensive needs and has, sooner or later, to be analyzed—tactfully, at the proper time, and yet not delayed too long, although I do not claim that I have always succeeded in analytically working it through at the right time.

## INNER CONFLICT AS THE MOST SPECIFIC FOCUS OF PSYCHOANALYTIC WORK AND THE DIALECTIC ABOUT INNER AND OUTER AUTHORITY

人 能 弘 道
非 道 弘 人

(Rén néng hóng dào, fei dào hóng rén)
Man can make the principles great; the principles cannot make man great.
—Confucius, Lun Yü, XV, 28

I have mentioned before that the question about the nature of the repetition compulsion inevitably changes to a problem that in the essential sense is metapsychological, even if we cannot agree anymore with the metapsychological program of Freud, Hartmann, or Rapaport. The problem of repetition compulsion reaches beyond what is psychological and points towards the encompassing worldview underlying the theories and determining them—hence willy nilly to something metaphysical. For even the scientific worldview adduced by Freud has presuppositions that are unprovable and are in the nature of faith; namely, that the logical categories are known and valid everywhere, that we know them fully and can use them to advantage for the insight into the phenomena, and that every claim for truth has to measure itself on these given criteria.

Furthermore, the exploration of what is singular is only then feasible when we have a model, a design, of the whole, and this design, or *Entwurf*, decides after all always again how we interpret the connections of the details—according to Gadamer's (1975) "hermeneutic circle," but now referring to the wholeness of everything scientific. These questions are studied in great detail in *Broken Reality* (Wurmser 1989a) and answered with the help of the experience here given, as far as it is possible to answer them.

In the same context I referred earlier to the significance of distinguishing description from explanation. Most of our theories entail a subtle shift from the claim of describing to that of explaining. It is then often overlooked that most of the theoretical concepts and considerations help surprisingly little in the understanding of the severe cases; their value may lie in describing, but they fail in their power to explain. However, if something is ineffective or insufficiently effective in certain illnesses it means that the causal explanations are not fitting, that it may not be sufficient in order to be transferable with sufficient clarity to the individual case and practically applicable, and that at least something is missing its completeness. The experiences with the illnesses presented here show that the habitual analytic explanations do not suffice. Where is the break? Or the gap?

Where these lacks become painfully conscious—with the therapeutic failure of the method—suggestion often has to leap into the breach, *using the superego transference* for the purpose of therapeutic alteration, instead of its analysis. Authority is being employed in the hope of using what Ferenczi called "*superego intropression*" (I owe the reference to Professor W. Loch) in order to effect the desired inner change where insight has fallen short.

This makes it necessary that the theoretical understanding of the dynamics as well as the theory of technique should systematically examine these questions—that is, the very major technical conflict between advancement of self-observation and suggestion (Busch 1997, cf. Gray 1994), and with that the questions of how far the technique itself may vitiate what we presume to be objective inner truth (Friedman 1997), and how far the theories are circular and self-confirming.

As repeatedly mentioned, I consider the traditional metapsychology, if taken as a scientific foundation, to be largely mistaken. Still, in contrast to many of its critics, I do not see in these models completely wrongheaded efforts (*Ansätze*) but more or less useful *auxiliary constructions of a metaphorical character*. Most of all, I assign, especially in treatment, much greater significance to the model of *intrapsychic conflict* (the dynamic theory) than many authors nowadays do (cf. e.g., Lichtenberg et al. 1996). Indeed, *inner conflict is* moment by moment *the one and most specific focus of all my psychoanalytic work*. More generally, I still see *inner* processes as having at least equal rights, and being just as worthy of careful study as the *interactional* ones. In particular it seems to me that the great merit of psychoanalysis has been to defend the autonomy and independent dignity of the inner world vis-à-vis all outside relationships and to have opened it to systematic exploration. The essential *standing-in-relation* of the human being does not preclude an equally essential *being-for-itself*. This fundamental dialectic can be traced, interestingly enough, not just in the philosophy of the Occident but of China as well (Fung Yu-lan).

Certainly, there is a steady back-and-forth between inner and outer conflict. Still, both are *complementary*; both have to be continually kept in mind, as dialectic interchange.

One of the main technical preconditions of my work as an analyst is, as I have stressed throughout, the joint, detailed observation of the patient's "inner authority": the efficacy of the superego and of its variegated aspects, as well as the exact study of the defensive processes within and outside of the transference. It succeeds to the extent that we renounce upon falling ourselves into the transference role of authority. It can never be entirely avoided, to be sure, but "as much as possible" is mostly already good enough.

Elazar says: "I don't know where my boundaries are!" The global quality of the anxieties and of the other "big feelings" means: not to have boundaries! It is essential then that also the superego does not know any boundaries. But what does that mean, not to have any boundaries? It means: to wish for total merger with an ideal figure. It means that the demands on oneself are boundless and without measure. And it means that the feelings and wants ever so often threaten to become overwhelming, to burst the ties of societal norms, to disregard the limitations of nature, and to circumvent the dictates of reason, slyly and with guile.

The more severe the neurosis, the more difficult it is to avoid the attitude of suggestive authority. As we have noticed, at times it is imperative to use interventions that have a superego meaning and lead to that "internalization of authority" that is avoided during optimal analytic proceeding. This raises many hard questions.

What influence upon transference and upon its analysis do recommendations for the choice of profession or for auxiliary therapeutic methods, like behavioral therapy, the prescription of an antidepressant, or the direct giving of Antabuse really have? All this can of course not be indifferent, and yet I was surprised that these interventions actually interfered relatively little with the analytic process. Perhaps part of the answer may lie in the fact that even in these instances I never play myself up as an authority, but explicitly come to an agreement with the ego of the patient: "We see that our approach up to now has not sufficed to help you with your intentions and plans or to prevent the overrunning by that demonic force within. What would you suggest as additional support?" In such and similar ways I believe that I submit the problem of self-control and affect and drive regulation to our common deliberation. This does not seem to me to deviate from the spirit of good analytic technique. My giving of Naltrexone (a narcotics antagonist) or of Antabuse, when agreed upon in the way just sketched, is then part of the routine, principally not so different from the arrangements about payment or punctuality.

Still, this does not fully solve the problem. The choice of such interventions has to be made in the clear consciousness of the dilemma. These two contradictory requirements of technique—*enhancement of insight versus the role as protective authority, that is, the dialectic about authority*—represent a technical conflict that cannot be solved once and for all. With both, however, the purpose ought to be the strengthening of the *rational alliance with the ego* of the patient, which in the continuation permits the gradual diminution of the inner conflicts. Lastly, probably both mutative factors, *insight and authority*, stand in a relation of *complementarity* to each other, not in a necessary conflict.

The reconceptualization that I have given in the theoretical part of this chapter gives a new understanding of the pathology specific to severe neuroses. It is compatible with the classical theory of neuroses (e.g., that of Freud himself, of Anna Freud, and of Fenichel) and with modern infant research, though at variance with the current theory of borderline and narcissistic pathology.

The practical consequences that result from the collected experiences in the treatment of the severe neuroses and lead mostly beyond what has been presented in Chapter 2 can now be summarized as follows:

1. Aggressive wishes and feelings are not treated primarily by confrontation nor direct drive interpretations, but by defense and superego analysis; the main access is sought from the side of the anxiety. Moreover, they are not understood as primary, but as expressions of deep threats to the self-esteem and the intactness of the person (Mitchell 1993, cf. Thomä and Kächele 1985, Wurmser 1981).

2. An essential focus is on the specific range of affects, especially those of anxiety and depression, and the defenses employed dealing with them.

3. There is no assumption of a "superego defect" or a "superego lacuna," nor is there an a priori assumption of visible, deep ego-defects, except for the intolerance toward certain specific affects (as disturbances in the form of affect regulation); only at the end of thorough conflict analysis is it possible to pinpoint ego defects.

4. There is continued emphasis on and deepened exploration of inner conflicts. It should not be given up in favor of alternate forms of intervention; these are at best "in addition, not instead."

5. Great care is being given not to assume much of a real superego role, but rather, as far as this is possible, to analyze the externalized or projected superego functions, as they are manifested in the transference. There exists however a dialectical relationship, since the recommendations of ancillary measures let the analyst occasionally appear as a protective superego figure in reality. Moreover the sympathetic, nonjudgmental listening is itself a powerful form of "corrective emotional experience," in Anna Freud's (1974b) words: ". . . today we observe that transference is sometimes useful as a 'corrective emotional experience'" (p. 46). In this it cannot fail to have

a direct impact upon the superego experience of the patient (Strachey 1934). Still it is preferrable to analyze, as far is possible, the externalized and projected superego functions, especially where they manifest themselves in the transference. The *superego transference* seems to me to be altogether of special and often overlooked importance.

6. Much importance is given to a rational alliance and hence to a therapeutic atmosphere of kindness and tact, which facilitates such an alliance; it requires great flexibility in the responses to the necessities of each moment (cf. Thomä and Kächele 1985).

7. In most cases, auxiliary measures are needed because of the severity of affect intolerance and flooding, and hence the severity of conflict and superego pressure. Almost without exception the severe neuroses require a treatment strategy combining several modalities simultaneously. Drugs (medicinal as well as illegal) appear to serve predominantly such affect regulation; addiction is by and large a form of self-treatment that fails in the long run.

While psychoanalysis concentrates upon the work on the conflicts—as its central focus, its main task, and its main methodological legitimation—it is often imperative to involve other treatment modalities for the regulation of those overwhelming affects. External structures and chemical substances offer themselves as such auxiliary regulators. Our function as therapists consists in integrating in our therapeutic strategy the conflict-centered with the auxiliary treatment, that is, the vertical with the horizontal approach. This should happen in such ways and forms that we are able to assist our patients in solving their neurotic core conflicts in a space that is as much protected against intolerable terror and despair as is possible.

For good analytic work it is necessary that most of these auxiliary methods are taken over by other therapists. The combination of several modalities in the same treatment compromises the transference analysis too much.

## CAUSALITY: CONFLICT AND COMPLEMENTARITY

I started out this book with general questions, some explicit, some implicit: Narrative or historic truth? Hermeneutics or causal explanation? Reconstruction or transference interpretation? External reality or internal conflict solution? Conflict or deficit? Self or object relations? Analysis or synthesis? Drive or reason? Intrapsychic or interpersonal?

I think all these are dichotomies, either-or positions; they fail to do justice to the enormous complexity of the human soul and hence the equally enormous complexity of our work as psychotherapists and analysts. Obviously both parts of the dilemmas are important. Only the judicious weighing, moment by moment, of their respective importance, the constant awareness of their *complementarity*, can be commensurate with our task of understanding and helping.

In what I have presented I was guided by such a complementary vision. I have shown specific and concrete forms of what Freud called *reconstruction*—the putting together of systems of motivations that can most parsimoniously explain the problems that brought these patients into treatment. Such reconstructions may be focused on supposed, though not clearly recoverable recollections of events, traumas, or experiences from early childhood—*historical truth*; on the defensive processes of how the ego dealt with some drive urges, like jealousy, revenge, or sexual wishes—an *ego psychological construction*; or on the plausible story, synthetically woven out of the problems encountered and giving them an acceptable, coherent meaning—*narrative truth*. I proposed a meaning of reconstruction implicit in Freud's concept that encompasses and transcends these: a systematic study of the *causality specific for the psychoanalytic method*. With that I meant to give a coherent picture of *core phenomena, core fantasies, core conflicts, and core affects, engendered by some delimited or chronic traumatizations*. The central, most specific factor among these five, the one most usefully approached by this specific method of psychoanalysis, is the third: the core conflicts. They are in the center of our vision; the others move to the periphery without their becoming irrelevant.

Behind the four layers of psychopathology described—*core phenomena, core fantasies, central conflicts, and main affects*—there looms like a monster, in every case of severe neurosis, the fatal power of *trauma*. It is as if the brutality of the trauma were living on in the cruelty of the conscience—like the devastating dragon of mythical "*Urzeit*" in his cave: that the trauma lives on in the severity and pitiless character of the conscience. Of course, analytically we know that it is just as much the patient's own aggression, mobilized by the massive helplessness, as the "aggression" perceived as coming from the outside, from "fate" and uncomprehending, unliving, shaming others, that have become invested in the superego. But the metaphor of that outer cruelty living on like a dragon in the draconic conscience (the demonic "inner judge"), that sadistic version of conscience a patient called "the borrowed monster" (*den geborgten Unhold*), severe and pitiless, has proven quite helpful in the analysis of such severe forms of masochism.

What I have presented is a *reconstruction of causality*, understood as giving an account of this path from description to explanation.

Conflict is never fully solvable. What we may reach however is a shift from the feeling of inner compulsion to that of inner freedom. This shift is due to the broadened and deepened access to inner conflict, and especially to that tragic "*Wissen um das Gewissen*"—the knowledge about conscience—that Nietzsche (1878–1880) refers to when he cites Byron: "Sorrow is knowledge; they who know the most / Must mourn the deepest o'er the fatal truth, / The tree of knowledge is not that of life" (I, III, 109, p. 100).

## CHANGE AND CONTINUITY

But it is nothing yet if one only *knows* these things; the essential step consists in *making them real.*

—Louis-Claude de St. Martin[4]

It always turns out after all that the soul is so much richer than can be shown by all the conceptual frameworks. Our increasing experience just with the hard and hardest cases induces us to resort to other, new ordering systems as valuable and useful; they themselves consist of encompassing, more general, and supra-individually valid metaphors. Usually, they enter additionally, not in place of the old systems, although these themselves may sometimes require certain modifications. Yet it is these encompassing metaphors that stand with those of poetry and the philosophy of culture in a relation of themes and variations.

Only what works and is fruitful is true—Goethe's "*Was fruchtbar ist, allein ist wahr.*" This is also valid for psychoanalysis. New demands bring new insights, but also new temptations. But only in this is its inner strength, its mettle, tested. Whether it shows itself up to these challenges and capable of growing on them or whether it withdraws into a bastion of faith and ritual, will determine its future as science and as an acceptable treatment form.

Yet, the new experiences mean also that suddenly the questions of value and truth of our individual life and of the cultures among and between which we move show up anew and in a blinding light of strangeness. In the testing of these new insights, psychoanalysis will be a discrete, but not a wordless companion. It holds up a mirror where we often see ourselves and our cultures in a distorted shape because this mirror unveils the hidden fissures in reality. Yet, the mirror itself also has cracks—because it lies in the nature of the soul that such rents occur. And the science of the psychic illnesses and their treatment cannot itself escape from the fractures of the time in which it finds itself, nor from the breaks in the nature of what is scientific, nor in the scientific method itself in which it partakes.

The breaks in our identity and the compulsion to repeat are finally nothing else but expressions of the encompassing dialectic of change and continuity. "Transformation is the life of life; it is the very mystery of creative nature; standing firm is freezing and death. Who wants to live must get beyond himself, has to transform himself; he has to forget. And yet all human dignity is tied to standing firm, to not-forgetting, to fidelity."[5]

Beyond knowing about the conflicts there lies therefore the understanding of their deep complementarity. And this complementarity of opposite truths that push toward reconciliation and yet never quite achieve it is reflected in the conflicts of the neuroses. The compulsion to repeat and the fractures in the inner life of every individual are attempts to reach beyond those conflicts to the great life-immanent complementarities, yet to keep failing in this endeavor. Is it hubris, if the art, the know-how (techne— τέχνη) refuses to capitulate in the face of this compulsion?

What we can hope as analysts is for the decrease of the compulsiveness and the increase of inner freedom, the reduction of the splitting and the growth of inner unity. But this too is only a more or less, not either-or. Compulsion and freedom are the complementary conditions of our destiny. "Like the whole in which we are contained, our life is in an incomprehensible way composed of freedom and necessity."[6]

At issue is the surmounting of absoluteness.

## ENDNOTES

1. Jacob's soul was thoughtfully and gravely solemn in the days when he, together with his brother, buried his father, because all the stories rose up in front of him and became present in his mind, as they had become again present in the flesh, after the stamped original image [archetype]; and it seemed to him as if he were walking on transparent ground which consisted of infinitely many crystal layers leading down into the unfathomable depth and was illuminated by lamps burning between those layers. (*Joseph and His Brothers*, p. 188).

2. In Kubie's (1958) succinct formulation: ". . . the behavior which results from a preponderance of conscious processes is . . . flexible, adaptable, satiable, capable of learning from experience, admonition, exhortation, and instruction; whereas at the other end of this same spectrum, where the identical act may be produced by a constellation of processes among which unconscious processes predominate, the resultant behavior will be rigid, stereotyped, and insatiable, unmodifiable by the experience of success or failure, by rewards and punishments, by admonition

or exhortation. Evidently at one end we have the essence of normal behavior; and at the other, the essence of sick behavior" (p. 29).

3. The biological baggage connected with this English term, lacking in the German *Trieb*, lets me express my reservations by quotation marks.

4. (*Aber es ist noch nichts, wenn man diese Dinge nur* weiß; *das Wesentliche ist, sie zu* verwirklichen) (Louis-Claude de St. Martin, quoted by G. K. Kaltenbrunner, *Neue Zürcher Zeitung*, February 8/9, 1986, p. 37.)

5. (*Verwandlung ist Leben des Lebens, ist das eigentliche Mysterium der schöpfenden Natur; Beharren ist Erstarren und Tod. Wer leben will, der muß über sich selbst hinwegkommen, muß sich verwandeln: er muß vergessen. Und dennoch ist ans Beharren, ans Nichtvergessen, an die Treue alle menschliche Würde geknüpft.*) (Hugo von Hofmannsthal [letter], quoted in M. Stern [1986], p. 269.)

6. (*Unser Leben ist, wie das Ganze, in dem wir enthalten sind, auf eine unbegreifliche Weise aus Freiheit und Notwendigkeit zusammengesetzt.*) (Goethe)

# References

Abelin, E. L. (1975). Some further observations and comments on the earliest role of the father. *International Journal of Psycho-Analysis* 56:293–302.

Abend, S. M., Porder, M. S., and Willick, M. S. (1983). *Borderline Patients: Psychoanalytic Perspectives.* New York: International Universities Press.

Adler, A. (1908). Der Aggressionstrtieb im Leben und in der Neurose. In: Fortschritte der Medizin.

Aeschylus. *Aeschyli septem quae supersunt tragoediae.* Recensuit Gilbertus Murray. Oxford, England: Oxford University Press, 1955.

Andreas-Salomé, L. (1921). Narzißmus als Doppelrichtung. In *Das 'zweideutige' Lächeln der Erotik: Psychoanalytic texts of Lou Andreas-Salomé,* ed. I. Weber and B. Rempp, pp. 191–222. Freiburg, Germany: Kore, 1990.

Aristotle. *Nicomachean ethics. I.iii.* Loeb edition, trans. H. Rackham. Cambridge, MA: Harvard University Press, 1926/1968.

Arlow, J. A. (1969a). Unconscious fantasy and disturbances of conscious experience. *Psychoanalytic Quarterly* 38:1–27.

——— (1969b). Fantasy, memory and reality testing. *Psychoanalytic Quarterly* 38:28–51.

——— (1972). The only child. *Psychoanalytic Quarterly* 41:507–536.

——— (1979). The genesis of interpretation. *Journal of the American Psychoanalytic Association* 27 (Suppl.):93–206.

Arlow, J. A., and Brenner, C. (1964): *Psychoanalytic Concepts and the Structural Theory.* New York: International Universities Press.

Asch, S. S. (1988). The analytic concepts of masochism: a reevaluation. In *Masochism: Current Psychoanalytic Perspectives,* ed. R. A. Glick and D. I. Meyers, pp. 93–116. Hillsdale, NJ: Analytic Press.

Bach, S. (1991). On sadomasochistic object relations. In *Perversions and Near-Perversions in Clinical Practice. New Psychoanalytic Perspectives,* ed. G. I. Fogel and W. A. Myers. pp. 75–92. New Haven, CT: Yale University Press.

Bak, R. C. (1968). The phallic woman. *Psychoanalytic Study of the Child* 23:37–46. New York: International Universities Press.

Balint, M. (1968). *The Basic Fault: Therapeutic Aspects of Regression.* London: Tavistock.

Balzac, H. de. *La Comédie Humaine. Vol. 7. La cousine Bette. Bibliothèque de la Pléiade.* Paris: Gallimard, 1977.

Barth, B. (1990). Die Darstellung der weiblichen Sexualität als Ausdruck männlichen Uterusneides und dessen Abwehr. *Jahrbuch der Psychoanalyse* 26:64–101.

Basch, M. F. (1974). Interference with perceptual transformation in the service of defense. *Annual of Psychoanalysis* 2:87–97.

——— (1983): The perception of reality and the disavowal of meaning. *Annual of Psychoanalysis* 11:125–154.

Bass, E., and Davis, L. (n.d.). *The Courage to Heal: A Guide for Women Survivors of Child Sexual Abuse.* New York: Harper Perennial.

Beebe, B., and Sloate, P. (1982). Assessment and treatment of difficulties in mother–infant attunement in the first three years of life. *Psychoanalytic Inquiry* 1:601–623.

Beres, D. (1965). Structure and function in psycho-analysis. *International Journal of Psycho-Analysis* 46:53–63.

——— (1974). *Character pathology and the "borderline" syndrome.* Unpublished manuscript.

Berlin, I. (1996). *The Sense of Reality.* New York: Farrar, Straus, & Giroux.

Berliner, B. (1940). Libido and reality in masochism. *Psychoanalytic Quarterly* 9:322–333.

——— (1947). On some psychodynamics of masochism. *Psychoanalytic Quarterly* 16:459–471.

Bibring, E. (1954). Psychoanalysis and the dynamic psychotherapies. *Journal of the American Psychoanalytic Association* 2:745–770.

Blos, P., Jr. (1991). Sadomasochism and the defense against recall of painful affect. *Journal of the American Psychoanalytic Association* 39:417–430.

Blum, H. P. (1976). Masochism, the ego ideal, and the psychology of women. *Journal of the American Psychoanalytic Association* 24 (Suppl.):157–192.

——— (1991). Sadomasochism in the psychoanalytic process, within and beyond the pleasure principle: discussion. *Journal of the American Psychoanalytic Association* 39:431–450.

Boesky, D. (1982). Acting out: a Reconsideration of the Concept. *International Journal of Psycho-Analysis* 63:39–56.

Böszörmenyi-Nagy, I., and Framo, J. L. (1965). *Intensive Family Therapy: Theoretical and Practical Aspects.* New York: Harper & Row.

Böszörmenyi-Nagy, I., and Spark, G. M. (1973). *Invisible Loyalties.* New York: Harper & Row.

Brenner, C. (1959). The masochistic character: genesis and treatment. *Journal of the American Psychoanalytic Association* 7:197–226.

——— (1976). *Psychoanalytic Technique and Psychic Conflict.* New York: International Universities Press.

——— (1982). *The Mind in Conflict.* New York: International Universities Press.

Breuer, J., and Freud, S. (1893–1895). Studies on hysteria. *Standard Edition* 2.

Brodey, W. (1965). On the dynamics of narcissism: I. Externalization and early ego development. *Psychoanalytic Study of the Child* 20:165–193. New York: International Universities Press.

Brody, S. (1982). Psychoanalytic theories of infant development and its disturbances: a critical evaluation. *Psychoanalytic Quarterly* 51:526–597.

Brouček, F. (1982). Shame and its relationship to early narcissistic developments. *International Journal of Psycho-Analysis* 65:369–378.

——— (1991). *Shame and the Self.* New York: Guilford.

Bulka, R. B. (1980). *Chapters of the Sages. A Psychological Commentary on Pirqey Avoth.* Northvale, NJ: Jason Aronson, 1993.

Busch, F. (1997). The patient's use of free association. *Journal of the American Psychoanalytic Association* 45:407–424.

Calef, V., and Weinshel, E. M. (1979). The new psychoanalysis and psychoanalytic revisionism. (Book review essay on Kernberg's *Borderline Conditions and Pathological Narcissism.*) *Psychoanalytic Quarterly* 48:470–491.

Cancrini, A. (1970). *Syneidesis. Il tema semantico della 'con-scientia' nella Grecia antica.* Rome: Edizioni dell'Ateneo.

Cassirer, E. (1923a, 1923b, 1929). *Philosophie der symbolischen Formen, Vols. I, II, III.* Darmstadt, Germany: Wissenschaftliche Buchgesellschaft, 1956 (Vol. I) and 1958 (Vols. II and III).

——— (1944). *An Essay on Man.* New Haven: Yale University Press, 1962.

Caws, P. (1986). The scaffolding of psychoanalysis. *Behavioral and Brain Sciences* 9:229–230.

Chasseguet-Smirgel, J. (1988a). A woman's attempt at a perverse solution and its failure. *International Journal of Psycho-Analysis* 69:149–161.

——— (1988b). From the archaic matrix of the Oedipus complex to the fully developed Oedipus complex. *Psychoanalytic Quarterly* 57:505–527.

——— (1991). Sadomasochism in the perversions; some thoughts on the destruction of reality. *Journal of the American Psychoanalytic Association* 39:399–415.

Class, M. (1964). *Gewissensregungen in der griechischen Tragödie.* Hildesheim, Germany (cit. by Cancrini; no publisher given).

Coen, S. J. (1981). Sexualization as a predominant mode of defense. *Journal of the American Psychoanalytic Association* 29:893–920.

——— (1985). Perversion as a solution to intrapsychic conflict. *Journal of the American Psychoanalytic Association* 33 (Suppl.):17–57.

——— (1988). Sadomasochistic excitement: character disorder and perversion. In *Masochism: Current Psychoanalytic Perspectives,* ed. R. A. Glick and D. I. Meyers, pp. 43–60. Hillsdale, NJ: Analytic Press.

Conrad, J. (1911). *Under Western Eyes.* London: Penguin, 1989.

Cooper, A. M. (1988). The narcissistic-masochistic character. In *Masochism: Current Psychoanalytic Perspectives,* ed. R. A. Glick and D. I. Meyers, pp. 117–139. Hillsdale, NJ: Analytic Press.

——— (1991). The unconscious core of perversion. In *Perversions and Near-Perversions in Clinical Practice: New Psychoanalytic Perspectives,* ed. G. I. Fogel and W. A. Myers, pp. 17–35. New Haven, CT: Yale University Press.

Cremerius, J. (1984). *Vom Handwerk des Psychoanalytikers: Das Werkzeug der psychoanalytischen Technik.* 2 vols. Stuttgart/Cannstadt, Germany: Frommann-Holzboog.

Crews, F. (1993). The unknown Freud. *New York Review of Books* 40(19):55–66.

——— (1994a). The revenge of the repressed, I. *New York Review of Books* 41(19):54–60.

———— (1994b). The revenge of the repressed, II. *New York Review of Books* 41(20): 49–58.

Dickens, C. (1846–48). *Dombey and Son*. New York: New American Library, 1964.

Dickes, R. (1974). The concept of borderline states: an alternative proposal. *International Journal of Psychoanalytic Psychotherapy* 3:1–27.

Edelson, M. (1984). *Hypothesis and Evidence in Psychoanalysis*. Chicago: University of Chicago Press.

———— (1985). The hermeneutic turn and the single case study in psychoanalysis. *Psychoanalysis and Contemporary Thought* 8:567–614.

Eickhoff, F.-W. (1986a). Identification and its vicissitudes in the context of the Nazi phenomenon. *International Journal of Psycho-Analysis* 67:33–44.

———— (1986b). Über das 'entlehnte unbewußte Schuldgefühl' als transgenerationellen Übermittler mißglückter Trauer. *Sigmund Freud House Bulletin* 10:14–20, Vienna.

Einstein, A. (1918). Motiv des Forschens. In *Zu Max Plancks 60. Geburtstag*. Müller, Karlsruhe (ref. in Holton 1973).

Eissler, K. R. (1958). Remarks on some variations in psychoanalytic technique. *International Journal of Psycho-Analysis* 39:222–229.

———— (1959). On isolation. *Psychoanalytic Study of the Child* 14:29–60. New York: International Universities Press.

Eliot, G. (1859). *Adam Bede*. New York: Penguin/Signet Classic, 1981.

———— (1862/3). *Romola*. Oxford, England: Oxford University Press, 1994.

———— (1871–1872). *Middlemarch*. New York: Signet Classic, New American Library, 1964.

———— (1876). *Daniel Deronda*. London: Penguin, 1982.

Emde, R. N. (1983). The prerepresentational self and its affective core. *Psychoanalytic Study of the Child* 38:165–192. New Haven, CT: Yale University Press.

Erard, R. E. (1983). New wine in old skins: a reappraisal of the concept "acting out." *International Review of Psycho-Analysis* 10:63–74.

Erikson, E. H. (1946). Ego development and historical change. *Psychoanalytic Study of the Child* 2:359–396. New York: International Universities Press.

Euripides. Quoted from Greek text of Loeb edition; trans. A. S. Way. Cambridge, MA: Harvard University Press, 1912.

Fenichel, O. (1941). Problems of psychoanalytic technique, trans. D. Brunswick. New York: *Psychoanalytic Quarterly*.

———— (1944). Remarks on the common phobias. In *Collected Papers, Vol II*, ed. Hanna Fenichel, pp. 278–287. New York: Norton, 1954.

———— (1945). *Psychoanalytic Theory of Neurosis*. New York: Norton.

Ferenczi, S. (1932). Sprachverwirrung zwischen den Erwachsenen und dem Kind (Die Sprache der Zärtlichkeit und der Leidenschaft). In *Bausteine zur Psychoanalyse*, ed. Vilma Kovács, pp. 511–525. Bern, Switzerland: Hans Huber, 1939.

Fingarette, H. (1969). *Self-Deception*. London: Routledge & Kegan Paul.

———— (1988). *Heavy Drinking. The Myth of Alcoholism as a Disease*. Berkeley, CA: University of California Press.

Fliess, R. (1956). *Erogeneity and Libido*. New York: International Universities Press.

Fraiberg, S. (1982). Pathological defenses in infancy. *Psychoanalytic Quarterly* 51: 612–635.

Freud, A. (1936). *The Writings of Anna Freud, Vol 2: The Ego and the Mechanisms of Defense.* New York: International Universities Press, 1971.

———— (1965). *The Writings of Anna Freud, Vol 6: Normality and Pathology in Childhood—Assessments of Development.* New York: International Universities Press.

———— (1974a). A psychoanalytic view of developmental psychopathology (Panel discussion, 1954). *Journal of the Philadelphia Association for Psychoanalysis* 1:7–17.

———— (1974b). The ego and the mechanisms of defense: a review. (Panel discussion, 1954). *Journal of the Philadelphia Association for Psychoanalysis* 1: 35–53.

———— (1974c). Problems of technique in adult analysis. *Journal of the Philadelphia Association for Psychoanalysis* 1:68–98.

Freud, S. (1892–1893). A case of successful treatment by hypnotism, with some remarks on the origin of hysterical symptoms through "counterwill." *Standard Edition* 1:115–128.

———— (1894). The neuro-psychoses of defence. *Standard Edition* 3:41–61.

———— (1896). The aetiology of hysteria. *Standard Edition* 3:189–224.

———— (1898). Sexuality in the aetiology of the neuroses. *Standard Edition* 3:259–285.

———— (1900). The interpretation of dreams. *Standard Edition* 4/5.

———— (1905). On psychotherapy. *Standard Edition* 7:255–268.

———— (1909). Analysis of a phobia in a five-year-old boy. *Standard Edition* 10:3–149.

———— (1910a). The psychology of love, I: a special type of object choice. *Standard Edition* 11:165–175.

———— (1910b). The psychology of love, II: on the universal tendency to debasement in the sphere of love. *Standard Edition* 11:179–190.

———— (1912). The dynamics of transference. *Standard Edition* 12:97–108.

———— (1913). Totem and taboo. *Standard Edition* 13:1–164.

———— (1914a). Remembering, repeating and working through. *Standard Edition* 12:145–156.

———— (1914b). On narcissism: an introduction. *Standard Edition* 14:69–102.

———— (1915). Instincts and their vicissitudes. *Standard Edition* 14:109–140.

———— (1916/7). Introductory lectures on psychoanalysis. *Standard Edition* 15/16.

———— (1918). Lines of advance in psycho-analytic therapy. *Standard Edition* 17:157–168.

———— (1919a). A child is being beaten. *Standard Edition* 17:175–204.

———— (1919b). The "uncanny." *Standard Edition* 17:217–256.

———— (1920). Beyond the pleasure principle. *Standard Edition* 18:3–64.

———— (1923). The ego and the id. *Standard Edition* 19:3–66.

———— (1924a). The dissolution of the Oedipus complex. *Standard Edition* 19:173–179.

———— (1924b). Neurosis and psychosis. *Standard Edition* 19:149–153.

———— (1924c). The economic problem of masochism. *Standard Edition* 19:157–170.

———— (1925). Negation. *Standard Edition* 19:235–242.

———— (1926). Inhibitions, symptoms, and anxiety. *Standard Edition* 20:77–175.

———— (1927). Fetishism. *Standard Edition* 21:147–157.

—— (1930). Civilization and its discontents. *Standard Edition* 21:57–145.

—— (1936). A disturbance of memory on the Acropolis. *Standard Edition* 22:237–248.

—— (1937). Analysis terminable and interminable. *Standard Edition* 23:209–254.

—— (1939). Moses and monotheism. *Standard Edition* 23:3–137.

—— (1940a). Splitting of the ego in the process of defence. *Standard Edition* 23:271–278.

—— (1940b). An outline of psychoanalysis. *Standard Edition* 23:141–207.

Friedman, L. (1985). Toward a comprehensive theory of treatment. *Psychoanalytic Inquiry* 5:589–599.

—— (1997). "Ferrum, ignis, and medicina: return to the crucible." *Journal of the American Psychoanalytic Association* 45:21–36.

Fromm, E. (1941). *Die Furcht vor der Freiheit. Vol. 1: Gesamtausgabe dtv*, ed. R. Funk, pp. 217–394. Munich: Deutscher Taschenbuch Verlag.

Gadamer, H.-G. (1975). *Wahrheit und Methode*. Tübingen, Germany: Mohr.

Gaensbauer, T. J. (1985). The relevance of infant research for psychoanalysis. *Psychoanalytic Inquiry* 5:517–530.

Galenson, E. (1986). Some thoughts about infant psychopathology and aggressive developments. *International Review of Psycho-Analysis* 13:349–354.

v. Gebsattel, V. E. (1954). *Prolegomena einer medizinischen Anthropologie*. Berlin: Springer.

Gedö, J. (1977). Notes on the psychoanalytic management of archaic transferences. *Journal of the American Psychoanalytic Association* 25:787–804.

—— (1979). *Beyond Interpretation*. New York: International Universities Press.

—— (1984). *Psychoanalysis and its Discontents*. New York: Guilford.

—— (1986). *Conceptual Issues in Psychoanalysis*. Hillsdale, NJ: Analytic Press.

—— (1988). Masochism and the repetition compulsion. *Masochism: Current Psychoanalytic Perspectives*, ed. R. A. Glick and D. I. Meyers, pp. 139–150. Hillsdale, NJ: Analytic Press.

Gill, M. M. (1976). Metapsychology is not psychology. In *Psychology versus Metapsychology. Psychoanalytic Essays in Memory of George S. Klein*, ed. M. M. Gill and P. S. Holzman, pp. 71–105. New York: International Universities Press.

—— (1991). Indirect suggestion. In *Interpretation and Interaction. Psychoanalysis or Psychotherapy*, ed J. D. Oremland, pp. 137–164. Hillsdale, NJ: Analytic Press.

—— (1994a). *Psychoanalysis in Transition*. Hillsdale, NJ: Analytic Press.

—— (1994b). Conflict and deficit: book review essay on "Conflict and Compromise. Therapeutic Implications." *Psychoanalytic Quarterly* 63:756–778.

—— (1996). Discussion. Interaction III. *Psychoanalytic Inquiry* 16(1):118–134.

Glenn, J. (1984). Psychic trauma and masochism. *Journal of the American Psychoanalytic Association* 32:357–386.

Goethe, J. W. v. (n.d.) *Dtv Gesamtausgabe*. Munich: Deutscher Taschenbuch Verlag, 1961.

Gottlieb, R. (1997). Does the mind fall apart in MPD? *Journal of the American Psychoanalytic Association* 45(3):907–932.

Grassi, E. (1979) *Die Macht der Phantasie*. Königstein, Germany: Syndikat/Athenäum.

—— (n.d.) Das heimatliche Unheimliche. In *Weimar am Pazifik*, ed. D. Borchmeyer and T. Heimeran. Tübingen, Germany: Niemeyer.

Gray, P. (1973). Psychoanalytic technique and the ego's capacity for viewing intra-psychic activity. *Journal of the American Psychoanalytic Association* 21:474–494.

—— (1982). "Developmental lag" in the evolution of technique for psychoanalysis of neurotic conflict. *Journal of the American Psychoanalytic Association* 30:621–656.

—— (1986). On helping analysands observe intra-psychic activity. In *Psychoanalysis: The Science of Mental Conflict. Essays in Honor of Charles Brenner*, ed. A. Richards and M. Willick, pp. 245–261. Hillsdale, NJ: Analytic Press.

—— (1987). On the technique of analysis of the superego—an introduction. *Psychoanalytic Quarterly* 56:130–154.

—— (1994). *The Ego and Analysis of Defense*. Northvale, NJ: Jason Aronson.

—— (1998). *On the receiving end: some consequences of Freud's concepts of aggression and a proposal for analyzing conflicts over aggressive drive derivatives without wounding the analyst's self-esteem*. Lecture at the Baltimore–Washington Psychoanalytic Society, June 13.

Grefe, J., and Reich, G. (1996). "Denn eben, wo Begriffe fehlen . . ." Zur Kritik des Konzeptes "Projektive Identifizierung" und seiner klinischen Verwendung. *Forum der Psychoanalyse* 12:57–77.

Grossman, W. I. (1986). Notes on masochism: a discussion of the history and development of a psychoanalytic concept. *Psychoanalytic Quarterly* 55:379–413.

—— (1991). Pain, aggression, fantasy, and concepts of sadomasochism. *Psychoanalytic Quarterly* 60:22–52.

Grünbaum, A. (1984). *The Foundations of Psychoanalysis*. Berkeley, CA: University of California Press.

—— (1986). *The validity of hidden motives in psychoanalytic theory*. Lecture at the Philosophy of Science Dept., Johns Hopkins University, April 9.

Grunberger, B. (1979). *Narcissism. Psychoanalytic Essays*. New York: International Universities Press.

Hartmann, H. (1964). *Essays on Ego Psychology. Selected Problems in Psychoanalytic Theory*. New York: International Universities Press.

Hartmann, H., Kris, E., and Loewenstein, R. M. (1949). Notes on the theory of aggression. *Psychoanalytic Study of the Child* 3/4:9–36. New York: International Universities Press.

Hartmann, H., and Loewenstein, R. M. (1962). Notes on the superego. *Psychoanalytic Study of the Child* 17:42–81. New York: International Universities Press.

Havens, L. (1997). Commentary to L. Friedman: "Ferrum, Ignis, and Medicina: Return to the Crucible." *Journal of the American Psychoanalytic Association* 45: 49–51.

Haynal, A. (1987). *La technique en question. Controverses en psychanalyse*. Paris: Payot, 1989.

Herman, J. L., Perry, J. C., and van der Kolk, B. A. (1989). Childhood trauma in borderline personality disorder. *American Journal of Psychiatry* 146(4):490–495.

Hesiod: *Works and Days* (*Erga kai hemerai*); *Theogonia*, ed. H. G. Evelyn-White. Greek text in Loeb Classical Library. Cambridge, MA: Harvard University Press, 1947. English trans. R. Lattimore. Ann Arbor: University of Michigan Press, 1959.

Hilgers, M. (1996). *Scham. Gesichter eines Affekts*. Göttingen, Germany: Vandenhoeck & Ruprecht.

Hoffer, A. (1985). Toward a definition of psychoanalytic neutrality. *Journal of the American Psychoanalytic Association* 33:771–796.

Holt, R. R. (1976). Drive or wish? A reconsideration of the psychoanalytic theory of motivation. In *Psychology versus Metapsychology*, ed. M. M. Gill and P. S. Holzman, pp. 158–197. New York: International Universities Press.

Holton, G. (1973). *Thematic Origins of Scientific Thought. Kepler to Einstein.* Cambridge, MA: Harvard University Press.

——— (1986). The advancement of science, and its burdens. *Daedalus* 115:75–104.

Ibsen, H. (1866). *Brand. Et dramatisk dikt.* Oslo: Gyldendal, 1991.

——— (1867). *Peer Gynt. Et dramatisk dikt*, ed. D. Haakonsen. Oslo: Gyldendal, 1988.

——— (1882). *En folkefiende. An Enemy of the People.* In *Nutidsdramaer 1877–1899*, pp. 157–216. Oslo: Norsk Forlag, Gyldendal, 1989. English trans. J. W. McFarlane. London: Oxford University Press, 1966.

Inderbitzin, L. B., and Levy, S. T. (1998). Repetition compulsion revisited: implications for technique. *Psychoanalytic Quarterly* 67:32–53.

Jacobson, E. (1964). *The Self and the Object World.* New York: International Universities Press.

——— (1971). *Depression: Comparative Studies of Normal, Neurotic and Psychotic Conditions.* New York: International Universities Press.

Janet, P. (1908–1911). *Les Obsessions et la Psychasthénie.* 2 vols. Paris: Alcan.

Jones, E. (1929). Fear, guilt, and hate. In *Papers on Psychoanalysis*, pp. 304–319. Boston: Beacon, 1961.

——— (1947). The genesis of the superego. In *Papers on Psychoanalysis*, pp. 145–152. Boston: Beacon, 1961.

——— (1961). *Papers on Psychoanalysis.* Boston: Beacon.

Josephs, L. (1997). The view from the tip of the iceberg. *Journal of the American Psychoanalytic Association* 45:425–464.

Jung, C. G. (1960). *Psychologische Typen.* Zürich: Rascher.

Kafka, F. (1919). *Letter to His Father.* Bilingual edition, trans. E. Kaiser and E. Wilkins. New York: Schocken, 1966.

——— (1935). *Der Prozeß.* ed. M. Brod. New York: Schocken, 1946.

Kafka, J. S. (1989). *Multiple Realities in Clinical Practice.* New Haven, CT: Yale University Press.

Karl, F. R. (1991). *Franz Kafka. Representative Man. Prague, Germans, Jews, and the Crisis of Modernism.* New York: Fromm, 1993.

——— (1995). *George Eliot: Voice of a Century. A Biography.* New York: Norton.

Kennedy, P. (n.d.) *Preparing for the Twenty-first Century.* New York: Random House. (Reviewed by A. Ryan, in *New York Review of Books* 40(9):20–23.)

Kernberg, O. F. (1975). *Borderline Conditions and Pathological Narcissism.* New York: Jason Aronson.

——— (1976). *Object-Relations Theory and Clinical Psychoanalysis.* New York: Jason Aronson.

——— (1984). *Severe Personality Disorders.* New Haven, CT: Yale University Press.

——— (1987). Projection and projective identification: developmental and clinical aspects. *Journal of the American Psychoanalytic Association* 35:795–820.

——— (1988). Clinical dimensions of masochism. In *Masochism. Current Psychoana-*

*lytic Perspectives*, ed. R. A. Glick and D. I. Meyers, pp. 61–80. Hillsdale, NJ: Analytic Press.

———— (1991a). Aggression and love in the relationship of the couple. In *Perversions and Near-Perversions in Clinical Practice. New Psychoanalytic Perspectives*, ed. G. I. Fogel and W. A. Myers, pp. 153–175. New Haven, CT: Yale University Press.

———— (1991b). Sadomasochism, sexual excitement, and perversion. *Journal of the American Psychoanalytic Association* 39:333–362.

Klauber, J. (1981). *Difficulties in the Analytic Encounter.* New York: Jason Aronson.

Klausmeier, F. (1978). *Die Lust, sich musikalisch auszudrücken.* Reinbek, Germany: Rowohlt.

Klein, G. S. (1976). Freud's two theories of sexuality. In *Psychology versus Metapsychology*, ed. M. M. Gill and P. S. Holzman, pp. 14–70. New York: International Universities Press.

Klein, M. (1932). *The Psycho-Analysis of Children.* London: Hogarth.

———— (1952a). *Development in Psycho-Analysis*, ed. J. Riviere. London: Hogarth.

———— (1952b). The mutual influences in the development of ego and id. [Discussion.] *Psychoanalytic Study of the Child* 7:51–53. New York: International Universities Press.

Kohut, H. (1971). *The Analysis of the Self.* New York: International Universities Press.

———— (1972). Thoughts on narcissism and narcissistic rage. *Psychoanalytic Study of the Child* 27:360–400. New Haven, CT: Yale University Press.

———— (1977). *The Restoration of the Self.* New York: International Universities Press.

Kris, A. O. (1983a). The analyst's conceptual freedom in the method of free association. *International Journal of Psycho-Analysis* 64:407–411.

———— (1983b). Determinants of free association in narcissistic phenomena. *Psychoanalytic Study of the Child* 38:439–458. New Haven, CT: Yale University Press.

———— (1984). The conflicts of ambivalence. *Psychoanalytic Study of the Child* 39:213–234. New Haven, CT: Yale University Press.

———— (1985). Resistance in convergent and in divergent conflicts. *Psychoanalytic Quarterly* 54:537–568.

———— (1987). Fixation and regression in relation to convergent and divergent conflicts. *Bulletin of the Anna Freud Centre* 10:99–117.

———— (1988). Some clinical applications of the distinction between divergent and convergent conflicts. *International Journal of Psycho-Analysis* 69:431–442.

Kris, E. (1951). Ego psychology and interpretation in psychoanalytic therapy. *Psychoanalytic Quarterly* 20:15–30.

———— (1952). *Psychoanalytic Explorations in Art.* New York: International Universities Press.

———— (1956). The recovery of childhood memories. *Psychoanalytic Study of the Child* 11:54–88. New York: International Universities Press.

———— (1975). *The Selected Papers.* New Haven, CT: Yale University Press.

Krystal, H. (1974). The genetic development of affects and affect regression. *The Annual of Psychoanalysis* 2:98–126. New York: International Universities Press.

———— (1975). Affect tolerance. *The Annual of Psychoanalysis* 3:179–219. New York: International Universities Press.

———— (1977). Self- and object-representation in alcoholism and other drug dependence: implications for therapy. In *Psychodynamics of Drug Dependence*, pp. 88–100. NIDA Research Monograph 12, U.S. Department of Health, Education and Welfare. Washington, DC: U.S. Government Printing Office.

———— (1978a). Trauma and affect. *Psychoanalytic Study of the Child* 36:81–116. New Haven, CT: Yale University Press.

———— (1978b). Self representation and the capacity for self care. *The Annual of Psychoanalysis* 6:209–246. New York: International Universities Press.

———— (1982). Adolescence and the tendencies to develop substance dependence. *Psychoanalytic Inquiry* 2:581–617.

———— (1988). *Integration and Self-Healing. Affect, Trauma, Alexithymia.* Hillsdale, NJ: Analytic Press.

———— (1997). Desomatization and the consequences of infantile psychic trauma. *Psychoanalytic Inquiry* 17:126–150.

Kubie, L. S. (1937). The Fantasy of Dirt. *Psychoanalytic Quarterly* 6:388–425.

———— (1947). The Fallacious Use of Quantative Concepts in Dynamic Psychology. *Psychoanalytic Quarterly* 16, 507–518.

———— (1950). *Practical and Theoretical Aspects of Psychoanalysis.* New York: Praeger.

———— (1954). The fundamental nature of the distinction between normality and neurosis. *Psychoanalytic Quarterly* 23:167–204.

———— (1958). *Neurotic Distortion of the Creative Process.* New York: Noonday Books, Farrar, Straus & Cudahy.

———— (1960). Psychoanalysis and the scientific method. *Journal of Nervous and Mental Disease* 131:495–512.

———— (1962). The fallacious misuse of the concept of sublimation. *Psychoanalytic Quarterly* 31:73–79.

———— (1963). The central affective potential and its trigger mechanisms. In *Counterpoint. Libidinal Object and Subject*, ed. H. S. Gaskill, pp. 106–120. New York: International Universities Press.

———— (1966). A reconsideration of thinking, the dream process and "the dream." *Psychoanalytic Quarterly* 35:191–198.

———— (1970). The retreat from patients. *International Journal of Psychiatry* 9:693–711.

———— (1974). The drive to become both sexes. *Psychoanalytic Quarterly* 43:349–426.

———— (1978). *Symbol and Neurosis. Selected Papers*, ed. H. J. Schlesinger. *Psychological Issues*, Monograph 44. New York: International Universities Press.

Lagerkvist, P. (1925). *Gäst hos verkligheten.* Stockholm: Bonniers, 1982.

———— (1944). *Dvärgen. (The Dwarf.)* Stockholm: Bonniers.

———— (1950). *Barabbas.* Stockholm: Bonniers, 1984.

———— (1966). *Pilgrimen* (last part: *Det Heliga Landet*). Stockholm: Bonniers.

Lagerlöf, S. (1891). *Gösta Berlings saga.* Stockholm: Delfinserien, Bonniers, 1978.

———— (1904). *Herr Arnes peningar.* Stockholm: Bonniers/Norbok, 1989.

Langer, S. K. (1953). *Feeling and Form. A Theory of Art.* London: Routledge & Kegan Paul.

Langs, R. (1976). *The Bipersonal Field.* New York: Jason Aronson.

Lansky, M. (1984). *The explanation of impulsive action.* Presented at the American Psychoanalytic Association meeting, New York, December.

———— (1992). The explanation of impulsive action. In *Fathers Who Fail. Shame and Psychopathology in the Family System*, pp. 93–112. Hillsdale, NJ: Analytic Press.

Laytner, A. (1990). *Arguing with God. A Jewish Tradition*. Northvale, NJ: Jason Aronson.

Levy, S. T., and Inderbitzin, L. B. (1997). Safety, danger, and analytic authority. *Journal of the American Psychoanalytic Association* 45:377–394.

Lewis, H. B. (1971). *Shame and Guilt in Neurosis*. New York: International Universities Press.

Lichtenberg, J. D. (1983). *Psychoanalysis and Infant Research*. Hillsdale, NJ: Analytic Press.

———— (1985). Response: in search of the elusive baby. *Psychoanalytic Inquiry* 5:621–648.

———— (1986). *The relevance of observations of infants for clinical work with adults*. Paper presented at the meeting of the Swiss Psychoanalytic Society, Zürich, May 26.

———— (1989). *Psychoanalysis and Motivation*. Hillsdale, NJ: Analytic Press.

Lichtenberg, J. D., Lachman, F. M., and Fosshage, J. L. (1996). *The Clinical Exchange*. Hillsdale, NJ: Analytic Press.

Lichtenberg, J. D., and Slap, J. W. (1973). Notes on the concept of splitting and the defense mechanism of the splitting of representations. *Journal of the American Psychoanalytic Association* 21:772–787.

Lipton, S. D. (1977a). The advantages of Freud's technique as shown in his analysis of the Rat Man. *International Journal of Psycho-Analysis* 58:255–274.

———— (1977b). Clinical observations on resistance to the transference. *International Journal of Psycho-Analysis* 58:463–472.

Loch, W. (1976). Psychoanalyse und Wahrheit. *Psyche* 30:865–898.

Loewald, H. W. (1980). *Papers on Psychoanalysis*. New Haven, CT: Yale University Press.

Loewenstein, R. M. (1957). A contribution to the psychoanalytic theory of masochism. *Journal of the American Psychoanalytic Association* 5:197–234.

Luborsky, L. (1984). *Principles of Psychoanalytic Psychotherapy. A Manual for Supportive-Expressive Treatment*. New York: Basic Books.

Luborsky, L., and Auerbach, A. H. (1969). The symptom-context method. *Journal of the American Psychoanalytic Association* 17:68–99.

Mahler, M. S. (1968). *On Human Symbiosis and the Vicissitudes of Individuation. Vol. I: Infantile Psychosis*. New York: International Universities Press.

Mahler, M. S., Pine, F., and Bergmann, A. (1975). *The Psychological Birth of the Human Infant: Symbiosis and Individuation*. New York: Basic Books.

Maleson, F. G. (1984). The multiple meanings of masochism in psychoanalytic discourse. *Journal of the American Psychoanalytic Association* 32:325–356.

Mann, T. (1933, 1936, 1943). *Joseph und seine Brüder*. Stockholm: Bermann-Fischer, 1966.

Meissner, W. W. (1970). Notes on identification. I. Origins in Freud. *Psychoanalytic Quarterly* 39:563–589.

———— (1971). Notes on identification. II. Clarification of related concepts. *Psychoanalytic Quarterly* 40:277–302.

———— (1972). Notes on identification. III. The concept of identification. *Psychoanalytic Quarterly* 41:224–260.

———— (1996). Empathy in the therapeutic interaction. *Psychoanalytic Inquiry* 16(1): 39–53.

Meyers, H. C. (1988). A consideration of treatment techniques in relation to the functions of masochism. In *Masochism. Current Psychoanalytic Perspectives*, ed. R. A. Glick and D. I. Meyers, pp. 175–188. Hillsdale, NJ: Analytic Press.

———— (1991). Perversion in fantasy and furtive enactments. In *Perversions and Near-Perversions in Clinical Practice. New Psychoanalytic Perspectives*, ed. G. I. Fogel and W. A. Myers, pp. 93–108. New Haven, CT: Yale University Press.

Michels, R. (1983). *Comments at the panel discussion on "Borderline."* Presented at the American Psychoanalytic Association meeting, New York, December.

Miller, S. (1993). *The Shame Experience.* Hillsdale, NJ: Analytic Press.

———— (1997). *Shame in Context.* Hillsdale, NJ: Analytic Press.

Mitchell, S. (1993). Aggression and the endangered self. *Psychoanalytic Quarterly* 62:351–382.

Modell, A. H. (1965). On having the right to a life: an aspect of the superego's development. *International Journal of Psycho-Analysis* 46:323–331.

———— (1984). *Psychoanalysis in a New Context.* New York: International Universities Press.

Moore, B. E., and Fine, B. (1968). *Psychoanalytic Terms and Concepts. American Psychoanalytic Association.* New Haven, CT: Yale University Press, 1990.

Müller-Pozzi, H. (1985). Identifikation und Konflikt. Die Angst vor Liebesverlust und der Verzicht auf Individuation. *Psyche* 39:877–904.

Nathanson, D. L. (1985). *Denial, projection and the empathic wall.* Paper presented at the International Conference on Denial, Jerusalem, January 26–31.

———— (1986). The empathic wall and the ecology of affect. *Psychoanalytic Study of the Child* 41:171–187. New Haven, CT: Yale University Press.

———— (1987). A timetable for shame. In *The Many Faces of Shame*, ed. D. L. Nathanson, pp. 1–63. New York: Guilford.

———— (1992). *Shame and Pride. Affect, Sex, and the Birth of the Self.* New York: Norton.

Nietzsche, F. (1873). *Unzeitgemäße Betrachtungen.* Stuttgart: Kröner, 1976.

———— (1878–1880). *Menschliches, Allzu-Menschliches. Der Wanderer und sein Schatten.* Stuttgart: Kröner, 1978.

———— (1880). *Sämtliche Werke. Kritische Studienausgabe in 15 Bänden.* ed. G. Colli and M. Montinari. Munich: DTV; Berlin: de Gruyter.

———— (1882). *Die fröhliche Wissenschaft.* Stuttgart: Kröner, 1976.

———— (1883–1885). *Also sprach Zarathustra.* Stuttgart: Kröner, 1988.

———— (1885). *Jenseits von Gut und Böse.* Stuttgart: Kröner, 1976.

———— (1886). *Morgenröte.* Stuttgart: Kröner, 1976.

———— (1887). *Zur Genealogie der Moral.* Stuttgart: Kröner, 1976.

———— (1888). *Götzendämmerung, Der Antichrist, Ecce Homo, Gedichte.* Stuttgart: Kröner, 1964.

Novick, K. K., and Novick, J. (1987). The essence of masochism. *Psychoanalytic Study of the Child* 42:353–384. New Haven, CT: Yale University Press.

———— (1991). Some comments on masochism and the delusion of omnipotence from a developmental perspective. *Journal of the American Psychoanalytic Association* 39:307–331.

―――― (1996a). *Fearful Symmetry. The Development and Treatment of Sadomasochism.* Northvale, NJ: Jason Aronson.

―――― (1996b). A developmental perspective on omnipotence. In *Journal of Clinical Psychoanalysis* 5:131–175.

Oliner, M. M. (1988). *Cultivating Freud's Garden in France.* Northvale, NJ: Jason Aronson.

Papoušek, H., and Papoušek, M. (1975). Cognitive aspects of preverbal social interaction between human infants and adults. In *Parent–Infant Interactions.* New York: Associated Scientific Publishers.

Parens, H. (1979). *The Development of Aggression in Early Childhood.* New York: Jason Aronson.

Person, E. S. (1995). *By Force of Fantasy.* New York: Penguin.

Person, E. S., and Klar, H. (1994). Establishing trauma: the difficulty distinguishing between memories and fantasies. *Journal of the American Psychoanalytic Association* 42:1055–1081.

Petschenig, M. (1940). *Der kleine Stowasser. Lateinisch-deutsches Schulwörterbuch.* Berlin: Freytag.

Plato. *Platonis Opera* (*in 5 vols.*), ed. J. Burnet. Oxford Classical Texts. Oxford: Clarendon, 1967; English: *Great Books of the Western World,* vol. 7, ed. R. M. Hutchins. trans. B. Jowell and J. Harward, "Phaedrus," pp. 115–141; "The Seventh Letter," pp. 800–814. Chicago: Encyclopaedia Britannica.

Pulver, S. (1970). Narcissism: the term and the concept. *Journal of the American Psychoanalytic Association* 18:319–341.

Rangell, L. (1963a). The scope of intrapsychic conflict: microscopic and macroscopic considerations. *Psychoanalytic Study of the Child* 18:75–102. New York: International Universities Press.

―――― (1963b). Structural problems in intrapsychic conflict. *Psychoanalytic Study of the Child* 18:103–138. New York: International Universities Press.

―――― (1967). Psychoanalysis, affects, and the "human core." *Psychoanalytic Quarterly* 36:172–202.

―――― (1968). A point of view on acting out. *International Journal of Psycho-Analysis* 49:195–201.

―――― (1974). A psychoanalytic perspective leading currently to the syndrome of the compromise of integrity. *International Journal of Psycho-Analysis* 55:3–12.

―――― (1976). Lessons from Watergate: a derivative for psychoanalysis. *Psychoanalytic Quarterly* 45:37–61.

―――― (1980). *The Mind of Watergate.* New York: Norton.

―――― (1981). Psychoanalysis and dynamic psychotherapy: similarities and differences twenty-five years later. *Psychoanalytic Quarterly* 50:665–693.

―――― (1982). The self in psychoanalytic theory. *Journal of the American Psychoanalytic Association* 30:863–892.

Rapaport, D. (1953). Some metapsychologial considerations concerning activity and passivity. In *Collected Papers of D. Rapaport,* ed. M. M. Gill, pp. 530–568. New York: Basic Books, 1967.

―――― (1967). *Collected Papers of D. Rapaport,* ed. M. M. Gill. New York: Basic Books.

Reed, G. S., and Baudry, F. (1997). Susan Isaacs and Anna Freud on fantasy. *Journal of the American Psychoanalytic Association* 45:465–490.

Reich, W. (1933). *Character Analysis*, trans. T. P. Wolfe. London: Vision, 1958.

Renik, O. (1995). The ideal of the anonymous analyst and the problem of self-disclosure. *Psychoanalytic Quarterly* 64:466–495.

——— (1996). The perils of neutrality. *Psychoanalytic Quarterly* 65:495–517.

Roiphe, H., and Galenson, E. (1981). *Infantile Origins of Sexual Identity*. New York: International Universities Press.

Rosenfeld, H. A. (1988). On masochism: a theoretical and clinical approach. In *Masochism: Current Psychoanalytic Perspectives*, ed. R. A. Glick and D. I. Meyers, pp. 151–174. Hillsdale, NJ: Analytic Press.

Rothstein, A. (1991). Sadomasochism in the neuroses conceived of as a pathological compromise formation. *Journal of the American Psychoanalytic Association* 39:363–376.

Rubinstein, B. (1983). Freud's early theories of hysteria. In *Physics, Philosophy and Psychoanalysis: Essays in Honor of Adolf Grünbaum*, ed. R. S. Cohen and L. Laudan, pp. 169–190. Dordrecht, Holland: D. Reidel.

Rubenstein, R. L. (1978). *The Cunning of History. The Holocaust and the American Future*. New York: Harper Colophon.

Sampson, H., and Weiss, J. (1983). Testing hypotheses: the approach of the Mount Zion Psychotherapy Research Group. In *The Psychoanalytic Process*, ed. L. Greenberg and W. Pinsof. New York: Guilford.

Sandemose, A. (1933). *En flykting korsar sitt spår* (*En flyktin krysser sitt spor*), trans. into Swedish by C. Johnson. Harrisonburg, VA: Donelley, 1980.

Sandler, J. (1960). On the concept of superego. *Psychoanalytic Study of the Child* 15:128–162. New York: International Universities Press.

Sandler, J., and Freud, A. (1985). *The Analysis of Defense: The Ego and the Mechanisms of Defense Revisited*. New York: International Universities Press.

Schafer, R. (1960). The loving and beloved superego in Freud's structural theory. *Psychoanalytic Study of the Child* 15:163–188. New York: International Universities Press.

——— (1976a). *A New Language for Psychoanalysis*. New Haven, CT: Yale University Press.

——— (1976b). Emotion in the language of action. In *Psychology versus Metapsychology*, ed. M. M. Gill and P. S. Holzman, pp. 106–133. New York: International Universities Press.

——— (1988). Those wrecked by success. In *Masochism: Current Psychoanalytic Perspectives*, ed. R. A. Glick and D. I. Meyers, pp. 81–92. Hillsdale, NJ: Analytic Press.

Scheler, M. (1915). Das Ressentiment im Aufbau der Moralen. In *Vom Umsturz der Werte. Gesammelte Werke*, 3, pp. 33–147. Bern: Francke, 1955.

Schiller, F. *Sämtliche Werke* (Complete works in 4 vols.). ed. P. Merker. Leipzig: Reclam, 1911.

Schottländer, F.(n.d.; c. 1959). Blendung durch Bilder. In *Entfaltung der Psychoanalyse*, ed. A. Mitscherlich, pp. 222–235. Stuttgart: Klett.

Schur, M. (1966). *The Id and the Regulatory Principles of Mental Functioning*. New York: International Universities Press.

Shengold, L. (1989). *Soul Murder. The Effects of Childhood Abuse and Deprivation*. New Haven, CT: Yale University Press.

———— (1991). *Father, Don't You See I'm Burning?* New Haven, CT: Yale University Press.

Slap, J. W., and Levine, F. J. (1978): On hybrid concepts in psychoanalysis. *Psychoanalytic Quarterly* 47: 499–523.

Snell, B. (1930). Review of F. Zucker, Syneidesis–Conscientia. In *Gesammelte Schriften*, pp. 9–17. Göttingen: Vandenhoeck & Ruprecht, 1966.

———— (1948). *Die Entdeckung des Geistes.* Hamburg: Claassen & Goverts. English: *The Discovery of the Mind. The Greek Origins of European Thought.* New York: Harper, 1960.

Sophocles. *Sophoclis Fabulae. Oxford Classical Texts,* ed. A. C. Pearson. Oxford: Clarendon.

Spence, D. P. (1982). *Narrative Truth and Historical Truth.* New York: Norton.

———— (1983). Narrative persuasion. *Psychoanalysis & Contemporary Thought* 6: 457–481.

Steinsaltz, A. (1989–1999). *The Talmud,* trans. I. Berman, D. Strauss, et al. New York: Random House.

Sterba, R. (1934). The fate of the ego in analytic theory. *International Journal of Psycho-Analysis* 15:117–126.

Stern, D. N. (1985). *The Interpersonal World of the Infant. A View from Psychoanalysis and Developmental Psychology.* New York: Basic Books.

Stern, M. (1986). Autobiographie und Identität. In *Ein Inuk sein. Interdisziplinäre Vorlesungen zum Problem der Identität,* ed. G. Benedetti and L. Wiesmann, pp. 257–270. Göttingen: Vandenhoeck & Ruprecht.

Stierlin, H. (1969). *Conflict and Reconciliation.* New York: Anchor.

———— (1974). *Separating Parents and Adolescents.* New York: Quadrangle.

Stoller, R. J. (1975). *Perversion: The Erotic Form of Hatred.* New York: Pantheon.

———— (1991). The term perversion. In *Perversions and Near-Perversions in Clinical Practice. New Psychoanalytic Perspectives,* ed. G. I. Fogel and W. A. Myers, pp. 36–56. New Haven, CT: Yale University Press.

Stone, L. (1984). *Transference and its Context.* New York: Jason Aronson.

Strachey, J. (1934). The nature of the therapeutic action of psychoanalysis. *International Journal of Psychoanalysis* 50:275–292, 1969.

Tabin, J. K. (1985). *On the Way to Self. Ego and Early Oedipal Development.* New York: Columbia University Press.

*Talmud: Hebrew/Aramaic edition of the Babylonian Talmud,* 1962, ed. Rabbi M. Zioni. Jerusalem, Bnei Brak. English trans. 1936, ed. Isidore Epstein. London: Soncino.

Thomä, H. (1993). Über einige therapeutische und wissenschaftliche Sackgassen im Zusammenhang mit Freuds Gold-Kupfer-Metapher. *Zeitschrift für psychosomatische Medizin* 39:238–245.

Thomä, H., and Kächele, H. (1973). Wissenschaftstheoretische und methodologische Probleme der klinisch-psychoanalytischen Forschung. *Psyche* 27:205–236, 309–355.

———— (1985). *Lehrbuch der psychoanalytischen Therapie. I. Grundlagen.* Berlin: Springer-Verlag. English trans. M. Wilson and D. Rosevaere. *Psychoanalytic Practice. I. Principles,* Berlin, Heidelberg, New York: Springer, 1987.

———— (1988). *Lehrbuch der psychoanalytischen Therapie. II. Praxis.* Berlin: Springer-

Verlag. English: *II. Clinical Studies*, trans. M. Wilson. Berlin, Heidelberg, New York: Springer, 1992.

Ticho, E. (1972). Termination of psychoanalysis: treatment goals, life goals. *Psychoanalytic Quarterly* 41:315–333.

Tomkins, S. S. (1962). *Affect/Imagery/Consciousness. Vol. 1: The Positive Affects.* New York: Springer.

——— (1963). *Affect/Imagery/Consciousness. Vol. 2: The Negative Affects.* New York: Springer.

——— (1979). Script theory: differential magnification of affects. In *Nebraska Symposium of Motivation 1978*, Vol. 26, ed. H. E. Howe and R. A. Dienstbier, pp. 201–236.

——— (1982). Affect theory. In *Emotion in the Human Face*, ed. P. Ekman, pp. 353–395. Cambridge, England: Cambridge University Press.

Trunnell, E. E., and Holt, W. E. (1974). The concept of denial or disavowal. *Journal of the American Psychoanalytic Association* 22:769–784.

Valenstein, A. F. (1973). On attachment to painful feelings and the negative therapeutic reaction. *Psychoanalytic Study of the Child* 28:365–392. New Haven, CT: Yale University Press.

van der Kolk, B.A. (1998). *Die sozialen und neurobiologischen Dimensionen des Zwanges, Traumata zu wiederholen.* Paper presented at the Congress, "Trauma und Kreative Lösungen," Cologne, Germany, March 5–7.

van der Kolk, B. A., Pelcovitz, D., Roth, S., et al. (1996). Dissociation, somatization, and affect dysregulation: the complexity of adaptation to trauma. *American Journal of Psychiatry* (Festschrift Suppl.) 153(7): 83–93.

Waelder, R. (1930). The principle of multiple function. In *Selected Papers*, ed. S. A. Guttman, pp. 68–83. New York. International Universities Press.

——— (1936). Zur Frage der Genese der psychischen Konflikte im frühen Kindesalter. *Internat. Zschr.f.Psychoanalyse* 22:513–570. English: The problem of the genesis of psychical conflict in earliest infancy: remarks on a paper by Joan Riviere. In *Selected Papers*, ed. S. A. Guttman, pp. 121–188. New York: International Universities Press.

——— (1951). The structure of paranoid ideas: a critical survey of various theories. In *Selected Papers*, ed. S. A. Guttman, pp. 207–228. New York: International Universities Press.

——— (1976). Psychoanalysis: observation, theory, application. In *Selected Papers*, ed. S. A. Guttman. New York: International Universities Press.

Wallerstein, R. S. (1986). Psychoanalysis as a science: a response to the new challenge. *Psychoanalytic Quarterly* 55:414–451.

——— (1997). Merton Gill, psychotherapy, and psychoanalysis. *Journal of the American Psychoanalytic Association* 45:233–256.

Wangh, M. (1962). The evocation of a proxy. *Psychoanalytic Study of the Child* 17:451–472. New York: International Universities Press.

——— (1985). *The evolution of psychoanalytic thought on negation and denial.* Paper presented at the International Conference on Denial, Jerusalem, Jan. 26–31.

Weiss, J., and Sampson, H. (1986). *The Psychoanalytic Process.* New York: Guilford.

Winnicott, D. W. (1965). *The Maturational Processes and the Facilitating Environment: Studies in the Theory of Emotional Development.* New York: International Universities Press.

Wright, L. (n.d.). *Remembering Satan.* New York: Knopf.

Wurmser, L. (1974). Psychoanalytic considerations of the etiology of compulsive drug use. *Journal of the American Psychoanalytic Association* 22:820–843.

——— (1977a). A defense of the use of metaphor in analytic theory formation. *Psychoanalytic Quarterly* 46:466–498.

——— (1977b). The Janus face of psychiatry. *Journal of Nervous and Mental Disease* 164:375–379.

——— (1978). *The Hidden Dimension: Psychodynamics in Compulsive Drug Use.* Northvale, NJ: Jason Aronson, 1995.

——— (1980). Phobic core in the addictions and the paranoid process. *International Journal of Psychoanalytic Psychotherapy* 8: 311–337.

——— (1981a). *The Mask of Shame.* Baltimore, MD: Johns Hopkins University Press; Northvale, NJ: Jason Aronson, 1994.

——— (1981b). Is psychoanalysis a separate field of symbolic forms? *Humanities and Society* 4:263–294.

——— (1984a). More respect for the neurotic process. *Journal of Substance Abuse Treatment* 1:37–45.

——— (1984b). The role of superego conflicts in substance abuse and their treatment. *International Journal of Psychoanalytic Psychotherapy* 10:227–258.

——— (1984c). Goethe's relevance for psychoanalysis. *Psychoanalytic Inquiry* 4:533–554.

——— (1987a). Shame: the veiled companion of narcissism. In *The Many Faces of Shame,* ed. D. L. Nathanson, pp. 64–92. New York: Guilford.

——— (1987b). *Flucht vor dem Gewissen. Analyse von Über-Ich und Abwehr bei schweren Neurosen* [Flight from Conscience: Analysis of Superego and Defense in the Severe Neuroses]. Heidelberg: Springer.

——— (1987c). *"My poisoned blood." The spirit of resentment: comments on Pär Lagerkvist's The Dwarf.* Paper presented at study group "Psychoanalysis and Creativity" (J. Lichtenberg), Jan. 24, and at the psychiatric hospital St. Sigfrid Sjukhuset, Växjö, Sweden, Jan. 31.

——— (1988). "The sleeping giant": a dissenting comment about "borderline pathology." *Psychoanalytic Inquiry* 8:373–397.

——— (1989a). *Die zerbrochene Wirklichkeit. Psychoanalyse als das Studium von Konflikt und Komplementarität* [Broken Reality. Psychoanalysis as the Study of Conflict and Complementarity]. Heidelberg: Springer.

——— (1989b). "Either-or": some comments on Professor Grünbaum's critique of psychoanalysis. *Psychoanalytic Inquiry* 9:220–248.

——— (1989c). Blinding the eye of the mind: denial, impulsive action, and split identity. In *Denial: A Clarification of Concepts,* ed. E. L. Edelstein, D. L. Nathanson, and A. M. Stone, pp. 175–201. New York: Plenum.

——— (1990a). *Die Maske der Scham. Die Psychoanalyse von Schamaffekten und Schamkonflikten* [The Mask of Shame. The Psychoanalysis of Shame Affects and Shame Conflicts]. Heidelberg: Springer, 1993, 1997.

—————— (1990b). The question of conflict in Chinese thought, specifically in Confucius: some psychoanalytic considerations. *Journal of the Korean Psychoanalytic Study Group* 1:115–130.

—————— (1990c). *Man of the most dangerous curiosity–Nietzsche's "fruitful and frightful vision" and his war against shame.* Paper presented at study group "Psychoanalysis and Creativity" (J. Lichtenberg), Bethesda, MD, April 7.

—————— (1990d). *The creative agon–Thomas Mann's overt dialogue with, and hidden trial against, Nietzsche.* Paper presented at study group "Psychoanalysis and Creativity" (J. Lichtenberg), Bethesda, MD, June 30.

—————— (1991a). The question of conflict in Lao Tzu: some psychoanalytic considerations. *Journal of the Korean Psychoanalytic Study Group* 2:112–133.

—————— (1991b). "Der goldleuchtende Dolch"—Masochistische Übertragung, Über-Ich- Übertragung und Gegenübertragung. *Forum der Psychoanalyse* 7:1–19.

—————— (1993, 1998). *Das Rätsel des Masochismus. Psychoanalytische Untersuchungen von Gewissenszwang und Leidenssucht* [The Riddle of Masochism: Psychoanalytic Studies of the Compulsion of Conscience and the Addiction to Suffering]. Heidelberg: Springer-Verlag.

—————— (1994). *The "prison of lies"—comments about Joseph Conrad's "Under Western Eyes."* Paper presented at study group "Psychoanalysis and Creativity" (J. Lichtenberg), July 9.

—————— (1997a). Nietzsche's war against shame and resentment. In *The Widening Scope of Shame,* ed. M. Lansky and A. Morrison, pp. 181–204. Hillsdale, NJ: Analytic Press.

—————— (1997b). The shame about existing—a comment about the analysis of "moral" masochism. In *The Widening Scope of Shame,* ed. M. Lansky and A. Morrison, pp. 367–382. Hillsdale, NJ: Analytic Press.

—————— (1999a). "Man of the most dangerous curiosity"—Nietzsche's "fruitful and frightful vision" and his war against shame. In *Scenes of Shame,* ed. J. Adamson and H. Clark, pp. 111–146. Albany: State University of New York Press.

—————— (1999b). Magische Verwandlung und tragische Verwandlung. Die Behandlung der schweren Neurose [Magic Transformation and Tragic Transformation. The Treatment of Severe Neurosis]. Göttingen: Vandenhoeck & Ruprecht.

Wurmser, L., and Gidion, H. (1999c). *Die eigenen verborgensten Dunkelgänge.* Göttingen: Vandenhoeck & Ruprecht.

Wurmser, L., and Zients, A. (1982). The "return of the denied superego"—a psychoanalytic study of adolescent substance abuse. *Psychoanalytic Inquiry* 2:539–580.

# Index

## ABOUT THE AUTHOR

Léon Wurmser, M.D., is Clinical Professor of Psychiatry at the University of West Virginia and Training and Supervising Analyst at the New York Freudian Society. Former Professor of Psychiatry and Director of the Alcohol and Drug Abuse Program at the University of Maryland, he has also taught extensively throughout Europe. Dr. Wurmser trained as a psychiatrist in his native Switzerland and received his psychoanalytic training in this country. Author of 300 articles and coeditor of the six-volume textbook *Psychiatric Foundations in Medicine,* he has written several books such as *The Hidden Dimension* and *The Mask of Shame.* Dr. Wurmser is a recipient of the 1997 Margrit Egnér Foundation Award in recognition of outstanding work in anthropologic psychology and philosophy. He maintains a private practice in psychotherapy in Towson, Maryland.